AF752220

PROTEIN BIOCHEMISTRY, SYNTHESIS, STRUCTURE AND CELLULAR FUNCTIONS

ADVANCES IN PROTEOMICS RESEARCH

PROTEIN BIOCHEMISTRY, SYNTHESIS, STRUCTURE AND CELLULAR FUNCTIONS

Additional books in this series can be found on Nova's website under the Series tab.

Additional E-books in this series can be found on Nova's website under the E-book tab.

PROTEIN SCIENCE AND ENGINEERING

Additional books in this series can be found on Nova's website under the Series tab.

Additional E-books in this series can be found on Nova's website under the E-book tab.

PROTEIN BIOCHEMISTRY, SYNTHESIS,
STRUCTURE AND CELLULAR FUNCTIONS

ADVANCES IN PROTEOMICS RESEARCH

YA LI HUANG
AND
ANGUÓ CHEN
EDITORS

Nova Science Publishers, Inc.
New York

For permission to use material from this book please contact us:
Telephone 631-231-7269; Fax 631-231-8175
Web Site: http://www.novapublishers.com

Library of Congress Cataloging-in-Publication Data

ISBN: 978-1-61942-227-8

Published by Nova Science Publishers, Inc. † New York

CONTENTS

PREFACE

This book presents recent advances in proteomics research. Topics discussed include redox proteomics approaches to the evaluation of UV-induced protein oxidative damage; decoding amino acid sequences of proteins using inter-residue average distance statistics to extract information on protein folding mechanisms and modelling of protein folding and prediction of rate based on nucleation mechanism.

Chapter 1 - UV-induced photomodification of proteins has been implicated in damage toa broad range of different protein-based substrates. Protein photo-oxidation has been linked to such diverse degenerative processes as human hair and skin damage, degradation of pharmaceuticals, reduced food quality and nutrition, discoloration of natural fibres, eye lens opacification, loss of enzymatic activity and crop damage. Ongoing ozone reduction in the stratosphere, with resultant increased exposurc to UVB, hasgenerated further impetus for advancing the understanding and controlling the complex protein degradation mechanisms and pathways underlying these damage processes.

For proteins, photo-oxidative damage is generally attributable to the generation and attack of reactive oxygen species (ROS) on amino acid residue sidechains and the protein backbone. Singlet oxygen and hydroxyl radicals, in particular, play a significant role in initiating protein modification.

This paper explores and discusses the complex cascade of modifications induced within proteins through exposure to irradiation, the effect of photo-oxidation on protein substrate properties from the protein primary level through to higher order structure, and the mechanisms underpinning protein photo-oxidation. It will also discuss exciting new approaches to the characterisation, location, tracking, and ultimately control of photo-oxidation within proteins.

Chapter 2 - One of the ultimate goals of bioinformatics is to discover the principles governing protein folding. However, information on folding mechanisms of proteins cannot be easily decoded from amino acid sequences using standard bioinformatics techniques such as multiple sequence alignment and so on. The authors do not sufficiently understand how the determinants of protein folding are encoded in amino acid sequences. In this review, the authors summarize how information about protein folding mechanisms can be extracted from amino acid sequences using inter-residue average distance statistics. The authors' kind of predicted contact map (Average Distance Map, ADM) pinpoints regions of possible folding nuclei for proteins. The amino acid sequence of a given protein suffice for construction of the ADM of a protein. An inter-residue effective potential is defined from the average distance statistics and is utilized to predict folding nucleation sites of a protein sequence. The authors review examples of the applications of these methods to the analyses of the protein folding of members of several protein families. The general possibility of predicting protein folding mechanisms from only sequences is also discussed.

Chapter 3 - The problem of protein self-organization is one of the most important problems of molecular biology nowadays. Despite the recent success in the understanding of general principles of protein folding, details of this process are yet to be elucidated. Moreover, the prediction of protein folding rates has its own practical value due to the fact that aggregation directly depends on the rate of protein folding. The time of folding and transition state ensembles for 67 proteins with known experimental data at the point of thermodynamic equilibrium between unfolded and native state have been calculated using a Monte Carlo method and Dynamic programming one where each residue is considered to be either folded as in the native state or completely disordered. The times of folding for 67 proteins which reach the native state within a limit of 10^8 Monte Carlo steps are in a good correlation with experimentally measured folding time at mid-transition point (the correlation coefficient is -0.82). A lower correlation was obtained if to use Dynamic programming approach (the correlation coefficient is -0.72). The capillarity model allows us to predict the folding rate at the same level of correlation as by Monte-Carlo simulations. The calculated model entropy capacity (conformational entropy per residue divided by the average contact energy per residue) for 67 proteins correlates by about 78% with the experimentally measured folding rate at the mid-transition point. Theoretical consideration of a capillarity model for the process of protein folding demonstrates that the difference in the folding rate for proteins sharing more ball-like and less ball-like folds is the result of differences in the conformational entropy due to a larger surface of the boundary between folded and unfolded phases in the transition state for proteins with more ball-like fold.

Chapter 4 - Despite much progress in molecular biology, biophysics, and biochemistry, the mechanisms by which unfolded polypeptide chains gain their native conformation are not yet fully understood. Likewise, the network of forces that stabilize folded proteins and prevent them from unfolding elude a thorough accounting so far. Such an accounting is, however, necessary to engineer protein stability, which is often required for enzymes in technical applications.

The folding process of proteins starts with a hydrophobic collapse or local events at so-called 'nuclei' or 'initiation sites' and proceeds stepwise to the natively folded protein. The occurrence of rate-limiting steps often leads to the population of folding intermediates. In contrast to the successive protein folding process, protein *un*folding is highly cooperative. Due to the principle of microscopic reversibility, unfolding must be a progressive process as well, which is postulated to start at a confined region—'unfolding region', 'critical region' or similar—of the tertiary structure of the native protein molecule.

The rate constants of the folding (k_f) and unfolding reaction (k_U), both of which determine the respective free energy of activation $\Delta G_f^\ddagger$ and $\Delta G_U^\ddagger$, provide information on the contribution of these reactions to the thermodynamic stability (Gibbs free energy $\Delta G = \Delta G_U^\ddagger - \Delta G_f^\ddagger$). The comparison of proteins with their chemically modified or, preferably, genetically engineered variants yields information on the involvement of specific residues in the folding or unfolding reaction.

RibonucleaseA (RNaseA) has been a model protein for half a century and is one of the most thoroughly studied examples concerning the protein folding problem. Whereas the folding reaction is complex due to proline isomerization reactions, the unfolding reaction can be described by a single-exponential reaction. Modifications by, *e.g.*, genetic engineering have revealed the importance of confined regions for the unfolding and refolding reaction, respectively.

Starting from basic principles of thermodynamics and kinetics, the effect of protein modifications on the stability and tools for protein stabilization are presented with special focus on work on RNase A.

Chapter 5 - Yeast is an important platform for the production of therapeutic proteins. It has principally been used for the production of relatively simple proteins that lack *N*-linked glycosylation. However, with recent developments in technologies focused on glycoengineering yeast to produce humanized *N*-glycans, its application to the field of human therapeutics becomes greatly potentiated. A constant challenge in the biotechnology industry is the production of recombinant proteins at high levels. Like other protein expression platforms, productivities in yeast depend on the host strain, its process of cultivation and the type of protein being expressed. In addition, it has been demonstrated that yeast lack some molecular chaperones found in higher eukaryotic cells. Protein folding in the endoplasmic reticulum is a key process that can influence the fate of a protein, directing it either to secretion or ER-associated degradation. Some proteins require specific molecular chaperones for their protein maturation and others require general protein folding chaperones. In this review, yeast folding machinery as well as attempts made to improve protein folding will be discussed.

Chapter 6 - Treatment options for cancer have increased in the last years due to the ongoing research and development of new therapeutics. A focus shift from formerly undirected cytostatic agents to more targeted therapies, mainly antibodies and protein kinase inhibitors has taken place. New agents directed against receptors which control proliferation, migration and angiogenesis of tumor cells have been developed. Mainly specific antibodies directed against the extracellular ligand binding domain of various receptor tyrosine kinases, and protein kinase inhibitors targeting the intracellular protein kinase domain of receptors or cytoplasmic signalling proteins have been increasingly developed in the past years. In this chapter the authors will address the current treatment options with protein kinase inhibitors exemplarily for hepatocellular carcinoma and renal cell cancer. The authors will further give an insight into the actual research perspectives and the conception of incorporating new drugs into clinical trials as single agent treatment or combined with "classical" chemotherapy. The first part elucidates the molecular pathways of carcinogenesis and depicts the mode of action of these new agents in the treatment of hepatocellular carcinoma, the second part illustrates the pathogenesis of renal cell cancer and the resulting therapeutic options by targeting these pathways.

Chapter 7 - The most abundant molecules in nature other than water are proteins, which are involved to stimulate or control virtually every chemical process. Majority of proteins must be converted into tightly folded compact structures in order to function and their ability to fold to a unique structure generate enormous selectivity and diversity in their functions. Conformational changes in proteins result in misfolding, aggregation, and intra- or extraneuronal accumulation of amyloid fibrils in many neurodegenerative disorders. Proteins appear to fold by diverse pathways, the rates of folding are largely determined by the topology of the native structure. In general, secondary structure is inherently unstable and its stability is enhanced by tertiary interactions. The most conspicuous feature of many neurodegenerative disorders, including Alzheimer's, Parkinson's, and Huntington's disease, is the occurrence of protein aggregates in ordered fibrillar structures known as amyloid found inside and outside of brain cells. The appearance of aggregates in diseased brains implies an underlying incapacity in the cellular machinery of molecular chaperones that normally functions to prevent the accumulation of misfolded proteins. Molecular chaperones provide a first line of defense against misfolded, aggregation-prone proteins, and are among the most potent suppressors of neurodegeneration known for animal models of human disease. A detailed understanding of the molecular basis of protection by chaperones against neurodegeneration might lead to the development of therapies for neurodegenerative disorders that are associated with protein misfolding and aggregation.

In this review, the advances on the protein folding in neurodegenrative disorder and unfolding the role of molecular chaperones in neuroprotection has been discussed.

Versions of these chapters were also published in *Proteomics Research Journal,* Volume 2, Numbers 1/2, published by Nova Science Publishers, Inc. They were submitted for appropriate modifications in an effort to encourage wider dissemination of research.

In: Advances in Proteomics Research
Editors: Ya Li Huang et al. pp. 1-31

ISBN: 978-1-61942-227-8

Chapter 1

REDOX PROTEOMICS APPROACHES TO THE EVALUATION OF UV-INDUCED PROTEIN OXIDATIVE DAMAGE

Jolon M. Dyer*

Team Leader, Protein and Structure,
Growth and Development Section
AgResearch Lincoln Research Centre,
Cnr Springs Rd and Gerald St, Lincoln
Christchurch 8140
New Zealand

ABSTRACT

UV-induced photomodification of proteins has been implicated in damage toa broad range of different protein-based substrates. Protein photo-oxidation has been linked to such diverse degenerative processes as human hair and skin damage, degradation of pharmaceuticals, reduced food quality and nutrition, discoloration of natural fibres, eye lens opacification, loss of enzymatic activity and crop damage.Ongoing ozone reduction in the stratosphere, with resultant increased exposure to UVB, hasgenerated further impetus for advancing the understanding and

* "Dyer, Jolon" <Jolon.Dyer@agresearch.co.nz>

controlling the complex protein degradation mechanisms and pathways underlying these damage processes.

For proteins, photo-oxidative damage is generally attributable to the generation and attack of reactive oxygen species (ROS) on amino acid residue sidechains and the protein backbone. Singlet oxygen and hydroxyl radicals, in particular, play a significant role in initiating protein modification.

This paper explores and discussesthe complex cascade of modifications induced within proteins through exposure to irradiation, the effect of photo-oxidation on protein substrate properties from the protein primary level through to higher order structure, and the mechanisms underpinning protein photo-oxidation. It will also discuss exciting new approaches to the characterisation, location, tracking, and ultimately control of photo-oxidation within proteins.

1. INTRODUCTION

1.1. Protein Photo-oxidative Damage

Understanding and controlling the photodegradation of complex protein-based systems represent significant goals in protein science and photobiology. These goals are also of considerable medical and commercial interest. Ultraviolet light (UV) induced photo-oxidation of proteins has been implicated in damage and degenerative processes within a diverse range of biological systems and protein-based substrates[1]. These include hair damage [2],cit_cit_af ref_bf(Ruetsch, S. B. 2003 ref_num189)ref_af skin carcinogenesis and ageing effects [3],cit_cit_af ref_bf(Wondrak, G. T. 2004 ref_num120)ref_af loss of structural or enzymatic functionality [4, 5],cit_bcit_af ref_bf(Sidorkina, O. M. 1999 rccit_af ref_bf(Dalle-Donne, I. 2005 ref_num483)ref_af deterioration in food quality [6, 7], eye lens opacification [8-10] and crop damage[11-13].cit_cit_af ref_bf(Stapleton, A. E. 1992 ref_nccit_af ref_bf(Gerhardt, K. E. 1999 ref_num122)ref Continuing ozone depletion in the stratosphere, with a resultingincrease in UVB intensity at the earth's surface [14],cit_bcit_af ref_bf(Frederick J. E. 1988 re have added further impetus to studies aimed at elucidating the complex protein photo-oxidation processes underlying this photodamage.

1.2. Initiation of Damage

Tryptophan and tyrosine are the two standard amino acid residues in proteins which can absorb light at wavelengths over 290nm[15, 16].When oxygen is present, tryptophan excited by UVB can generate singlet oxygen and superoxide anions. Tyrosine can similarly generate ROS through photo-excitation, but this process is less efficient and often results in electron transfer to proximal cystine residues and subsequent cleavage of the disulfide bond [17].

Overall, however, proteins have low absorbance in the solar UV range. Most protein photodamage is therefore the consequence, not of direct UV absorption, but of the attack of reactive oxygen species (ROS) generated through photo-excitation of sensitisers within the proteinaceous substrate [17]. The photoproducts of protein photo-oxidation themselves, such as *N*-formylkynurenine or dityrosine, also act as photosensitisers for production of ROS, such as hydroxyl radicals, thereby promoting further degradation [18, 19]. In addition to tryptophan and tyrosine, crosslinked amino acids, such as desmosine, characteristic of proteins such as collagen and elastin, are also able to absorb UVB radiation, and it is thought that these may also act as photosensitisers [20].

1.3. Underpinning Oxidative Mechanisms

ROS may be generated during protein photo-oxidation throughboth Type and Type II processes, with Type I reactions yielding free radicals via electron transfer and hydrogen abstraction,and Type II photo-oxidation occurring through energy transfer with molecular oxygen to yield the reactive excited state, singlet oxygen [17, 21].

Singlet oxygen is a highly reactive, electrophilic, non-radical moleculethatmay be formed on irradiation of triplet oxygenin the presence of photosensitisers[22].It reacts with proteins to form hydroperoxides, which decompose and oxidise further to form a variety of photoproductson protein residue side chains. In addition, where proteins are in proximity to lipids, lipid hydroperoxides formed through initial ROS attack may contribute to secondary protein damage. This lipid-mediated damage is thought to occur both through the triggering of radical chains and via the by-products of free radical lipid oxidation, including electrophilic aldehydes [20].

Hydroxyl radicals are a highly reactive free radical oxygen species that form *in vitro*through initial production of superoxide and hydrogen peroxide [23]. These radicals can attack any protein residue through abstraction of the α-hydrogen or direct oxidation of residue side chains, but have a particular affinity for attacking electron rich moieties, notably aromatic rings and sulfur species [24].

More recently, the characterisation of nitrated photoproducts in irradiated protein substrates has also implicated reactive nitrogen species such as peroxynitrite in contributing to protein photo-oxidation in some systems [25, 26]. Peroxynitrite is similar to the hydroxyl radical in its reactivity, including its affinity for aromatic species [27, 28].

2. Protein Damage Hierarchies

Protein oxidative damage at the primary structural level can be induced through backbone cleavage [29], scission of the residue side chain [30], modification of a terminus [31] or reaction of the side chain [32]. Within intact proteins, it has been shown that peptide α- or β- positions are not the primary site of attack for UV-generated reactive oxygen species, which means that side-chain modification is an important component of photo-oxidative damage[33].

2.1. Residue Specific Modification

Although all amino acid residues are susceptible to ROS attack, the most photosensitive residues in proteins are typically aromatic and sulfur-containing amino acids[34].Model studies on the photodegradation of free amino acids have characterised the highest levels of photo-oxidationproducts within solutions of tryptophan, tyrosine, histidine, phenylalanine, and cysteine. This correlates well with the observation that these residues are also those which degrade the most significantly when whole proteins are exposed to UV[35-39].

2.1.1. Aromatic Residues

With respect to photomodifications leading to chromophore formation in proteins, tryptophan and tyrosine photoproducts in particular have been observed to be the chief contributors[40, 41]. Hydroxyl radicals, in particular,have a characteristic affinity for aromatic ring structures[42-45]. Recent studies have revealed a wide range of photoproducts formed within intact proteins from these residues [19, 25, 46-48]. In both cases, photo-oxidation of tryptophan and tyrosine side chains results in a cascade of oxidation products forming progressively more coloured chromophores. Figures 1 and 2 outline some of the key photoproducts and pathways involved in tryptophan and tyrosine photo-oxidation respectively. The dominant photo-oxidation pathway for tryptophan is through the formation of kynurenine derivatives, while for tyrosine, dopa and topa derivatives predominate. It should be noted that photo-oxidation of phenylalanine leads to the same general profile of products as tyrosine, through initial ring hydroxylation[49], while the most notable histidine residue photoproducts are hydroxylated derivatives and degradation to asparagines and aspartic acid[40, 50].

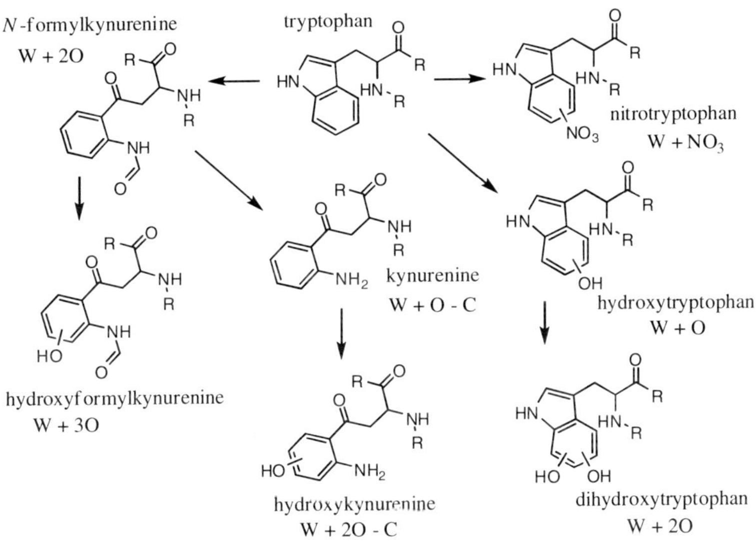

Figure 1. Keyinitial pathways in the photo-oxidation of the tryptophan residue side-chain, showing notable photoproducts.

When tyrosine and phenylalanine residues are in close proximity to tryptophan residues, energy transfer to tryptophan can occur, with associated fluorescence quenching [51-53] This energy transfer contributes to the preferential oxidation of tryptophan residues within proteins. In our recent studies characterising photoproducts within UVB irradiated tryptophan-free collagen, a much wider range of phenylalanine, tyrosine and histidine photoproducts was observed than is usual when tryptophan is present, including the formation of nitrated products [25].

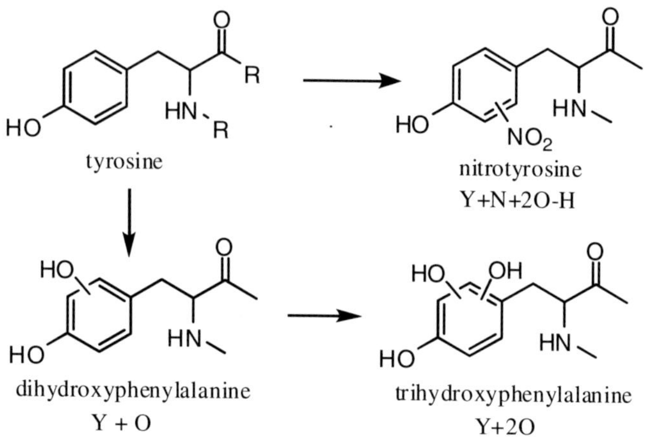

Figure 2. Key initial pathways in the photo-oxidation of the tyrosine residue side-chain, showing notable photoproducts.

2.1.2. Sulfur-containing Residues

The sulfur-containing residues are also particularly susceptible to photodamage. Photo-oxidation of methionine leads predominantly to the formation of methionine sulfoxide, which is a reversible oxidative modification within living systems, but generally accumulates in structural proteins and other proteins particularly affected by solar radiation [54].

Cysteine residues in proteins are found as free thiols or in disulfide bonds (cystine), and are critical to the structural integrity and mechanical properties of the substrate [55-57]. These two forms are redox interconvertible and the relative ratio of these within the protein therefore has a correlation to the degree of photo-oxidative damage. High levels of disulfides can have a protective effect on other protein sites, acting as efficient quenchers [58]. Once cysteine is oxidised to sulfonic acid, the modification is irreversible. Cystine can also be photomodified to lanthionine [59, 60].

2.1.3. Other Modifications

As a cyclic species, proline is also susceptible to photomodification through hydroxylation, with the main products being hydroxyproline and dihydroxyproline [25, 61]. These photoproducts are particularly relevant in the photodegradation of collagen, when proline residues are present in high abundance [62]. Other photodegradation products of proline include glutamic semialdehyde and pyroglutamic acid [30].

Although not residue-specific, other photomodifications of note include deamidation and decarboxylation, which are particularly abundant where photo-induced generation of ROS has initiated Fenton chemistry (hydroxyl radical production) within the protein substrate [63]. Deamidation particularly affects asparagine and glutamine residues, but also occurs at the protein or peptide *N*-terminus. Decarboxylation can occur in tandem with deamidation, and particularly affects terminal residues.

As all residue side-chains can be photo-oxidatively modified, there is a wide array of further photoproducts which have been characterised in addition to those highlighted [38, 47, 64]. However, most of these are believed to play a relatively minor role in the overall protein damage.

2.2. Structural Damage

2.2.1. Carbonylation

The level of formation of carbonyl groups in proteins is generally significantly higher than other oxidative modifications and is an irreversible modification [30]. Therefore, the formation of carbonyl groups has long been associated with protein photodamage [65, 66]. Carbonyl moieties may be generated on residue side chains, notably proline, threonine, arginine and lysine, after these residues are photo-oxidatively aldehyde or ketone derivatised [67].

2.2.2. Backbone Cleavage and Side-chain Scission

ROS, in particular hydroxyl radicals, can extract α-hydrogen atoms, leading to the generation of carbon-centred radicals within the protein [68]. These in turn react with molecular oxygen to form peroxy radicals, and subsequently peroxides and alkoxyl derivatives. Peptide bond cleavage can then occur through two different pathways, namely the diamide and α-amidation pathways [30]. The key difference between the two pathways is that the diamide pathways produces peptide fragments with diamide and isocyanate terminal moieties, while the α-amidation pathway leads to peptide fragments with amide and α-ketoacyl terminal moieties. Significantly, the α-amidation pathway therefore provides another route for the introduction of carbonyl functionality.

Exposure of proteins to ionising radiation also results in residue side-chain scission, with cleavage occurring at the β-position [30, 40]. Side chain scission results in the formation within the protein of small carbonyl containing molecules as side-chain derivatives, including formaldehyde and acetone, from alanine and valine respectively. This can therefore lead indirectly to protein modifications such as formylation. Scission also results in the introduction of a carbon centred radical into the protein backbone.

2.2.3. Crosslinking

UV irradiation of proteins also results in crosslinking between peptide chains [13, 34]. Once again, a wide and complex array of photoproducts can result, and crosslinking can be both inter- and intramolecular [30].

One key crosslinked photoproduct of tyrosine is dityrosine. Dityrosine formation is generated oxidatively in proteins through attack by ROS, such as hydroxyl or peroxynitrite radicals, on tyrosine to form tyrosyl radicals, followed by radical-radical combination of proximal oxidised residues [46] As well as directly contributing to the coloration changes in proteins, dityrosine formation is also believed to play an important role in initiating secondary photochemical reactions in proteins [69].

Other residues with a propensity to form crosslinks on photo-oxidation include lysine, arginine and histidine [70].

3. Effect on Functional Attributes

Accumulation of photo-oxidative modifications at the primary residue level translates to secondary, tertiary and quaternary protein level damage through denaturation, breakdown and re-ordering of the native protein conformation [40], and ultimately to the ultrastructuralbreakdown of the proteinaceous material. For many protein substrates, the details of these modifications behind the observed deterioration in performance, condition and quality of the protein material are not yet particularly well understood.A summary of the effects of photo-oxidation on the functional attributes of selected protein-based materials of particular interest either medically or commercially is presented.

3.1. Human Health and Wellbeing

Proteins comprise a critical component of the body's external structure and defences. Photodamage to these proteins is therefore of significant concern.

3.1.1. Skin

Photodamage to skin is arguably the most concerning consequence of increasing UV levels around the globe. Photo-oxidation of proteins within the skin contributes directly or indirectly to photo-ageing and the development of skin disease, notably carcinogenesis [71].

Skin is composed of three major layers – the outermost epidermis, the dermis and the hypodermis[72]. The outermost sub-layer of the epidermis is the stratum corneum (SC), a highly crosslinked proteinaceous matrixwhich is comprised of plate-like envelopes filled with keratin. The keratin contained within the SC plays a key role in preventing moisture loss and keeping the skin hydrated. The dermis consists largely of connective tissue, with high levels of collagen[71].Collagens are a key protein component of all the skin layers[73].

UVB, associated with erythema and carcinoma development, is primarily absorbed in the epidermis, while UVA, associated with skin photo-ageing, can pass through to the dermal layer [74].UV exposure results in the introduction of carbonyl groups into the SC proteins, with protein oxidation levels increasing towards the outer layers [75].Collagen and keratin photodamagecontributes tothe progressive loss of structural integrity and therefore cosmetic damage, including wrinkling and line formation[76]. As skin ages, it becomes thinner and more susceptible to photodamage.

There is increasing evidence for the generation of ROS in skin upon UVexposure. Chronic and acute photodamage is mediated by depleted antioxidant enzyme expression within the SC and in the epidermis,and increased levels of oxidisedproteins[77]. Importantly, oxidatively modified proteins have been found to accumulate specifically within the upper dermis of photo-aged skin[77]. This correlation between overall skin photodamage and protein oxidation is considered a key pathophysiologic factor in photo-ageing and carcinogenesis.

3.1.2. Hair

Human hair is a proteinaceous material composed of an inner cortex of keratins enveloped in overlapping cuticle cells [78]. Intermediate filament proteins represent the major structural proteins in hair, and these are arranged into filamentous bundles within a protein matrix [79]. Hair has a high sulfur content, with extensive disulfide crosslinking within the cortex. The cuticle is also highly crosslinked, with both disulfide and isopeptide bonds [80]. Photo-oxidation of proteins within hair, therefore, can dramatically affect inherent fibre properties.

Photo-oxidation affects important perception attributes of hair such as colour, moisture retention and lustre [81, 82].The effect of sun exposure is related to the amount of melanin present in the hair, which has a protective effect [82]. The formation of chromophores within hair proteins leads to changes in the base coloration.Manageability is also affected through changes in the physical and mechanical properties of the fibres, particularly an increase in brittleness. Photodegradation can exacerbate damage caused by cosmetic treatments, such as bleaching and dyeing. Bleaching, in particular, results in residual peroxides, which contribute to further damage with light exposure [83]. The most common protection utilised is the incorporation of UV blockers into hair-care products, however, as with UV blockers utilised in skin-care applications, these can act as photosensitisers to generate ROS and promote protein damage.

3.1.3. Eyes

The outer structures of the eye, particularly the cornea, absorb most incident UVB under typical sunlight exposure, with little reaching the lens [18]. UVA radiation, however, is strongly implicated in lens photodamage.

The proteins within the eye lens are not subject to the typical removal and replacement protective mechanisms occurring elsewhere in the body, and diffusion of the proteins becomes progressively more limited with ageing [84] Therefore, accumulation of oxidative damage to lens crystallins is a serious concern, particularly with increasing exposure to solar UV. Cataracts result from ongoing photo-oxidation of lens proteins, which leads to loss of light transmission, sight impairment and in the worst cases blindness [38, 84].

Natural protective filters in the young lens, including kynurenine and hydroxykynurenine, absorb about 95% of light >300nm, with the remainder chiefly absorbed by tryptophan residues in the lens proteins. It has been shown the build-up of tryptophan photo-oxidation products, in particular, acts to photosensitise the lens to further damage [18, 38, 85-87]. Some photosensitisation is believed to come directly from the filter compounds, which can end up covalently bound to lens proteinsthrough addition to nucleophilic protein sites, such as cysteine, lysine and histidine [88]. Advanced glycation endproducts have also been implicated in photosensitisation [89].

3.1.4. Pharmaceuticals and Cosmaceuticals

There are many protein- and peptide-based pharmaceutical and cosmaceutical products on the market, with more constantly in further development. It is critical that protein pharmaceuticals maintain their native structure and activity during long-term storage.While photo-oxidation has been recognised as a major contributor to protein degradation in other systems, the effects of photo-induced damage have not yet been widely studied for biopharmaceuticals [21]. This is particularly important since photodegradation can lead to changes in primary, secondary, and tertiary structures of protein and these changes could lead to differences in long-term stability, bioactivity, or immunogenicity. Photostability is therefore a key issue for these products in terms of packaging, shelf-life, efficacy, and particularly with respect to the potential formation of harmful side-products [90, 91]. With pharmaceuticals, solid state photostability is often the key concern, and there is still significant work required to explore underlying photodegradation mechanisms in the absence of water [92]. With protein-based cosmetic products also, often designed for topical application, the photo-oxidative breakdown products are important with respect to efficacy and toxicity.

3.2. Foods

Photo-oxidation is one means by which oxidative degradation is induced in foodstuffs during production, processing, storage, retail, and after purchase[22].Generally speaking, the effects of photo-oxidation will be additive to other forms of oxidative degradation, but are an important consideration when determining food handling protocols. Protein photomodification is of particular concern in the following food categories.

3.2.1. Meat and Seafood

Flavour, colour, texture, nutritional value and functionality comprise essential quality parameters for all meat and seafood products, with direct correlation to product value and consumer perception[93]. These critical attributes are all directly or indirectly affected by protein, and associated lipid, photo-oxidation[94].

For meat and meat products, particularly, lipid oxidation must be considered in parallel to protein oxidation. Aldehyde-derived secondary products of lipid oxidation are associated with the formation of proteinaceous chromophores and fluorophores, and therefore coloration changes[95].Oxidative degradation also leads to deterioration of the nutritional value of meat, through protein damage such as protein-protein crosslinks, protein-lipid crosslinks, protein cleavage and residue specific damage [96, 97], and is particularly important in determining meat colour [98], a characteristic to which consumers are very sensitive. The texture of meat is directly affected by the effects of photo-oxidation, with structural changes resulting from protein backbone cleavage and crosslinking [99]. These structural modifications in turn affect performance properties such as moisture retention and protein solubility [100].

Protein oxidative degradation in seafood products is generally less well studied than meat, however it is of equal concern [101-103].Fish and seafood products are often exposed to light during retail, and photodegradation contributes to tainting and spoilage[104].

3.2.2. Dairy

Proteins represent a critical nutritional and functional component of dairy products. The major milk protein classes are caseins, albumins and globulins[105].

Light-induced degradation reactions in milk and dairy products create a serious problem for the dairy industry because of the development of off-flavours, the decrease in nutritional quality and functionality, and the speed and severity atwhich these phenomena can develop [7, 106-108].Flavour changes are quickly noticeable in milk exposed to sunlight. In tandem with protein photodegradation, riboflavin and vitamin A gradually degrade, milk fat is photo-oxidised, oxygen dissolved in the milk is consumed, and the sensorial quality decreases significantly [106].

Off flavour development in dairy products, such as milk and cheeses, after exposure to light is thought to be mediated by the conversion of riboflavin into a highly reactive, triplet-excited state, enabling it to oxidise proteins [109]. After photo-oxidation, there is an increase in protein carbonyl content in tandem with the specific oxidation of tryptophan, histidine, and methionine residues, as well as the formation of dityrosine. Loss of tryptophan through photo-oxidation has been well-correlated with the formation of *N*-formylkynurenine and kynurenine[110]. The protein structure of all the major milk proteins changes in response to photo-oxidation[111].Caseins are particularly susceptible to photodegradation, with photo-oxidation of tryptophan leading to observed conformational changes in the micro-environment of the residues. Formation of dityrosines is also notably high in caseins. Changes at the secondary and tertiary protein structural levelsoccurinthe globular milk proteins, with protein unfolding noted particularly for lactalbumin and lactoglobulin. This can be accompanied by quaternary protein damage in the form of protein polymerisation[110].

Photo-oxidation also affects the hydrolysis of milk proteins.Changes are observed in the formation of peptides by chymosin after photo-oxidation, with decreased accessibility of chymosin to oxidised proteins reflected in a lower overall level of free amino-terminal groups[112].

3.2.3. Crops

Rising levels of UV exposure are becoming a concern for crop growth and yield, with increased levels of photodegradation observed [11, 113]. This affects proteins within the growing plant, due in some cases to the photo-oxidation of key enzymic tryptophan residues [12, 114]. Specific proteins appear to be particularly vulnerable to oxidative carbonylation in the matrix of plant mitochondria; these include several enzymes of the Krebs cycle, glycine decarboxylase, superoxide dismutase and heat shock proteins [113]. Photo-oxidative insults also affect the quality of high protein plant-derived foods, such as cereals. As with other foodstuffs, oxidative deterioration results in off-flavours and decreased nutritional value [115]. Increasingly, cereal and other proteinaceous plant derivatives are being utilised as additives and ingredients in formulations and processed food, and photo-oxidative stability is a key factor in the final product performance.

3.3. Materials

3.3.1. Wool and Silk Textiles

Wool and other natural animal fibres are keratinous materials with an anatomy comparable to human hair, with a central cortical region comprised largely ofIFP filaments within a matrix, and an outer cuticle region with high levels of crosslinking. Animal fibres are generally >90% proteinaceous in composition. Whereas human hair typically has multiple layers of cuticle cells, many wool types, such as Merino, have only one cuticle layer [116]. Silk, on the other hand,is an extracellular fibrous material comprised mostly of fibroins [117].

Appearance retention is a critical determinant of quality and value for furnishing and apparel textile products, and is directly related to the degree and nature of protein degradation.Photodegradation correlates to several deleterious effects of commercial significance.

Firstly, coloration is severely affected through competing processes of photoyellowing and photobleaching [118]. Photoyellowing is the progressive increase in yellowness generally associated with exposure to UVB and shorter wavelength UVA. There is also an associated decrease in brightness. This phenomenon is particularly significant for apparel textiles which are exposed directly to solar radiation. UVB radiation has been shown to produce a wide range of protein-derived chromophores within wool, with ongoing exposure leading to increasingly coloured species [46, 47]. A correlation has been established between photoyellowing and the carbonyl content in silk [119].Fluorescent whitening agents (FWA), also known as optical brightening agents (OBA), which are now commonly a component of laundry detergents, have been shown to significantly accelerate photoyellowing in wool and silk [120, 121]. These additives act as photosensitisers, generating increased ROS, hydroxyl radicals in particular, and directly cause considerable enhancement in the levels of protein photoproducts [25, 121, 122].Bleaching is also often incorporated into fibre and textile processing, and this has also been shown to exacerbate subsequent photoyellowing. Photobleaching is the progressive decrease in the base yellowness of the fibre generally associated with exposure to blue light or longer wavelength UVA. This is a key concern for interior textiles, where window glass filters out most UVB, and results in uneven photofading [121].

Additionally, fibre protein photo-oxidation results in phototendering, the process by which the proteins progressively lose their structural integrity. This results in increased brittleness and lowered strength, thereby leading to enhanced wear in the textile product [121].

3.3.2. Other

Other protein-based materials where protein photo-oxidation is a significant issue include biomaterials, feathersand artworks/objects of historical and cultural importance, particularly those utilising paints derived from egg-based materials[123]. With an escalating move away from oil-derived materials towards biomaterials, the photostability of protein and peptide components of these is likely to take on increasing importance.

4. Evaluation of Photo-oxidation – New Proteomic Approaches

The complex array, location and interaction of modifications induced within proteins on irradiative exposure make characterisation and evaluation of photodamage very difficult in real biological systems. For this reason, holistic assessment techniques, such asfluorescence mapping and protein extractability have traditionally been used to try to study these systems.

The development and application of powerful new proteomic tools, based around mass spectrometry (MS), promise to revolutionise our understanding of protein photo-oxidation and assist significantly with the development and validation of new strategies for the control of photodamage.

4.1. Redox Proteomics

Redox proteomics is an emerging discipline centred on the study of key reduction and oxidation events occurring within proteins [68]. Application and customisation of techniques adapted from classical proteomics have enabled protein oxidation to be studied and understood in far greater detail than was previously possible. This field therefore provides an ideal set of tools for evaluating the photo-oxidation of proteinaceous systems.

4.1.1. Characterisation and Location

Protein MS is the underpinning tool in proteomics. The two most common modes of MS utilised for protein analysis are electrospray ionisation mass spectrometry (ESI-MS) and matrix assisted laser desorption ionisation mass spectrometry (MALDI-MS) [46, 124, 125], which differ in the means by which the sample is introduced. ESI-MS involves ionising the sample with an applied potential directly from an injected solution, while in MALDI-MS the sample is co-crystallised with a matrix on a plate and is then ionised using a laser.

With respect to studying photo-oxidation directly within proteins, two aspects, in particular, make evaluation challenging –

- Any given protein is likely to have a different pattern of damage
- Any given photomodification at a particular primary location in the protein is likely to be present in extremely low abundance within the sample as a whole

These two factors are often further complicated by extensive protein crosslinking in the substrate.In addition, any effective analytical technique must not induce any further oxidative modification. Mass spectrometry offers a significant advantage over other analytical technologies by enabling the characterisation of what is essentially an array of environmentally-induced post-translational modifications within a complex mixture without the need for complete purification.Typically, the protein sample is enzymatically digested and the generated peptides analysed. Detailed analysis of low abundance peptides within the sample is achieved through liquid chromatography (LC)-ESI or LC-MALDI, where chromatographic fractionation of the peptide mixture is performed prior to MS analysis. Where multiple chromatographic media are utilised in tandem, this approach is referred to as MudPIT (Multi-dimensional Protein Identification Technology)[126].

Through tandem mass spectrometric (MS/MS) analysis, specific peptides can be selected and fragmented through post-source decay or collision with an inert gas to generate fragment ions which provide structural information. Photomodified residues can be determined qualitatively through MS/MS comparison with native non-modified peptides. An example of this is shown in Figure 3[47].

The location of modifications within the primary sequence of proteins is determined through bioinformatic analysis, using software such as Mascot or SEQUEST. Where unknown proteins are involved, BLASTsoftware can be used to find homologous sequences [127]. Where extensive crosslinking inhibits complete enzymatic digestion, such as in the evaluation of hair or wool cuticle, combination chemical/enzymic digestion strategies can be employed. One example is the utilisation of 2-nitro 5-thiocyanobenzoic acid (NTCB) in tandem with trypsin. NTCB cleaves on the N-terminal side of cysteine residues to produce a characteristic terminal modification, allowing selective searching.

4.1.2. Profiling and Tracking

The levels of specific photoproducts provide important information regarding the biological or commercial significance of any given photomodification. Tracking the rates of formation, and the relative levels of specific photoproducts within peptides and proteins generates a protein degradation profile: a useful tool in understanding photodegradative mechanisms, allowing the development of targeted amelioration strategies[41, 128].

Photo-oxidation typically generates a range of products in susceptible protein regions.The formation of these products may be individually detected withMS ion abundance data. MS abundance profiling gives an indication of the relative abundance of each photoproduct.

MS-based profiling can be further progressed to track the progressive degradation of parent peptides, and the corresponding formation of photomodifications, through the changes in their relative abundance. An example is shown in Figure 4 [129].

Tracking the variation in this profile allows the formation of specific peptide modifications to be monitored over time, or over variation in any other parameter.

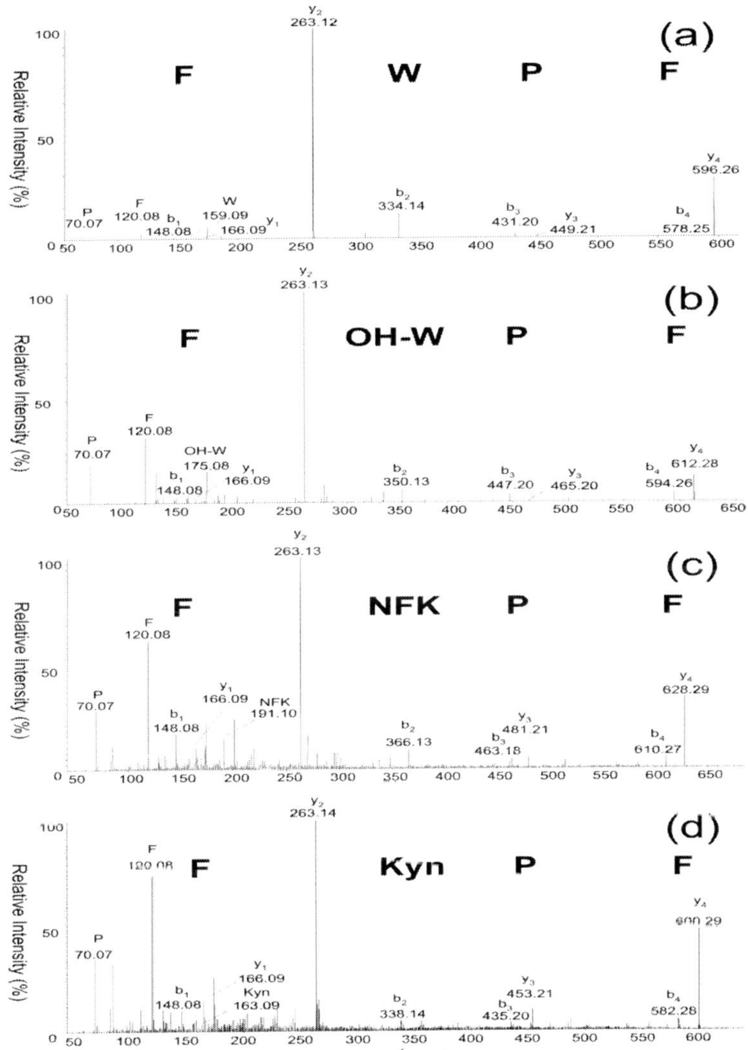

Figure 3. ESI-MS/MS spectra of the wool peptide of native sequence FWPF, (a) unmodified andwith the tryptophan residue photo-oxidisedto (b) hydroxykynurenine (OH-W), (c) N-formylkynurenine (NFK), and (d) kynurenine (Kyn) [47].

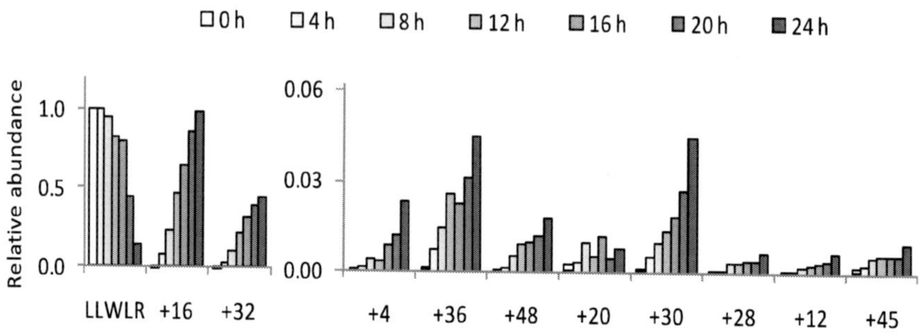

Figure 4. Relative abundance profiling of tryptophan photo-oxidation products formed duringprogressive UVA irradiation of the peptide,LLWLR[129]. Legend: unmodified peptide; +16) W+O modification; +32) W+2O; +4) W+O-C; +36) W+3O; +48) W+4O; +20) W+2O-C; +30) W+2O-2H; +28) W+2O-4H; +12) W+C; +45) W+N+2O-H

For instance, specific ROS can be either blocked or amplified to provide mechanistic information. This approach can be utilised to explore the relative contributions of singlet oxygen and hydroxyl radicals to the formation of specific photoproducts. The current limitations to this strategy revolve around the variation in ion abundances ratios between MS runs. Stable isotope labelling techniques, such as ICAT and iTRAQ, are currently being utilised to effectively quantitate relative protein abundance in a wide range of proteomic studies [130, 131]. We envisage the development and application of related approaches to overcome the currently limitation of MS relative abundance profiling.

A related emerging approach to evaluating protein photo-oxidation involves the characterisation and tracking of marker peptides. Marker peptides are selected through a range of criteria, including reproducible extraction and the presence of a residue which is sensitive to specific photodamage or a specific reactive species [129]. These marker peptides are then utilised to evaluate the overall profile of damage in the protein substrate. This is envisaged to be a particularly effective approach to testing and validating photoprotection treatments.

4.1.3. Carbonylated Proteins

Protein carbonyl content is a good indicator of overall photo-oxidation. Traditionally, overall protein carbonylation has been evaluated through initial derivitisation with 2,4-dinitrophenylhydrazine (DNPH), and subsequent immuno- or spectrophotometric assay [126]. However, two key goals of redox proteomics, as applied to photo-oxidation, are the identification of proteins susceptible to photomodification, and the characterisation and location of specific residues where damage occurs. Recently, affinity purification has been coupled with LC-MS/MS to directly identify and locate carbonylation within a range of oxidised proteins simultaneously. This form of affinity purification involves reaction of biocytin hydrazide with the carbonyl groups in oxidatively modified proteins to induce hydrazone conjugate formation [126]. These are then affinity purified using streptavidin immobilised on agarose, and analysed using MudPIT. This approach offers promise in the evaluation of protein photo-oxidative damage.

It is anticipated that as the field of redox proteomics advances, further developed technologies will be applied and customised to better understand protein photodegradation.

4.2. Crosslink Elucidation

Photo-induced protein-protein crosslinks are particularly difficult to characterise and locate. Not only are any specific crosslinks likely present in very low abundance within the protein substrate, but digestion must be performed in such a way that the crosslinked peptides remain intact during extraction and solubilisation. Novel proteomic approaches are also emerging for the elucidation of crosslinks, which offer routes to advancing progress in this area.

These approaches centre on the utilisation of partial digestion strategies, followed by isotopic labeling [132, 133]. ^{18}O from isotopically enriched water is incorporated into the C-termini of proteolytic peptides [134]. Since crosslinked peptides have two C-termini, two ^{18}O atoms are incorporated where a crosslink is present. These are then combined with peptides from a parallel sample digested in ^{16}O water. Mass spectrometric analysis of the resultant modified peptides can then distinguish and select for crosslinks through searching for a characteristic mass shift of 8 amu relative to the unlabelled peptide [133].

Application of these techniques to detecting photo-induced crosslinks is significantly more complex than for elucidation of native crosslinks, however, this approach provides a potential means to identify and locate specific crosslinked photoproducts.

4.3. Directions

To fully understand each of the protein-based systems affected by photo-oxidation, it is critical that protein primary level information be linked and correlated to damage observed at higher orders of protein and cellular structure. Initial progress has been made in this direction, but there is substantially more progress required.

An enhanced understanding of protein photodegradative mechanisms through the characterisation and location of low abundance photomodifications, in parallel with the development of protocols to examine the pattern and relative abundance of these modifications, represent important goals in protein science. New proteomic approaches to the characterisation and understanding of protein photo-oxidation are revealing significant new levels of detail. We envisage further application and customisation of tools derived from redox proteomics to specific protein-based systems will facilitate the optimisation and validation of new targeted photoprotection treatments.

Acknowledgements

I would like to gratefully acknowledge the assistance of Anita Grosvenor for her critical review and editing of this chapter.

References

[1] Kochevar, IE. Molecular and cellular effects of UV radiation relevant to chronic photodamage. In: Gilchrest, BA, editor. *Photodamage*; 1999, p. 51-67.

[2] Ruetsch, SB; Yang, B; Kamath, YK. Chemical and photo-oxidative hair damage studied by dye diffusion and electrophoresis. *Journal of Cosmetic Science* 2003;54,379-94.

[3] Wondrak, GT; Roberts, MJ; Jacobson, MK, et al. 3-hydroxypyridine chromophores are endogenous sensitizers of photo-oxidative stress in human skin cells. *Journal of Biological Chemistry* 2004;279,30009-20.

[4] Sidorkina, OM; Kuznetsov, SV; Blais, JC, et al. Ultraviolet-B-induced damage to Escherichia coli Fpg protein. *Photochemistry and Photobiology* 1999;69,658-63.

[5] Dalle-Donne, I; Scaloni, A; Giustarini, D, et al. Proteins as biomarkers of oxidative/nitrosative stress in diseases: The contribution of redox proteomics. *Mass Spectrometry Reviews* 2005;24,55-99.

[6] O'Sullivan, MG; Kerry, JP. Sensory and quality properties of packaged meat. In: Kerry, JP; Ledward, D, editors. *Improving the Sensory and Nutritional Quality of Fresh Meat.* Cambridge: Woodhead Publishing Limited; 2009, p. 595-7.

[7] Østdal, H; Weisbjerg, MR; Skibsted, LH, et al. Protection against photo-oxidation of milk by high urate content. *Milchwissenschaft* 2008;63,119-22.

[8] Reddy, GB; Bhat, KS. Protection against UVB inactivation (in vitro) of rat lens enzymes by natural antioxidants. *Molecular and Cellular Biochemistry* 1999;194,41-5.

[9] Kubiak, K; Kowalska, M; Nowak, W. Molecular dynamics study of early events during photo-oxidation of eye lens protein γβ-crystallin. *Journal of Molecular Structure (Theochem)* 2003;630,315-25.

[10] Fujii, N; Uchida, H; Saito, T. The damaging effect of UV-C irradiation on lens alpha-crystallin. *Molecular Vision* 2004;10,814-20.

[11] Stapleton, AE. Ultraviolet radiation and plants: Burning questions. *Plant Cell* 1992;4,1353-8.

[12] Caldwell, CR. Ultraviolet-induced photodegradation of cucumber (*Cucumis sativus* L.) microsomal and soluble protein tryptophanyl residues in vitro. *Plant Physiology* 1993;101,947-53.

[13] Gerhardt, KE; Wilson, MI; Greenberg, BM. Tryptophan photolysis leads to a UVB-induced 66 kDa photoproduct of ribulose-1,5-bisphosphate carboxylase/oxygenase (rubisco) in vitro and in vivo. *Photochemistry and Photobiology* 1999;70,49-56.

[14] Frederick, JE; Lubin, D. Possible long-term changes in biologically active ultraviolet radiation reaching the ground. *Photochemistry and Photobiology* 1988;47,571-8.

[15] Creed, D. The photophysics and photochemistry of the near-UV absorbing amino acids - II. Tyrosine and its simple derivatives. *Photochemistry and Photobiology* 1984;39,563-75.

[16] Creed, D. The photophysics and photochemistry of the near-UV absorbing amino acids - I. Tryptophan and its simple derivatives. *Photochemistry and Photobiology* 1984;39,537-62.

[17] Girotti, AW; Giacomoni, PU. Lipid and protein damage provoked by ultraviolet radiation: Mechanisms of indirect photo-oxidative damage. In: Giacomoni, PU, editor. *Biophysical and Physiological Effects of*

Solar Radiation on Human Skin. Cambridge, UK: RSC Publishing; 2007, p. 271-91.

[18] Mizdrak, J; Hains, PG; Truscott, RJW, et al. Tryptophan-derived ultraviolet filter compounds covalently bound to lens proteins are photosensitizers of oxidative damage. *Free Radical Biology and Medicine* 2008;44,1108-19.

[19] Davies, MJ. Reactive species formed on proteins exposed to singlet oxygen. *Photochemical and Photobiological Sciences* 2004;3,17-25.

[20] Trautinger, F. Damaged proteins: Repair or removal? In: Giacomoni, PU, editor. *Biophysical and Physiological Effects of Solar Radiation on Human Skin*. Cambridge, UK: RSC Publishing; 2007, p. 311-9.

[21] Kerwin, BA; Remmele, RLJ. Protect from light: Photodegradation and protein biologics. *Journal of Pharmaceutical Sciences* 2007;96,1468-79.

[22] Min, DB; Boff, JM. Chemistry and reaction of singlet oxygen in foods. *Comprehensive Reviews in Food Science and Food Safety* 2002;1,58-72.

[23] Lee, J; Koo, N; Min, DB. Reactive oxygen species, aging, and antioxidative nutraceuticals. *Comprehensive Reviews in Food Science and Food Safety* 2004;3,21-33.

[24] Nukuna, BN; Goshe, MB; Anderson, VE. Sites of hydroxyl radical reaction with amino acids identified by 2H NMR detection of induced 1H/2H exchange. *Journal of the American Chemical Society* 2001;123,1208-14.

[25] Dyer, J; Clerens, S; Cornellison, C, et al. Photoproducts formed in the photoyellowing of collagen in the presence of a fluorescent whitening agent. *Photochemistry and Photobiology* 2009;85,1314-1321.

[26] Thiagarajan, G; Lakshmanan, J; Chalasani, M, et al. Peroxynitrite reaction with eye lens proteins: a-crystallin retains its activity despite modification. *Investigative Ophthalmology and Visual Science* 2004;45,2115-21.

[27] Yamakura, F; Ikeda, K. Modification of tryptophan and tryptophan residues in proteins by reactive nitrogen species. *Nitric Oxide Biology and Chemistry* 2006;14,152-61.

[28] Beckman, JS; Beckman, TW; Chen, J, et al. Apparent hydroxyl radical production by peroxynitrite: implications for endothelial injury from nitric oxide and superoxide. *Proceedings of the National Academy of Sciences of the United States of America* 1990;87,1620-4.

[29] Davies, MJ. Singlet oxygen-mediated damage to proteins and its consequences. *Biochemical and Biophysical Research Communications* 2003;305,761-70.

[30] Stadtman, ER; Levine, RL. Chemical modification of proteins by reactive oxygen species. In: Dalle-Donne, I; Scaloni, A; Butterfield, DA, editors. *Redox Proteomics - From Protein Modifications to Cellular Dysfunctions and Diseases*. Hoboken: John Wiley and Sons, Inc.; 2006, p. 3-23.

[31] Gill, AC; Ritchie, MA; Hunt, LG, et al. Post-translational hydroxylation at the N-terminus of the prion protein reveals presence of PPII structure *in vivo*. *EMBO Journal* 2000;19,5324-31.

[32] Bender, DA; Barrett, GC. *Chemistry and biochemistry of the amino acids*. London: Chapman and Hall; 1985.

[33] Goshe, MB; Chen, YH; Anderson, VE. Identification of the sites of hydroxyl radical reaction with peptides by hydrogen/deuterium exchange: prevalence of reactions with the side chains. *Biochemistry* 2000;39,1761-70.

[34] Berlett, BS; Stadtman, ER. Protein oxidation in aging, disease, and oxidative stress. *Journal of Biological Chemistry* 1997;272,20313-6.

[35] Schäfer, K; Goddinger, D; Höcker, H. Photodegradation of tryptophan in wool. *Journal of the Society of Dyers and Colourists* 1997;133,350-5.

[36] Asquith, RS; Hirst, L; Rivett, DE. *Effects of ultraviolet radiation as related to the yellowing of wool*. Applied Polymer Symposium; 1971 1971; 1971. p. 333-5.

[37] Asquith, RS; Rivett, DE. The photolysis of tyrosine and its possible relationship to the yellowing of wool. *Textile Research Journal* 1969;39,633-7.

[38] Davies, MJ; Truscott, RJW. Photo-oxidation of proteins and its role in cataractogenesis. *Journal of Photochemistry and Photobiology B: Biology* 2001;63,114-25.

[39] Boreen, AL; Edhlund, BL; Cotner, JB, et al. Indirect photodegradation of dissolved free amino acids: The contribution of singlet oxygen and the differential reactivity of DOM from various sources. *Environmental Science and Technology* 2008;42,5492-8.

[40] Dean, RT; Fu, S; Stocker, R, et al. Biochemistry and pathology of radical-mediated protein oxidation. *Biochemical Journal* 1997;324,1-18.

[41] Davies, MJ; Fu, S; Wang, H, et al. Stable markers of oxidant damage to proteins and their application in the study of human disease. *Free Radical Biology and Medicine* 1999;27,1151-63.

[42] Asquith, RS; Rivett, DE. Studies on the photo-oxidation of tryptophan. *Biochimica et Biophysica Acta* 1971;252,111-6.

[43] Simat, TJ; Steinhart, H. Oxidation of free tryptophan and tryptophan residues in peptides and proteins. *Journal of Agricultural and Food Chemistry* 1998;46,490-8.

[44] Maskos, J; Rush, JD; Koppenol, WH. The hydroxylation of tryptophan. *Archives of Biochemistry and Biophysics* 1992;296,514-20.

[45] Żegota, H; Kołodziejczyk, K; Król, M, et al. o-Tyrosine hydroxylation by $OH^{\cdot}$ radicals.2,3-DOPA and 2,5-DOPA formation in γ-irradiated aqueous solution. *Radiation Physics and Chemistry* 2005;72,25-33.

[46] Dyer, JM; Bringans, S; Bryson, WG. Characterisation of photo-oxidation products within photoyellowed wool proteins: tryptophan and tyrosine derived chromophores. *Photochemical and Photobiological Sciences* 2006;5,698-706.

[47] Dyer, JM; Bringans, SD; Bryson, WG. Determination of photo-oxidation products within photoyellowed bleached wool proteins. *Photochemistry and Photobiology* 2006;82,551-7.

[48] Guedes, S; Vitorino, R; Domingues, Rr, et al. Oxidation of bovine serum albumin: identification of oxidation products and structural modifications. *Rapid Communications in Mass Spectrometry* 2009;23,2307-15.

[49] Maskos, Z; Rush, JD; Koppenol, WH. The hydroxylation of phenylalanine and tyrosine: A comparison with salicylate and tryptophan. *Archives of Biochemistry and Biophysics* 1992;296,521-9.

[50] Wei, C; Song, B; Yuan, J, et al. Luminescence and Raman spectroscopic studies on the damage of tryptophan, histidine and carnosine by singlet oxygen. *Journal of Photochemistry and Photobiology A: Chemistry* 2007;189,39-45.

[51] Teale, WWJ. The ultraviolet fluorescence of proteins in neutral solution. *Biochemical Journal* 1960;76,381-8.

[52] Chiu, HC; Bersohn, R. Electronic energy transfer between tyrosine and tryptophan in the peptides trp-$(pro)_n$-Tyr. *Biopolymers* 1977;16,277-88.

[53] Simpson, WS. *Origins of variation in the fluorescence patterns of wool and wool proteins*. Proceedings of the 9th International Wool Textile Research Conference; 1995 1995; Biella, Italy; 1995. p. 429-39.

[54] Garner, MH; Spector, A. Selective oxidation of cysteine and methionine in normal and senile cataractous lenses. *Proceedings of the National Academy of Sciences of the United States of America* 1980;77,1274-7.

[55] Hearle, JW. A critical review of the structural mechanics of wool and hair fibres. *International Journal of Biological Macromolecules* 2000;27,123-38.

[56] Parbhu, AN; Bryson, WG; Lal, R. Disulfide bonds in the outer layer of keratin fibers confer higher mechanical rigidity: correlative nano-indentation and elasticity measurement with an AFM. *Biochemistry* 1999;38,11755-61.

[57] Katsumi, A; Tuley, EA; Bodo, I, et al. Localization of disulfide bonds in the cystine knot domain of human von Willebrand factor. *Journal of Biological Chemistry* 2000;275,25585-94.

[58] Li, Z; Bruce, A; Galley, WC. Temperature dependence of the disulfide perturbation to the triplet state of tryptophan. *Biophysical Journal* 1992;61,1364-71.

[59] Earland, C; Raven, DJ. Lanthionine formation in keratin. *Nature* 1961;191,384-.

[60] Bessems, GJ; Rennen, HJ; Hoenders, HJ. Lanthionine, a protein crosslink in cataractous human lenses. *Experimental Eye Research* 1987;44,691-5.

[61] Sionkowska, A; Kaminska, A. Thermal helix-coil transition in UV irradiated collagen from rat tail tendon. *International Journal of Biological Macromolecules* 1999;24,337-40.

[62] Kato, Y; Uchida, K; Kawakishi, S. Oxidative degradation of collagen and its model peptide by ultraviolet irradiation. *Journal of Agriculture and Food Chemistry* 1992;40,373-9.

[63] Stadtman, ER; Berlett, BS. Fenton chemistry. Amino acid oxidation. *Journal of Biological Chemistry* 1991;266,17201-11.

[64] Gieseg, S; Simpson, JA; Charlton, TS, et al. Protein-bound 3,4-dihydroxyphenylalanine is a major reductant formed during hydroxyl radical damage to proteins. *Biochemistry* 1993;32,4780-6.

[65] Holt, LA; Milligan, B. The formation of carbonyl groups during irradiation of wool and its relevance to photoyellowing. *Textile Research Journal* 1977;47,620-4.

[66] Stadtman, ER. Protein oxidation and aging. *Free Radical Research* 2006;40,1250-8.

[67] Scaloni, A. Mass spectrometry approaches for the molecular characterisation of oxidatively/nitrosatively modified proteins. In: Dalle-Donne, I; Scaloni, A; Desiderio, DM; Nibbering, NM, editors. *Redox Proteomics*; 2006.

[68] Dalle-Donne, I; Scaloni, A; Butterfield, DA, editors. *Redox Proteomics - From Protein Modifications to Cellular Dysfunctions and Diseases*. Hoboken: John Wiley and Sons, Inc.; 2006.

[69] Vazquez, S; Aquilina, JA; Jamie, JF, et al. Novel protein modification by kynurenine in human lenses. *Journal of Biological Chemistry* 2002;277,4867-73.

[70] Taylor, CM; Wang, W. Histidinoalanine: a crosslinking amino acid. *Tetrahedron* 2007;63,9033-47.

[71] Giacomoni, PU, editor. *Biophysical and Physiological Effects of Solar Radiation on Human Skin.* Cambridge, UK: RSC Publishing; 2007.

[72] Song, HK; Wehrli, FW; Ma, J. *In vivo* MR microscopy of the human skin. *Magnetic Resonance in Medicine* 1997;37,185-91.

[73] Epstein, EH, Jr.; Munderloh, NH. Human skin collagen. Presence of type I and type III at all levels of the dermis. *Journal of Biological Chemistry* 1978;253,1336-7.

[74] Duval, C; Regnier, M; Schmidt, R. Distinct melanogenic response of human melanocytes in mono-culture, in co-culture with keratinocytes and in reconstructed epidermis, to UV exposure. *Pigment Cell Research* 2001;14,348-55.

[75] Thiele, JJ; Schroeter, C; Hsieh, SN, et al. The antioxidant network of the stratum corneum. *Current Problems in Dermatology* 2001;29,26-42.

[76] Gilchrest, BA. A review of skin ageing and its medical therapy. *British Journal of Dermatology* 1996;135,867-75.

[77] Sander, CS; Chang, H; Salzmann, S, et al. Photoaging is associated with protein oxidation in human skin in vivo. *Journal of Investigative Dermatology* 2002;118,618-25.

[78] Hashimoto, K. The structure of human hair. *Clinics in Dermatology* 1988;6,7-21.

[79] Popescu, C; Höcker, H. Hair - the most sophisticated biological composite material. *Chemical Society Reviews* 2007;36,1282-91.

[80] Bringans, SD; Plowman, JE; Dyer, JM, et al. Characterization of the exocuticle a-layer proteins of wool. *Experimental Dermatology* 2007;16,951-60.

[81] Nogueira, ACS; Richena, M; Dicelio, LE, et al. Photo yellowing of human hair. *Journal of Photochemistry and Photobiology B: Biology* 2007;88,119-25.

[82] Nogueira, ACS; Diceliob, LE; Joekes, I. About photodamage of human hair. *Photochemical and Photobiological Sciences* 2006;5,165-9.

[83] Dawber, R. Hair: Its structure and response to cosmetic preparations. *Clinics in Dermatology* 1996;14,105-12.

[84] Williams, DL. Oxidation, antioxidants and cataract formation: a literature review. *Veterinary Ophthamology* 2006;9,292-8.

[85] Dillon, J; Spector, A; Nakanishi, K. Identification of β-carbolines isolated from fluorescent human lens proteins. *Nature* 1976;259,422-3.

[86] Balasubramanian, D; Du, X; Zigler, JS. The reaction of singlet oxygen with proteins, with special reference to crystallins. *Photochemistry and Photobiology* 1990;52,761-8.

[87] Finley, EL; Dillon, J; Crouch, RK, et al. Identification of tryptophan oxidation products in bovine α-crystallin. *Protein Science* 1998;7,2391-7.

[88] Parker, NR; Jamie, JF; Davies, MJ, et al. Protein-bound kynurenine is a photosensitizer of oxidative damage. *Free Radical Biology and Medicine* 2004;37,1479-89.

[89] Fuentealba, D; Friguet, B; Silva, E. Advanced glycation endproducts induce photocrosslinking and oxidation of bovine lens tissue through Type-I mechanism. *Photochemistry and Photobiology* 2009;85,185-94.

[90] Piechocki, JT; Thoma, K, editors. *Pharmaceutical Photostability and Stabilization Technology*: Informa HealthCare; 2006.

[91] Manning, MC; Patel, K; Borchardt, RT. Stability of protein pharmaceuticals. *Journal Pharmaceutical Research* 1989;6,903-18.

[92] Byrn, SR; Xu, W; Newman, AW. Chemical reactivity in solid-state pharmaceuticals: formulation implications. *Advanced Drug Delivery Reviews* 2001;48,115-36.

[93] Kerry, JP; Ledward, D, editors. *Improving the Sensory and Nutritional Quality of Fresh Meat*. Cambridge: Woodhead Publishing Limited; 2009.

[94] Spanier, AM; Flores, M; Toldra, F, et al. Meat flavor: contribution of proteins and peptides to the flavor of beef. In: Shahidi, F, editor. *Quality of fresh and processed foods*: Kluwer Academic/Plenum Publishers; 2004, p. 33-49.

[95] Sun, Q; Faustman, C; Senecal, A, et al. Aldehyde reactivity with 2-thiobarbituric acid and TBARS in freeze-dried beef during accelerated storage. *Meat Science* 2001;57,55-60.

[96] Erickson, MC. Lipid oxidation: Flavor and nutritional quality deterioration in frozen foods. In: Erickson, MP; Hung, YC, editors. *Quality in Frozen Food*: Springer; 1997.

[97] Love, JD; Pearson, AM. Lipid oxidation in meat and meat products - a review. *Journal of the American Oil Chemists' Society* 1971;48,547-9.

[98] Møller, JKS; Bertelsen, G; Skibsted, LH. Photo-oxidation of nitrosylmyoglobin at low oxygen pressure. Quantum yields and reaction stoechiometries. *Meat Science* 2002;60,421-5.

[99] Kan, CW; Chan, K; Yuen, CWM, et al. Wool modification. *Textile Asia* 1997;28,39-45.

[100] Xiong, YL. Protein oxidation and implications for muscle food quality. In: Decker, E; Faustman, C; Lopez-Bote, CJ, editors. *Antioxidants in Muscle Foods - Nutritional Strategies to Improve Quality*: Wiley Interscience; 2000, p. 85-112.

[101] Kinoshita, Y; Sato, T. Proteomic studies on protein oxidation in bonito (*Katsuwonus pelamis*) muscle. *Food Science and Technology Research* 2007;13,133-8.

[102] Kjaersgard, IVH; Jessen, F. Two-dimensional gel electrophoresis detection of protein oxidation in fresh and tainted rainbow trout muscle. *Journal of Agricultural and Food Chemistry* 2004;52,7101-7.

[103] Baron, CP; KjÃ†rsgÃ¥rd, IVH; Jessen, F, et al. Protein and lipid oxidation during frozen storage of rainbow trout (*Oncorhynchus mykiss*). *Journal of Agricultural and Food Chemistry* 2007;55,8118-25.

[104] Tokur, B; Korkmaz, K. The effects of an iron-catalyzed oxidation system on lipids and proteins of dark muscle fish. *Food Chemistry* 2007;104,754-60.

[105] Farrell, HM, Jr.; Jimenez-Flores, R; Bleck, GT, et al. Nomenclature of the proteins of cows' milk - Sixth revision. *Journal of Dairy Science* 2004;87,1641-74.

[106] Mestdagh, F; De Meulenaer, B; De Clippeleer, J, et al. Protective influence of several packaging materials on light oxidation of milk. *Journal of Dairy Science* 2005;88,499-510.

[107] Havemose, MS; Weisbjerg, MR; Bredie, WLP, et al. Influence of feeding different types of roughage on the oxidative stability of milk. *International Dairy Journal* 2004;14,563-70.

[108] Jung, MY; Yoon, SH; Lee, HO, et al. Singlet oxygen and ascorbic acid effects on dimethyl disulfide and off-flavor in skim milk exposed to light. *Journal of Food Science* 1998;63,408-12.

[109] Becker, EM; Cardoso, DR; Skibsted, LH. Deactivation of riboflavin triplet-excited state by phenolic antioxidants: mechanism behind protective effects in photo-oxidation of milk-based beverages. *European Food Research and Technology* 2005;221,382-6.

[110] Dalsgaard, TK; Otzen, D; Nielsen, J, et al. Changes in structures of milk proteins upon photo-oxidation. *Journal of Agricultural and Food Chemistry* 2007;55,10968-76.

[111] Dalsgaard, TK; Heegaard, CW; Larsen, LB. Plasmin digestion of photooxidized milk proteins. *Journal of Dairy Science* 2008;91,2175-83.

[112] Dalsgaard, TK; Larsen, LB. Effect of photo-oxidation of major milk proteins on protein structure and hydrolysis by chymosin. *International Dairy Journal* 2009.

[113] Møller, IM; Kristensen, BK. Protein oxidation in plant mitochondria as a stress indicator. *Photochemical and Photobiological Sciences* 2004;3,730-5.

[114] Rinalducci, S; Murgiano, L; Zolla, L. Redox proteomics: basic principles and future perspectives for the detection of protein oxidation in plants. *Journal of Experimental Botany* 2008;59,3781-801.

[115] Heinio, R-L; Lehtinen, P; Oksman-Caldentey, K-M, et al. Differences between sensory profiles and development of rancidity during long-term storage of native and processed oat. *Cereal Chemistry* 2002;79,367.

[116] MacKinnon, PJ; Powell, BC; Rogers, GE. Structure and expression of genes for a class of cysteine-rich proteins of the cuticle layers of differentiating wool and hair follicles. *Journal of Cell Biology* 1990;111,2587-600.

[117] Jianzhong, S; Jinqiang, L; Jinhuan, Z, et al. X-ray photoelectron spectroscopic study of silk fibroin surface. *Polymer International* 2002;51,1479-83.

[118] Duffield, PA; Lewis, DM. The yellowing and bleaching of wool. *Review of Progress in Coloration* 1985;15,38-51.

[119] Baltova, S; Vassileva, V. Photochemical behaviour of natural silk--II. Mechanism of fibroin photodestruction. *Polymer Degradation and Stability* 1998;60,61-5.

[120] Dyer, JM; Cornellison, CD; Bringans, SD, et al. The photoyellowing of stilbene-derived fluorescent whitening agents—mass spectrometric characterization of yellow photoproducts. *Photochemistry and Photobiology* 2008;84,145-53.

[121] Millington, KR. Photoyellowing of wool. Part 1: Factors affecting photoyellowing and experimental techniques. *Coloration Technology* 2006;122,169-86.

[122] Millington, KR; Maurdev, G. The generation of superoxide and hydrogen peroxide by exposure of fluorescent whitening agents to UVA radiation and its relevance to the rapid photoyellowing of whitened wool. *Journal of Photochemistry and Photobiology A: Chemistry* 2004;165,177-85.

[123] Nevin, A; Anglos, D. Assisted interpretation of laser-induced fluorescence spectra of egg-based binding media using total emission fluorescence spectroscopy. *Laser Chemistry* 2006;Article ID 82823,5.

[124] Domingues, MR; Domingues, P; Reis, A, et al. Identification of oxidation products and free radicals of tryptophan by mass spectrometry. *Journal of the American Society for Mass Spectrometry* 2003;14,406-16.

[125] Abello, N; Kerstjens, HAM; Postma, DS, et al. Protein tyrosine nitration: Selectivity, physicochemical and biological consequences, denitration and proteomics methods for the identification of tyrosine-nitrated proteins. *Journal of Proteome Research* 2009;8,3222-38.

[126] Thomas, SN; Lu, B-W; Nikolskaya, T, et al. MudPIT (multidimensional protein identification technology) for identification of post-translational protein modifications in complex biological mixtures. In: Dalle-Donne, I; Scaloni, A; Butterfield, DA, editors. *Redox Proteomics - From Protein Modifications to Cellular Dysfunctions and Diseases*. Hoboken: John Wiley and Sons, Inc.; 2006, p. 233-52.

[127] BLAST software. Available from: http://blast.ncbi.nlm.nih.gov/Blast.cgi?PROGRAM=blastpand BLAST_PROGRAMS=blastpandPAGE_TYPE=BlastSearchandSHOW _DEFAULTS=onandLINK_LOC=blasthome

[128] Gracanin, M; Hawkins, CL; Pattison, DI, et al. Singlet-oxygen-mediated amino acid and protein oxidation: Formation of tryptophan peroxides and decomposition products. *Free Radical Biology and Medicine* 2009;47,92-102.

[129] Grosvenor, AJ; Morton, JD; Dyer, JM. Profiling of residue-level photo-oxidative damage in peptides. *Amino Acids* 2009 In Press. (doi: 10.1007/s00726-009-0440-7).

[130] Wiese, S; Reidegeld, KA; Meyer, HE, et al. Protein labeling by iTRAQ: A new tool for quantitative mass spectrometry in proteome research. *Proteomics* 2007;7,340-50.

[131] Wu, WW; Wang, G; Baek, SJ, et al. Comparative study of three proteomic quantitative methods, DIGE, cICAT, and iTRAQ, using 2D gel- or LC-MALDI TOF/TOF. *Journal of Proteome Research* 2006;5,651-8.

[132] Chen, X; Chen, YH; Anderson, VE. Protein crosslinks: Universal isolation and characterization by isotopic derivatization and electrospray ionization mass spectrometry. *Analytical Biochemistry* 1999;273,192-203.

[133] Back, JW; Notenboom, V; De Koning, LJ, et al. Identification of crosslinked peptides for protein interaction studies using mass spectrometry and 18O labeling. *Analytical Chemistry* 2002;74,4417-22.

[134] Mirza, SP; Greene, AS; Olivier, M. ^{18}O labeling over a coffee break: A rapid strategy for quantitative proteomics. *Journal of Proteome Research* 2008;7,3042-8.

In: Advances in Proteomics Research
Editors: Ya Li Huang et al. pp. 33-62
ISBN: 978-1-61942-227-8

Chapter 2

DECODING AMINO ACID SEQUENCES OF PROTEINS USING INTER-RESIDUE AVERAGE DISTANCE STATISTICS TO EXTRACT INFORMATION ON PROTEIN FOLDING MECHANISMS

Takeshi Kikuchi*
Department of Bioinformatics,
College of Biosciences, Ritsumeikan University, Japan.

ABSTRACT

One of the ultimate goals of bioinformatics is to discover the principlesgoverning protein folding. However, information on folding mechanisms of proteins cannot be easily decoded from amino acid sequences using standard bioinformatics techniques such as multiple sequence alignment and so on. We still do not sufficiently understand how the determinants of protein folding are encoded in amino acid sequences. In this review, we summarize how information about protein folding mechanisms can be extracted from amino acid sequences using inter-residue average distance statistics. Our kind of predicted contact

* Corresponding author: e-mail: tkikuchi@sk.ritsumei.ac.jp1-1-1 Nojihigashi, Kusatsu, Shiga575-8577, JAPAN

map (Average Distance Map, ADM) pinpoints regions of possible folding nuclei for proteins. The amino acid sequence of a given protein suffice for construction of the ADM of a protein. An inter-residue effective potential is defined from the average distance statistics and is utilized to predict folding nucleation sites of a protein sequence. We review examples of the applications of these methods to the analyses of the protein folding of members of several protein families. The general possibility of predicting protein folding mechanisms from only sequences is also discussed.

INTRODUCTION

A remarkable property of a protein is the approximate two-state transition from disorder to a folded state. [1] Thus, it is very interesting and significant to elucidate how a protein folds into a 3D structure in the two-state manner and how information on the folding mechanism is contained in the amino acid sequence. Predicting the protein 3D structure from the amino acid sequence and elucidating how the information on protein folding mechanism is coded in the amino acid sequence are still unsolved problems in molecular biophysics today. Development of new techniques for protein 3D structure prediction in the last decade is remarkable, but it is still not sufficient as seen in the CASP contests. [2, 3] The prediction of folding mechanism is usually based on its native structure. [4-7] Few studies have addressed the challenge of predicting folding mechanism from only sequence. Advances in predicting folding rate of proteins have been made in recent years. [8-11].

There are several remarkable properties of protein 3D structures and folding including the following examples.

1. There are some common folds of proteinswith low sequence identity. These folds are called superfolds. [12]
2. Some proteins whose sequences share high sequence identity show different folds. [13-16]
3. Some proteins sharing a same fold exhibit different folding mechanisms. [17]

It is commonly accepted that a pair of sequences with more than 30% identity shares a similar fold, and less than 20% is associated with 3D structures with no similarity. In the range 20–30%, predictability of the 3D structure similarity is difficult (twilight zone). However, there are some proteins that do not fit these criteria. The protein folding principle should explain the above remarkable phenomena 1-3.

The main problem, of course, is how we extract the various kinds of information on the3D structure of a protein from its amino acid sequence. Predicting the folding mechanism of a protein relates to the questionsof where and how a folding transition state or a folding intermediateis encoded in the sequence of a protein.Thus, the first question to be solved should be how such regionsin a protein are coded on its sequence. It is rather difficult to get such information from standard bioinformatics techniques such as multiple alignments, sequence motif, sequence profile, and so on. Here, we try to review some recent techniques to decode folding information from an amino acid sequence based on inter-residue average distance statistics of proteins.

The methods we explain here are based on the statistics of inter-residue average distances in protein with known 3D structures. A key method involves constructing a kind of contact map based on inter-residue average distances. We refer to this map as the Average Distance Map, or ADM. ADM is constructed from sequence only, and the method can be applied to a protein with unknown 3D structure. Another technique is an unfolding state simulation using a bead model of a protein with a potential derived from the inter-residue average distance statistics. This method also does not require any information on the 3D structure. That is, we can say that information in a protein sequence is translated to ADM or other data, and we try to extract the information of 3D structure formation from them.

AVERAGE DISTANCE MAP, ADM

In this section, the essence of this method is described. For the details of the method, see Refs. [18] and [19].

1. Calculation of Inter-Residue Average Distances in Proteins with Known 3D Structures

In the calculations of inter-residue average distances, an interval between residues i and j on a sequence isclassifiedbased on proximity ranges with k as $1 \leqq k \leqq 8$, $9 \leqq k \leqq 20$, $21 \leqq k \leqq 30$, $31 \leqq k \leqq 40$ and so on where $k=|i-j|$, and inter-residue average distances are calculatedin each interval. Each group of k is referred to as the range M, i.e., M=1 when $1 \leqq k \leqq 8$, M=2 when $9 \leqq k \leqq 20$,

M=3 when $21 \leqq k \leqq 30$ and so on. (Refer to Ref. [18] for proteins used in the calculations of average distances.) In this article, an inter-residue distance means an inter-Cα atomic distance.

2. Construction of a Predicted Contact Map (ADM) with the Amino Acid Sequence of a Protein with 3D Structure Unknown

ADM is constructed in a fashion similar to the usual contact map based on 3D coordinates of a protein [20-21], but unlike the usual contact map, a plot is made on the map to indicate when a pair of residues has an average distance less than cutoff distance.For a protein under study, a set of cutoff distances is determined to reproduce a ratio of the number of plots to the whole area (the whole area corresponds to N(N-1)/2 when N is the total number of residues in a protein). This ratio is referred to as density of plots. A density of plots on a map constructed from the known 3D structure of a protein is approximated to be inversely proportional to the residue number if we assume that residues in a protein packed into a globule shape in an ideal case. [18]

That is, the contact number for a residue is regarded roughly as constant and thus the total number of contacts is approximately proportional to N. The whole area includes roughly $N^2/2$ of pair of residues when N is large. The density of plot can be roughly estimated as constant × (1/N).

A cutoff distance is defined for each range of intervals of a pair of residues on a sequence. A set of cutoff distances are determined to reproduce the predicted density of plots on a contact map along the same consideration. That is, the number of pairs of residues to be plotted on ADM is set to be proportional to 1/M. [18] A map constructed in this way is referred to as an Average Distance Map or ADM

3. Analysis of ADM

Thearea with a high density of plots on a map is considered as indicating thatmany contacts occurred between two segments in a given protein. Such a region on a map can be detected as a sudden change of the density of plots. When a map is divided into two parts by a line parallel to the ordinate of a map, the difference in densities of plots between two parts, i.e., triangle part and trapezoid part, can be calculated (see Figure 1(a)). The same procedure is applied by a line parallel to the abscissa (see Figure 1(b)).

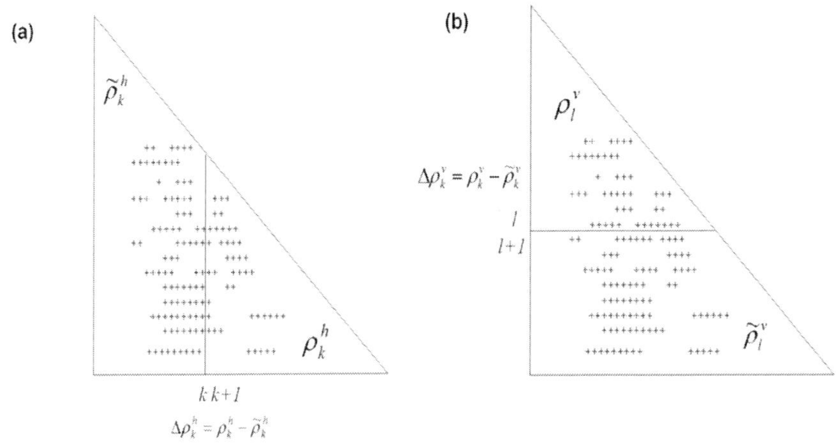

Figure 1. Schematic drawing of a fictitious ADM. (a) The map is divided by a line parallel to the ordinate. The ratio of the number of plots to the whole area in the trapezoid is $\tilde{\rho}_k^h$. The ratio of the number of plots to the area in the whole area in the triangle is ρ_k^h, and $\Delta\rho_k^h = \rho_k^h - \tilde{\rho}_k^h$. (b) The map is divided by a line parallel to the abscissa. The ratio of the number of plots to the whole area in the trapezoid is $\tilde{\rho}_l^v$. The ratio of the number of plots to the area in the whole area in the triangle is ρ_l^v, and $\Delta\rho_l^v = \rho_l^v - \tilde{\rho}_l^v$.

In Figure 1 (a), the density of plots of the trapezoid part is denoted as $\tilde{\rho}_k^h$ and that of the triangle part is ρ_k^h, and the difference in the densities is expressed as $\Delta\rho_k^h = \rho_k^h - \tilde{\rho}_k^h$. (h means the horizontal scanning of $\Delta\rho_k^h$.) The line showing highest difference in densities suggests the boundary of a compact region on a map as seen in the schematic drawing in Figure 2(a). The line denoting the plot of $\Delta\rho_k^h$ shows the peak at m and the valley at n and the peak and the valley indicate the boundary of the compact region at m and n in Figure 2(a). The same procedure can be performed with the line parallel to the abscissa (Figure 2(a)), and $\Delta\rho_k^v = \rho_k^v - \tilde{\rho}_k^v$. (v denotes the vertical scanning of $\Delta\rho_k^v$.) The boundary of the compact region can be indicated by the valley at o and the peak at p.

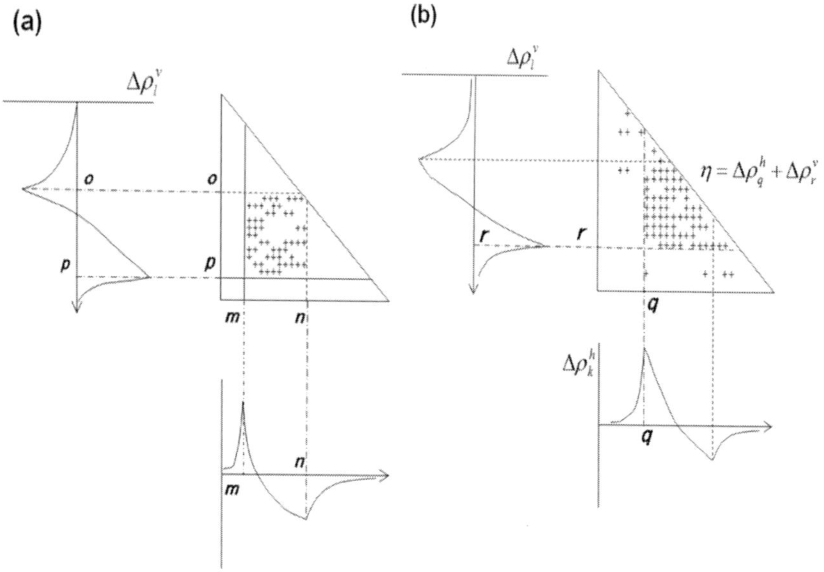

Figure 2. (a) A peak and a valley appear at the boundaries of a high dense region of plots. This fictitious map suggests the interaction between the segments m-n and o-p. (b)A compact region or a domain in a given protein can be observed as a highly dense region of plots along the diagonal of a map. This map shows a schematic drawing of a domain at q-r. We define η as a measure of the compactness of the region, i.e., $\eta = \Delta\rho_r^h + \Delta\rho_q^v$.

In Figure 2(a), we detect that the segments *m-n* and *o-p* in a given protein interact with each other. Acompact region in a given protein is observed as a highly dense region of plots along the diagonal of a contact map. In this case as schematically shown in Figure 2(b), two lines parallel to the ordinate and abscissa atthe peaks of the changes of densities (q and r in Figure 2(b)) in the ADM suggest the existence of a compact region q-r in a given protein. The summation of the differences in densities defined by lines parallel to the ordinate and the abscissa is called η value and this value is considered to be a measure of compactness of the region. ($\eta = \Delta\rho_r^h + \Delta\rho_q^v$ in the example of Figure 2(b)) We regard a compact region predicted by ADM as a folding initiation site.

F VALUE, CONTACT FREQUENCY OF RESIDUES IN UNFOLDED STATES

In this article, an F value is defined as a measure of a contact frequency of a residue during the structural sampling in unfolded states using a potential which can reproduce average distances and standard deviations in the inter-residue average distance statistics of the present work assuming the Gaussian distribution. [22]The F value is derived from a z value in the statistics of contact frequencies. [23]

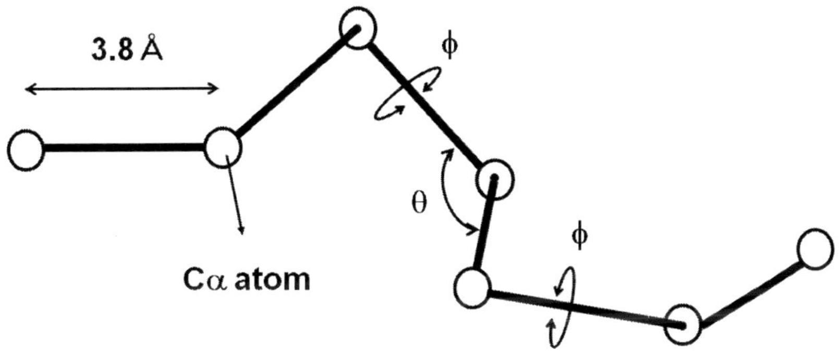

Figure 3. A bead model for a protein. A bead is located at a Cα atom of a residue and a peptide bond is expressed as a virtual bond of 3.8Å. A bead represents a residue and its details are ignored. A bond angle, θ, and a dihedral angle, ϕ, are variable.

A protein is modeled as a simple chain of beads which are located at Cα atoms and the detailed structure of each amino acid is ignored. A peptide bond is represented as a virtual bond with the fixed length of 3.8Å, and only each bond angle θ and each dihedral angle ϕ are variables as shown in Figure 3.

Let $\varepsilon_{ij}^{M}(r_{ij})$ be the inter-residue (Cα atom) effective potential between the residues i and j, where r_{ij} is the distance between Cα atoms of the residues i and j. $\varepsilon_{ij}^{M}(r_{ij})$ is expressed as Eq. (1), where $\bar{r}_{AB}^{M}$ denotes an average distance between Cα atoms of residue types A and B in the range M and σ_{AB}^{M} is the standard deviation [23]

$$\varepsilon_{ij}^{M}(r_{ij}) = kT\frac{(r_{ij}-\bar{r}_{AB}^{M})^2}{2\sigma_{AB}^{M}} - kT\ln Z + \frac{kT}{2}\ln 2\pi\sigma_{AB}^{M} \quad (1)$$

Z, k and T stand for the partition function, the Boltzmann constant and temperature respectively. A and B specify the names of amino acids of the i-thand j-th residues. The constant terms in Eq. (2) can be regarded as the zero point. $\varepsilon_{ij}^{M}(r_{ij}) = \varepsilon_{HC}$ when $\bar{r}_{ij}^{M} \le r_{cut}$. We set r_{cut} = 1.9Å and ε_{HC} = 50kcal/mol. These values were obtained empirically.[23]

We perform random sampling of structures of a protein using this potential by the standard Metropolis Monte Carlo (MC) method,[24] i.e., this simulation can be regarded as a simulation of an unfolded state. Each dihedral angleϕ and bond angle θ of a residue are varied within $-\gamma\pi \leqq \phi, \theta \leqq \gamma\pi$ during a MC simulation. γandthe temperature parameter T were adjusted in order that the acceptance ratio in the Monte Carlo routine is around 0.5. This procedure is iterated for all residues. For a whole simulation, this routine is iterated by 60000 times.

The contact frequency between a residue pair in the sequence is calculated. Let g(i, j)be the contact frequency between residues i and j ina sequence. g(i, j) can be regarded as a contact probability. When the distance between Cα atoms of the residues i and j, r_{ij}, is less 10Å, we regard this pair of residues as forming a contact. A measure of high contact frequency Q(μ, ν) is defined as the following equation.

$$Q(\mu,\nu) = \frac{(g(\mu,\nu) - g(m))}{D(m)} \quad (2)$$

Thus, Q(μ, ν) is a kind of a z value in the field of statistics. Here, D(m) and g(m) are defined as Eqs. (3) and (4).

$$D(m) = \sqrt{\frac{\sum_{|i-j|=m}(g(m)-g(i,j)_{|i-j|=m})^2}{\sum_{|i-j|=m}}} \quad (3)$$

$$g(m) = \frac{\sum_{|i-j|=m} g(i,j)}{\sum_{|i-j|}} \tag{4}$$

$F(\mu) = \sum_{\nu} Q(\mu,\nu)$ denotes a contact frequency of the residue μ with other residues and this value corresponds to a so-called Φ value. [25] We took average values of 10 simulations for each protein. A Φ value is an experimentally observed value defined for each residue and this value denotes the measure of the involvement of each residue for native structure formation in its folding transition state [25].

THE CASE OF PROTEINS WITH THE SAME FOLD SHARING RELATIVELY LOW SEQUENCE IDENTITY

In this section, we treat some proteins with the same 3D scaffold but which fold through different pathways. We specify proteins by the PDB codes.

1. Fatty Acid Binding Protein-like Family [26]

The 3D scaffold in this family is a β barrel structure with 10 β strands,β1–β10 of which β1-β5 and β6- β10 constitute respective faces of the sandwich, and the protein being globular as a whole. Here, we take the following 3 proteins in this family, i.e., retinoic acid binding protein I (PDB:1CBI), retinoic acid binding protein II (PDB:1OPA), and fatty acid binding protein (PDB:1IFC). The backbone 3D structures of these proteins and their sequences are presented in Figure 4(a)-(c) and Figure 5.

The pairwise alignments for these three proteins have moderate sequence identity, i.e., 36% for 1OPA and 1CBI, 28% for 1IFC and 1CBI, and 31% for 1IFC and 1OPA.The ADMs for these proteins are shown in Figure 6(a)-(c).

Also in Figure 6, locations of predicted compact regions are indicated. The details of the map analyses show that the predicted domains are 21-128 for 1IFC, 4-131 for 1OPA and 1-136 for 1CBI. That is, all proteins are predicted as one-domain proteins (Figure 6(a), 6(b) and 6(c)). This is consistent with the visual observations of these proteins. When we take the second highest peaks of the differences of density of plots of the maps, the following regions are also predicted to be compact regions; 21-41 (α2,β2) and 47-128 (β3-β10) for 1IFC, 4-43 (β1, α1, α2, β2) and 64-131 (β4-β10) for 1OPA, and 1-52 (β1, α1, α2, β3) and 93-136 (β7-β10) for 1CBI. The compact region in the C-terminal site of 1IFC contains the main part of the β–sandwich structure.

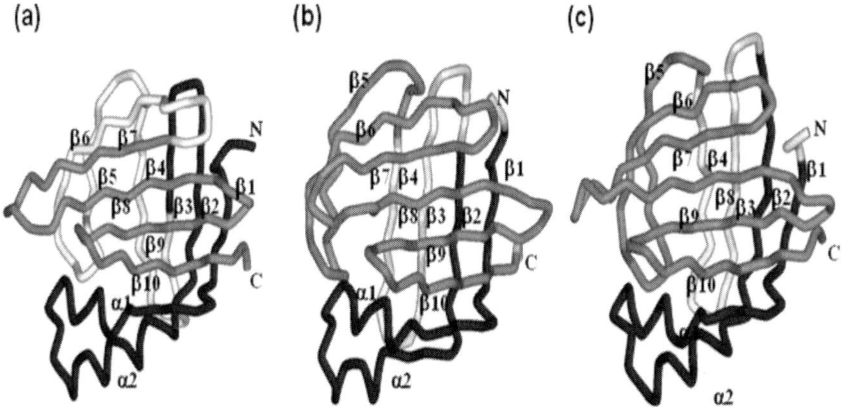

Figure 4. Backbone 3D structures of (a) retinoic acid binding protein I (PDB:1CBI), (b) retinoic acid binding protein II (PDB:1OPA), and (c) fatty acid binding protein (PDB:1IFC) The dark and grey portions correspond to the predicted compact regions by ADMs. See text.

```
Retinoic acid binding protein I(1CBI)    -PNFAGTWKMRSSENFDELLKALGVNAMLRKVAVAAASKPHVEIRQDGDQFYIKTSTTVR
Retinoic acid binding protein II(1OPA)   TKDQNGTWEMESNENFEGYMKALDIDFATRKIAVRLTQT--KIIVQDGDNFKTKTNSTFR
Fatty acid binding protein(1IFC)         --AFDGTWKVDRNENYEKFMEKMGINVVKRKLGAHDNLK--LTITQEGNKFTVKESSNFR
                                              ***::  .**::  :: :.::   **:..     .     * *:*::*  * .:..*

Retinoic acid binding protein I(1CBI)    TTEINFKVGEGFEEET--VDGRKCRSLPTWENENKIHCTQTLLEGDGPKTYWTRELANDE
Retinoic acid binding protein II(1OPA)   NYDLDFTVGVEFDEHTKGLDGRNVKTLVTWEG-NTLVCVQ---KGEKENRGWKQWVEGDK
Fatty acid binding protein(1IFC)         NIDVVFELGVDFAYSL--ADGTELTGTWTMEGNKLVGKFKR--VDNGKELIAVREISGNE
                                         . :: * :*  *         ** :      * *. : :    :    .:  :    : : .::

Retinoic acid binding protein I(1CBI)    LILTFGADDVVCTRIYVRE
Retinoic acid binding protein II(1OPA    LYLELTCGDQVCRQVFKKK
Fatty acid binding protein(1IFC)         LIQTYTYEGVEAKRIFKKE
                                         *          .  . ::: ::
```

Figure 5. Multiple alignment of retinoic acid binding protein I (PDB:1CBI), retinoic acid binding protein II (PDB:1OPA), and fatty acid binding protein (PDB:1IFC) by clustal W.

Each C-terminal compact region in the other two proteins corresponds to one-half of the β–sheet in the β–sandwich structure. These three ADMs show common features, e.g., the N terminal 2 α helix bundle with 2 β strands and the parts of the C terminal β sheet are predicted as two folding cores. It is confirmed that the plot patterns of these ADMs are also similar each other. [26]

The folding processes of these proteins were extensively investigated by Burns *et al.* [27-29]The following summarizes of the folding mechanisms elucidated by these works.

(1) The 1IFC folds with no intermediate, while 1OPA folding shows one intermediate (I), and 1CBI two intermediates (I_1 and I_2) are recognized in the folding pathway as expressed as:

$$1IFC : U \rightarrow N$$
$$1OPA : U \rightarrow I \rightarrow N$$
$$1CBI : U \rightarrow I_1 \rightarrow I_2 \rightarrow N.$$

Here U, N and I_l mean the unfolded state, the native structure and l-th intermediate, respectively. The order of the folding rates was also reported as 1IFC $\geqq$ 1OPA $\gg$ 1CBI. [26]

(2) The roles of the N-terminal two helices on the folding mechanisms were also investigated experimentally. Liu *et al.* [30] reported that the two helices are regarded as the folding initiation sitesin 1OPA, while the essence of the folding mechanism does not change after truncation of these helices in the folding of 1IFC as elucidated by Kim *et al.* [31]

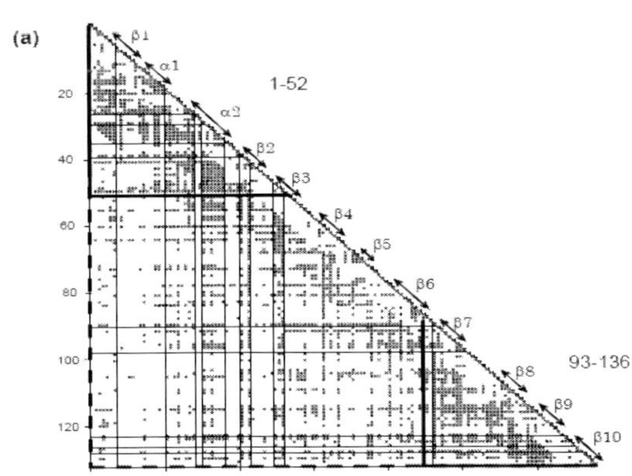

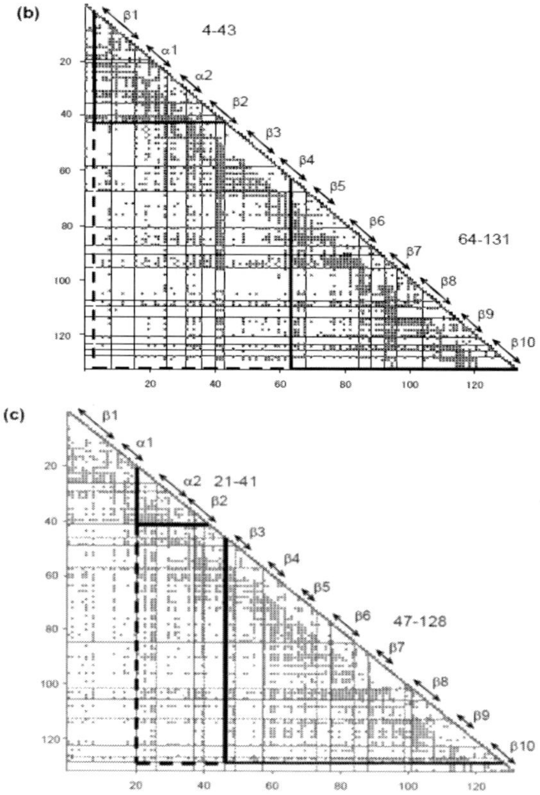

Figure 6. ADMs for(a) retinoic acid binding protein I (PDB:1CBI), (b) retinoic acid binding protein II (PDB:1OPA), and (c) fatty acid binding protein (PDB:1IFC) . In each figure, a double arrow denotes a location of a regular structure. αorβ means an α-helix or β-strand. A region enclosed by thick black lines denotes a predicted compact region by ADM. A region enclosed by broken lines implies the final assignment of the domain in a protein. Thin solid and thin broken lines denote a peak and a valley of plots of Δρ.

As indicated above, the predicted compact regions by the ADMs of these proteins are similar. However, in the present review we focus on the differences in these ADMs. Let us examine the ratio of the total size of the compact regions to the whole predicted domain region, i.e., these are 103/108 = 0.952 for 1IFC, 108/128 = 0.844 for 1OPA, and 96/136 = 0.706 for 1CBI The order of magnitude is 1IFC > 1OPA > 1CBI, and this order matches the experimental folding rates qualitatively. That is, the longer intervening region between two compact regions corresponds to a slower folding rate and more intermediates. Because a predicted compact region by an ADM can be regarded as a nucleus of folding at an early stage, the structural formation of the region between two compact regions in the present case is probably a rate-determining step of the folding. Thus, the longer intervening region denotes that this part tends to be trapped by an intermediate during the folding.

It is also interesting to note that the ADMs of 1IFC and 1OPA reflect the differences in the involvement of the two α helices of the respective N termini in the folding pathways. The ADM of 1IFC predicts the region 21-128 as the core of the 3D structure. This protein contains two helices at 14-20 (α1) and 25-33 (α2). That is, the first helix in this protein is not included in this core region as indicated in Figure 6(a)suggesting the insignificance of the first helix for the folding of 1IFC. In 1OPA and 1CBI, the two α-helices of the N termini are included in the first compact region, which suggests a strong involvement of these two α-helices in folding. These facts are consistent with the experimental results [29, 30].

2. Globin-like Fold [26, 32]

It is well-known that some of the proteins in the globin-like fold show the fairly low sequence identity (about 15%, see Figure 8), in spite of their common 3D structure. From this fact, it is considered that a protein fold is more conserved than a sequence. Thus, the folding principle of proteins in this fold is very interesting and significant. What finally we want to identify are the key residues to form this fold. On the other hand, it has been reported that some proteins in this fold form their 3D structures through different folding mechanisms. [33-35]This fold contains helices A-H (Figure 7).

First of all, let us examinethe differences in the folding mechanisms between sperm whale myoglobin (PDB ID:1MBN) and soybean leghemoglobin (PDB ID: 1FSL).It has been observed by Jennings and Wright [33] and Cavagnero *et al.* [34] that 1MBN folds via almost simultaneous structural formation(< 5msec) of helices A and B, and G and H. On the other hand, the early stage of the folding of 1FSL shows formation of helices E-H as investigated by Nishimura *et al.*[35] In Figure 7, we present the 3D structures of these hemoglobons. The alignment of these proteins shows only 16.9 % sequence identity (Figure 8).

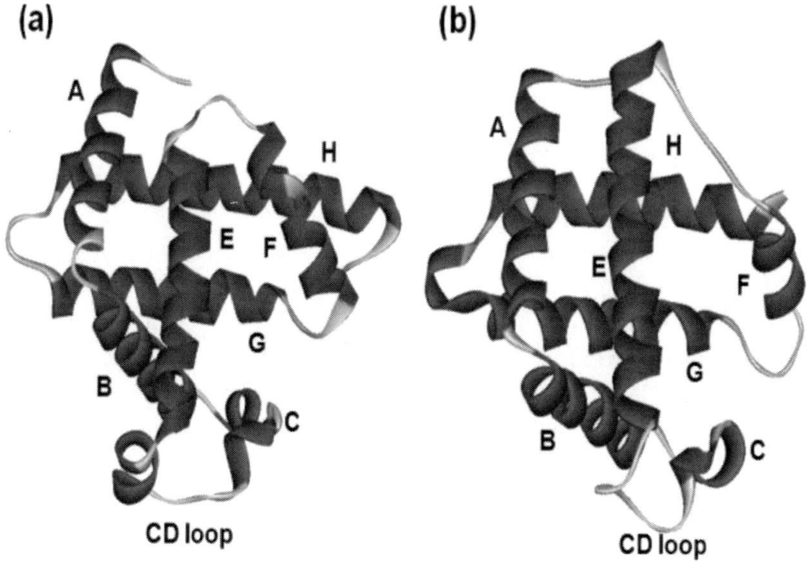

Figure 7. An example of the globin fold. (a) Myoglobin from sperm whale; 1MBN. (b) Leghemoglobin from soybean; 1FSL. Each helix is labeled by A-H.

As presented in Figure 9, the ADMs for 1MBN and 1FSL predict that both proteins are one-domain proteins. The subcompact regions can be assigned as 6-33 and 98-153, respectively, as shown in Figure 9(a). Thus, these regions are predicted as early stage folding sites. These regions correspond to helices A and B, and helices G and H. The η values of these regions are 0.273 for 6-33 and 0.255 for 98-158, respectively.The fact that these η values are comparable each other corresponds to the observation by Jennings and Wright[33], especially the fact that the A-B part and the G-H part fold simultaneously. The ADM for 1FSL (Figure 8(b)) predicts the existence of subcompact regions at 9-51 and 65-140 corresponding to helices A-C and helices E-H. The η value of 9-51is 0.220, whereas that of 65-140 is 0.324. This result can be interpreted to mean that the folding intermediate corresponding to 65-140 is more stable, and corresponds well to the observation by Nishimura *et al.* [35], i.e., the A and B helices are not stable in the early phase of the folding.

```
Sperm Whale Myoglobin (1MBN)      -VLSEGEWQLVLHVWAKVEADVAGHGQDILIRLFKSHPETLEKFDRFKHL
Soybean Leghemoglobin (1FSL)      VAFTEKQDALVSSSFEAFKANIPQYSVVFYTSILEKAPAAKDLFSFLANG
                                   .::* :  **   :  .:*::. :.  :   :::. * : : *. : :

Sperm Whale Myoglobin (1MBN)      KTEAEMKASEDLKKHGVTVLTALGAILKKKGHHEAELKPLAQSHATKHKI
Soybean Leghemoglobin (1FSL)      VDPTNPKLTGHAEKLFALVRDSAG-QLKASGTVVADAA-LGSVHAQK-AV
                                     :: * : . :*  . *  : *  ** .*   *:   *.. ** *  :

Sperm Whale Myoglobin (1MBN)      PIKYLEFISEAIIHVLHSRHPGDFGADAQGAMNKALELFRKDIAAKYKEL
Soybean Leghemoglobin (1FSL)      TDPQFVVVKEALLKTIK----AAVGDKWSDELSRAWEVAYDELAAAIKKA
                                  .   : .:.**::..::    . .* . .. :.:* *:  .::**  *:

Sperm Whale Myoglobin (1MBN)      GYQG
Soybean Leghemoglobin (1FSL)      ----
```

Figure 8. Clustal W alignment of sperm whale myoglobin and soybean leghemoglobin. The sequence identity is 16.9%.

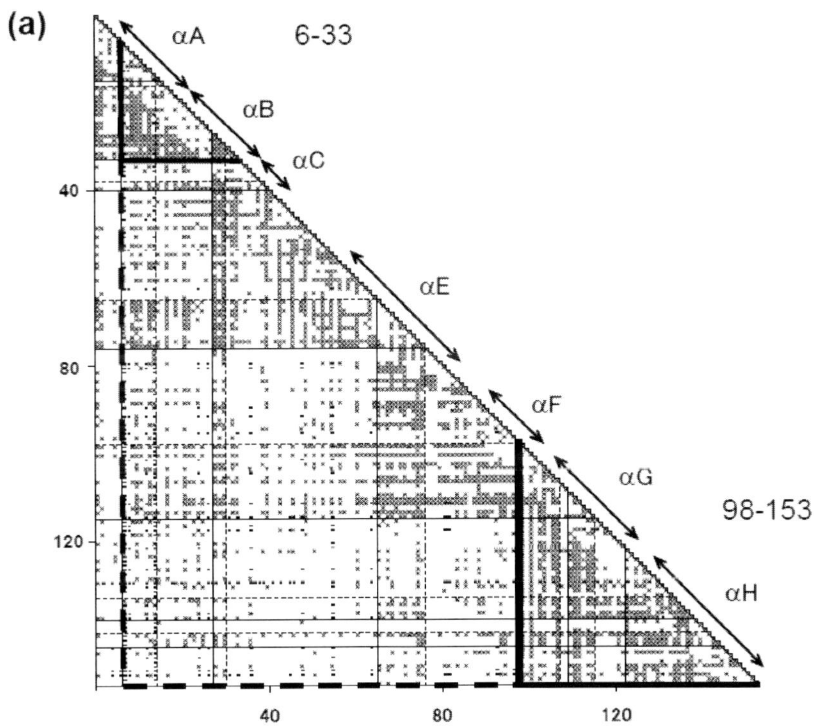

Figure 9. Continued on next page.

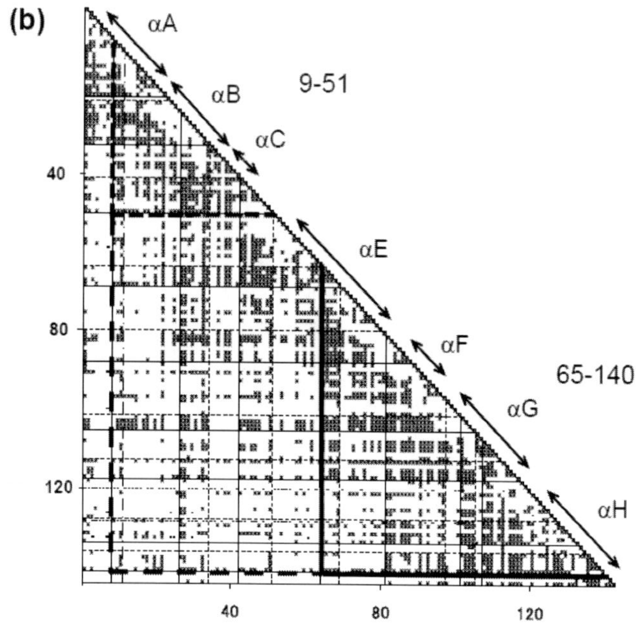

Figure 9. ADMs for(a) sperm whale myoglobin (PDB:1MBN) and (b) soybean leghemoglobin (PDB:1FSL). In each figure, a double arrow denotes a location of a regular structure. α means an α-helix. A region enclosed by thick black lines denotes a predicted compact region by ADM. A region enclosed by broken lines implies the final assignment of the domain in a protein. Thin solid and thin broken lines denote a peak and a valley of plots of αρ The α values of the regions 6-33 and 98-153 in 1MBN are 0.273 and 0.255. The α value of 9-51is 0.220whereas that of 65-140 is 0.324 in 1FSL.

In our previous research, [32] primitive plant hemoglobins like moss hemoglobin(*Ceratodon* hemoglobin) show the leghemoglobin-like ADM (Figure 10), and it is predicted that their folding initiates at the E-H part. [32].

Ancient globins, such as the bacterial tHbs have sequences truncated at the N-terminus. When the 3D structure of such a globin is examined, we notice that the part corresponding to the E-H unit is rather conserved. As an example, the 3D structures of the *M. tuberculosis*HbO and the 1FSL are shown in Figure 11, wherethe conservation of corresponding E-H unit structures in both globins can be seen. Thus, we make the speculation that the E-H unit might be an ancient tertiary structure in plant Hbs. [32]

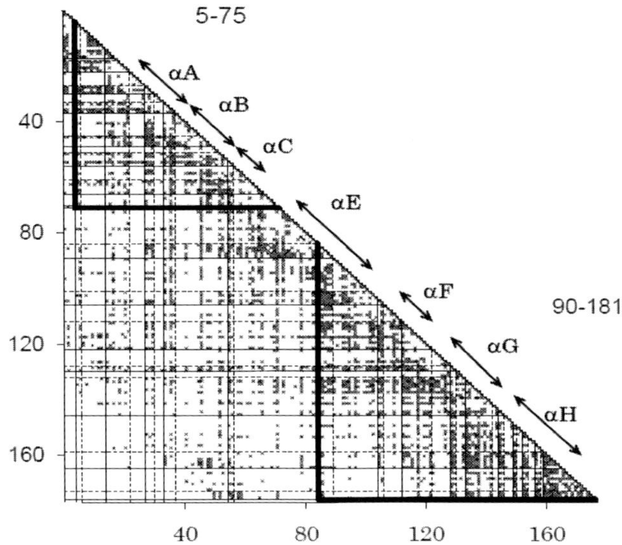

Figure 10. ADMs for moss hemoglobin(Ceratodon hemoglobin) In this figure, a double arrow denotes a location of a regular structure. α means an α -helix. A region enclosed by thick black lines denotes a predicted compact region by ADM. A region enclosed by broken lines implies the final assignment of the domain in a protein. Thin solid and thin broken lines denote a peak and a valley of plots of α ρThe α values of the regions 5-75 and 90-180 are 0.180 and 0.247.

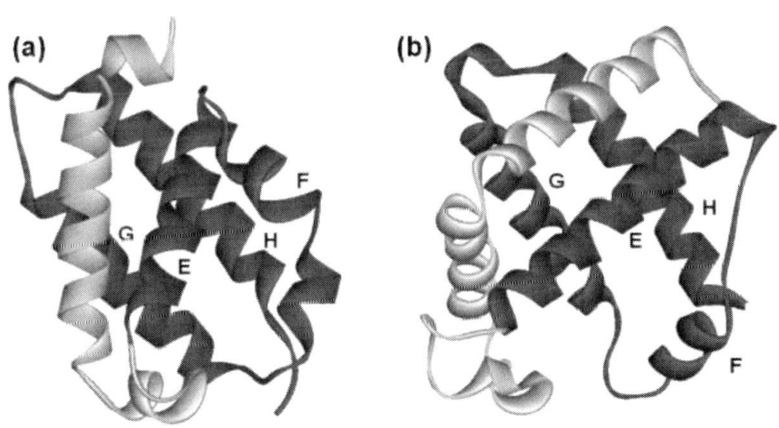

Figure 11. 3D structures of (a) HbO (Hemoglobin from *M. tuberculosis*, PDB:1NGK)(b) leghemoglobin from soybean (PDB:1FSL) Each part colored by dark gray denotes the E-H helix unit. The 3D structures of the E-H units are conserved.

3. c-Type Lysozyme Superfamily [36]

The third example is the c-type lysozyme superfamily. For example, the function of α-lactalbumin, a member of c-type lysozymes, is basically different from that of other members in spite of the fact that the 3Dstructure andsequence of the former are similar to those of latter. In this article, we focus on bovine α-lactalbumin (PDB ID: 1HFZ) and human lysozyme (PDB ID: 1LZ1). The 3D structures of these proteins are presented in Figure 12. The fold is the well-known (α+β) type and consists of a domain with α-helices A-D and three or five β-strands. The pairwise alignment of these proteins (Figure 13) reveals the 36% sequence identity.

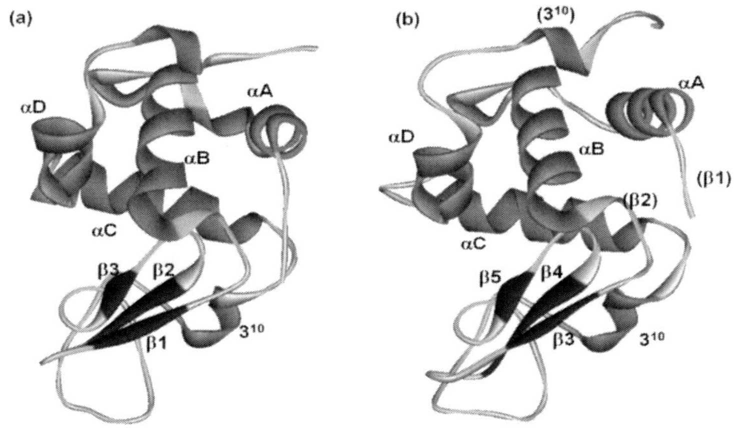

Figure 12. 3D structures of (a) bovine α-lactalbumin (PDB: 1HFZ) and (b) human lysozyme (PDB: 1LZ1)The regular structures are labeled by αA, α1 and so on.

```
Bovine α-Lactalbumin(1HFZ)   MEQLTKCEVFRELKDL--KGYGGVSLPEWVCTTFHTSGYDTQAIVQNND-
Human lysozyme(1LZ1)         -KVFERCELARTLKRLGMDGYRGISLANWMCLAKWESGYNTRATNYNAGD
                              : : :**: * ** *  .** *:**.:*:* :    ***:*:*   * .

Bovine α-Lactalbumin(1HFZ)   -STEYGLFQINNKIWCKDDQNPHSSNICNISCDKFLDDDLTDDIVCVKKI
Human lysozyme(1LZ1)         RSTDYGIFQINSRYWCNDGKTPGAVNACHLSCSALLQDNIADAVACAKRV
                              **:**:****.: **:*.:.* : * *::**. :*:*:::* :.*.*::

Bovine α-Lactalbumin(1HFZ)   L-DKVGINYWLAHKALCSEKLDQWLCEKL-
Human lysozyme(1LZ1)         VRDPQGIRAWVAWRNRCQNRDVRQYVQGCGV
                             : *  **. *:* :  *.::  :    :
```

Figure 13. Clustal W alignment of bovine α-lactalbumin and human lysozyme. The sequence identity is 36%.

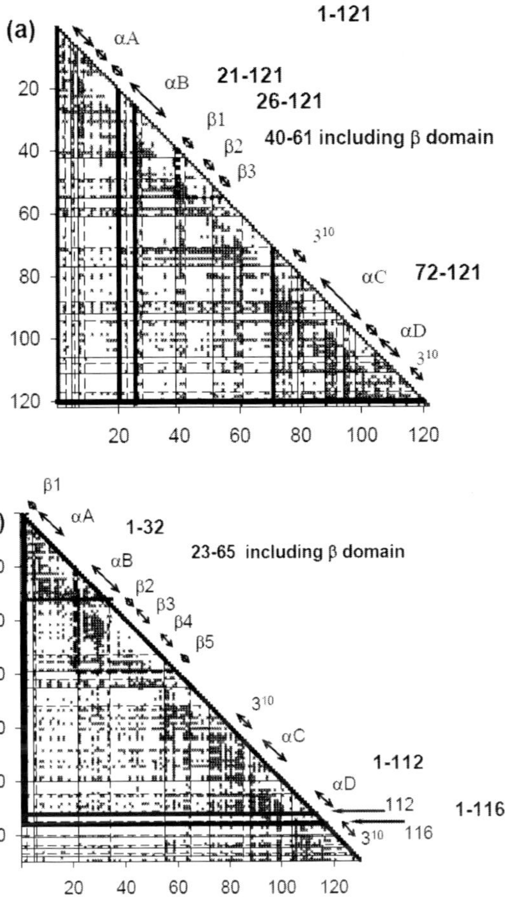

Figure 14. ADMs for(a) bovine α -lactalbumin(PDB:1HFZ) and (b) human lysozyme (PDB:1LZ1). In each figure, a double arrow denotes a location of a regular structure. α or α means an α -helix or α -strand. A region enclosed by thick black lines denotes a predicted compact region by ADM. A region enclosed by broken lines implies the final assignment of the domain in a protein. Thin solid and thin broken lines denote a peak and a valley of plots of α ρ In the ADM for 1HFZ, the α values of the region 1-121 is the highest, i.e, 0.493. The regions, 21-121, 26-121, 72-121 show the same α value of 0.366. The region enclosed by broken lines includes the α -sheet with an α value. Of 0.171. In the ADM for 1LZ1, the α values of the region 1-32 is the highest, i.e., 0.537. The two regions 1-112 and 1-116 show similar α values, i.e., 0.350 and 0.339. The region enclosed by broken lines includes the α -sheet with an α value of 0.177.

From the experiments by NMR for human lysozyme folding [37], we know that the A, B and C-terminal 3^{10}helics are involved in the initial folding event and that these regions interact with 112-Trp and 109-Trp. On the other hand, the amide protection measurement by NMR for α-lactalbumin [38] shows the strongest protection is at the C helix in both the molten globule and native state, but only small protection was observed at the A and B helices. Thus, the folding processes are slightly different between these proteins.

The ADM for 1HFZ (α-lactalbumin) (Figure 14(a)) shows almost the whole sequence forms a strong folding unit (η = 0.493). According to the ADM, the regions 21-121, 26-121, 72-121 can be regarded as possible folding units (η = 0.366 for each). The region 72-121 includes the C, D and the C-terminal 3^{10} helices, and this region might be a candidate for a folding unit. This prediction corresponds to the experimental result, i.e., the high stability of the C helix in the molten globule state of 1HFZ.

On the other hand, the ADM for 1LZ1 (human lysozyme) predicts that the regions 1-32 and 1-112 have similar η values, 0.357 and 0.350 as shown in Figure 14(b). These regions are included in a domain 1-116 with anη value of 0.339 and which is close to the regions mentioned above. Hence, the folding of 1LZ1 is predicted as that the initial event involving folding of the part 1-112 which includes helices A and B (see Figure 14(b)) and this part extends to 1-116, not like the case of α-lactalbumin. In the comparison with the experimental results, the predicted region 1-32 corresponds to helices A and B, and the ADM predicts that helices A and B are involved in the initial folding process. The prediction that the region 1-112 is also considered as the folding initiation site corresponds to the interaction between helices A and B and Trp-112. Thus, the results from the ADM well correspond to the experimental folding results.

The Case of Proteins Sharing High Sequence Identity but Having Different Folds

It is already well accepted that when a pair of proteins shares the sequence identity of more than 30%, this pair of proteins exhibits the same fold. However, recent research has revealed proteins share that 59% sequence identity yet possess different 3D structures. [13, 14] The native structure of the IgG binding domain from Staphylococcus (protein A) is the 3α-helix bundle structure, whereas the IgG binding domain of Streptococcus (protein G) shows the (α+β)-structure (Figure 15). These proteins have only 11% sequence identity (see Figure 16).

Two mutants were made from the wild types of proteins A and G strains with the phage display technique. These two proteins show 59% sequence identity but maintain the original 3D structures, i.e., the 3α–helix bundle structure and the (α+β)-structure, respectively. These mutants are referred to as protein A219 and protein G311 respectively. [13, 14] The question arises of whether we can detect the differences in the 3D structures between A219 and G311 from their sequences.

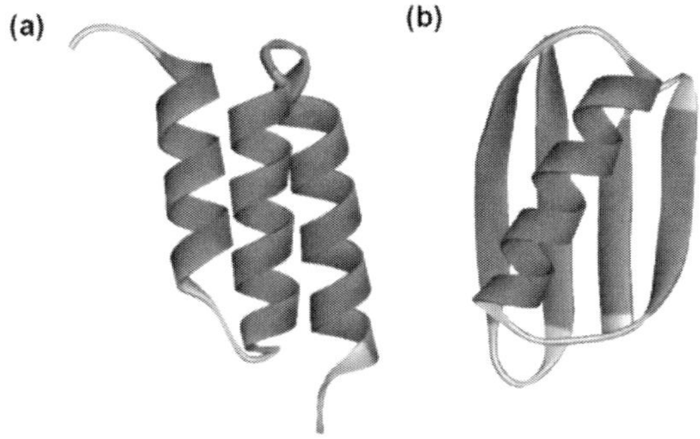

Figure 15. 3D structures of (a) Staphylococcal protein A (PDB: 1EDI) and (b)Streptococcal protein G (PDB: 1PGA).

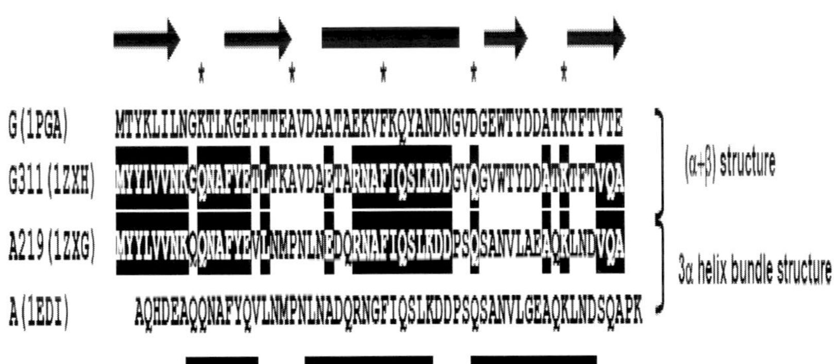

Figure 16. Sequence alignment of protein G (PDB: 1PGA), protein G311 (PDB: 1ZXH), protein A219 (PDB: 1ZXG) and protein A (PDB: 1EDI). A bar and an arrow denote the location of α helix and β strand respectively. The sequence identity between protein G311 and Protein A219 is 59% while that between protein A and protein G is 11%.

Figure 17 shows the ADMs for protein A219 and protein G311. The location of the predicted compact regions for Protein A219, i.e., 3α bundle proteins, is 16-56 including a part of the first helix plus all or most of the second and third helices. On the other hand, the compact region in protein G311 is predicted as 29-45, which contains the central α helix and β strand located in the C terminal region of the sequence. Thus, these ADMs predict that the 3helices are involved in the folding of 3α bundle protein, whereas the (α+β) proteinstart its folding in the C terminal part. That is, some differences are detected from the ADMs.

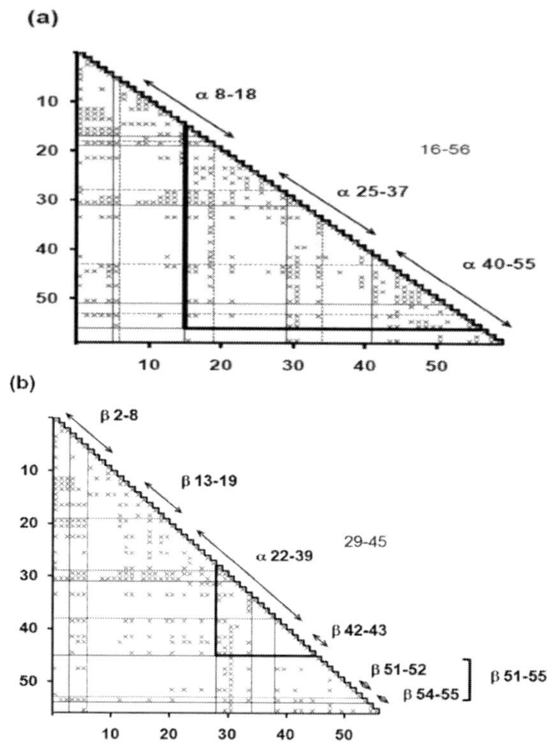

Figure 17. ADMs for(a) protein A219 (PDB: 1ZXG) and (b) protein G311 (PDB: 1ZXH)In each figure, a double arrow denotes a location of a regular structure. α means anα-helix. A region enclosed by thick black lines denotes a predicted compact region by ADM. Thin solid and thin broken lines denote a peak and a valley of plots of Δρ.

Figure, 18(a) presents the plots of the F values, as described earlier in this review for protein A219. The peaks of the F values for protein A219 correspond to 16-V, 30-F and 44-V. It is interesting to note that the residues at the peaks are totally conserved and these 3 residues located on the first, second and third helices. Furthermore, these residues form hydrophobic packing in the native structures as shown in Figure 19(a). It is inferred from the height of the peaks that the N-terminal helix is deeply involved in the folding. The experimentally observed ϕ values for protein A of Sato *et al.* [39] are included in Figure 18(a) (see also Sato *et al.*, [40]; Sato and Fersht, [41]), suggesting a good correspondence of the location of peaks of the F values and the ϕ values.

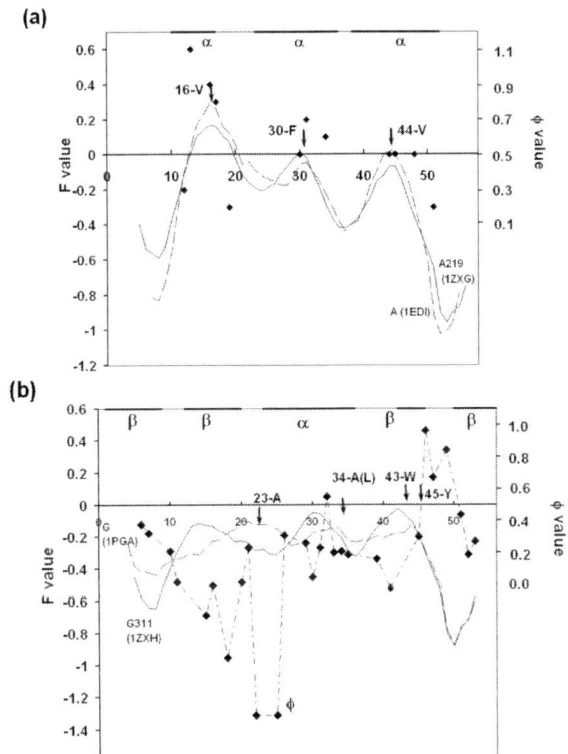

Figure 18. F value plots for (a) protein A219 (PDB: 1ZXG) and (b) protein G311 (PDB: 1ZXH). The F plots for protein A (PDB: 1EDI) and protein G (PDB: 1PGA) are also presented in (a) and (b) respectively. The experimentally observed Φ values are also plotted by dianmonds ([41, 42]). The location of the regular structures is denoted by α and β at the upper parts of the figures.

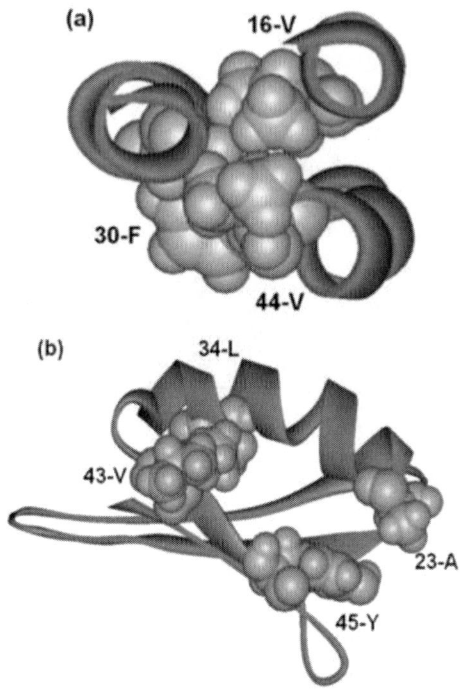

Figure 19. The residues forming hydrophobic packing in the native structures of (a) protein A219 (PDB: 1ZXG) and (b) protein G311 (PDB: 1ZXH) are shown in space-filling representation.

The F values for protein G311 are plotted in Figure 18(b). The F values tend to be higher at the central α helix and the third β strand compared to the case of the 3α bundle proteins. In the native structure of protein G311, 34-L and 43-W, and 23-A and 45-Y pack the hydrophobicly. These residues are included in the central α helix and the third β strand as indicated by the F value plot. The Φ values obtained by McCallister*et al.* [42] also indicate the role of the C-terminal region and the α helix on the folding, although detailed analysis suggests an involvement of the β-turn between β3 and β4.

We are interested in how to decode the difference in the 3D structures of protein A219 and protein G311 from their sequences. We seek information about the key residues in the sequences that determine the 3D motifs. Although we do not identify exactly such key residues for each protein, it is interesting to describe the following attempts. We focus on only the local sequences close to the peaks of the F value profiles. The highest peak in the F profile for protein A219 is at residue 16-V and that for G311 is at residue 42-V. As an attempt, ±5 window is taken as a local sequence, i.e., a sequence with i±5 where i denotes the residue number of a highest peak. Thus, residues 11-21 of protein A219 are compared to the corresponding local sequence of protein A (see Figure 20). Only one residue deffers between these two local sequences. (The sequence identity between these regions is 90.9%.) On the other hand, when we perform the same procedure using the sequence of protein G instead of protein A, the sequence identity drops all the way to 9%. When the residue 37-48, i.e., the local sequence around 42-V, is compared to the corresponding region in protein G (Figure 20), the amino acid identity is 81.8%, whereas the amino acid identity with the corresponding region 37-48 in protein A is just 18%. We notice that the local sequences of proteins with the same fold show high amino acid identity. This consideration leads us to think that a local sequence around a peak in an F profile may contain information on the key residues for 3D structure determination.

DECODING PROTEIN FOLDING INFORMATION FROM AMINO ACID SEQUENCES

What we want to do in general is to extract information on the 3D structure of a protein from its sequence. We think that it is rather difficult to extract such information from the usual bioinformatics sequence analyses. Hence, we propose to translate the sequence of a protein into an average distance map, and then we extract information about the native structure and folding mechanism. We believe that our methodology can help shed light on some of the principle determining the 3D architecture of proteins.

Our experiences described in this review lead us to the following considerations. The overall plot patterns in the ADMs are similar when two proteins share the same fold. However, some differences in local detail in the ADMs suggest differences in the folding process. That is, such information coded implicitly in amino acid sequences can be decoded with ADMs. Furthermore, a region predicted as compact by ADM can be regarded as a folding unit. From the analyses for globin family, such compact folding units may have varied during evolution, and we come to the interesting thought that ancestor proteins might contain a basic segment for folding as the E-H helix unit of globin proteins. Such ancestor folding units may be observed in a 3D structure database, and these units may play a role as folding intermediates or folding transition state structures.

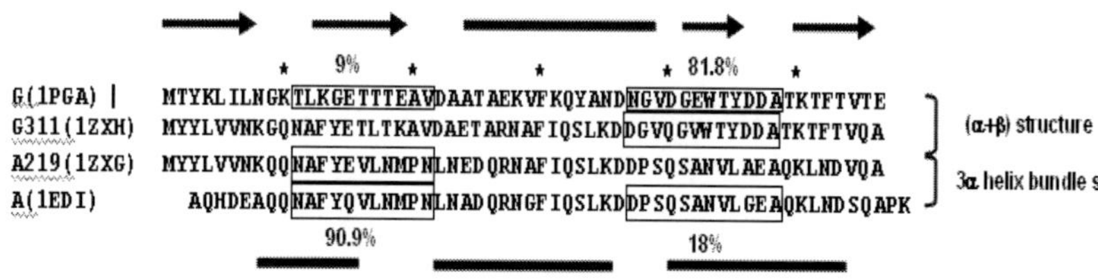

Figure 20. Comparison of local sequences around the peaks of the F value profiles. A local sequence enclosed by a rectangle is compared with the corresponding sequences of protein A and protein G.

As seen in the structural differences in IgG binding domains, ADM analyses can detect such differences. The analyses can be refined in combination with the F value analyses. That is, an F value analysis narrows the possible residues involved in folding, i.e., residues forming hydrophobic packing in a folding unit.

Let us conclude with our perspective on the prediction of protein 3D structures and folding mechanisms. It is well accepted that the number of folds is finite. If this is true, the number of the folding transition states may be also finite. If key residues for determination of the 3D structure, or sequence motif, for a folding intermediate or a folding transition state structure can be defined by development of the present methodology, the number of such structural motifs may be small beyond expectation. Also, the location and the 3D structure of the folding transition state for a given sequence may be predictable from the amino acid sequence.

ACKNOWLEDGMENT

The works presented here were partly supported by a Grant-in-Aid for Scientific Research on Priority Area (C)"Genome Information Science" and a Grant-in-Aid for Scientific Research (C) from the Ministry of Education, Culture, Sports, Science and Technology of Japan.

REFERENCES

[1] Anfinsen, CB; Scheraga, HA. Experimental and theoretical aspects of protein folding,*Adv. Protein Chem.*, 1975, 29, 205-300.

[2] Zhang, Y. Protein structure prediction: when is it useful?, *Curr. Opin. Struct. Biol.,* 2009,19,145-155.

[3] Ben-David, M; Noivirt-Brik, O; Paz, A; Prilusky, J; Sussman, JL; Levy, Y. Assessment of CASP8 structure predictions for template free targets, *Proteins*, 2009, 77, 50-65.

[4] Shakhnovich, E. Protein folding thermodynamics and dynamics: where physics, chemistry, and biology meet, *Chem. Rev.*, 2006, 106, 1559-1588.

[5] Karanicolas, J; Brooks, CL III. The origins of asymmetry in the folding transition states of protein L and protein G, *Protein Sci.*, 2002, 11, 2351-2361.

[6] Clementi, C; Nymeyer, H; Onuchic, JN. Topological and energetic factors: what determines the structural details of the transition state, *J. Mol. Biol.*, 2000, 298, 937-953.

[7] Zong, C; Eilson, CJ; Shen, T; Wolynes, PG; Wittung-Stafshede, P. ϕ-Value analysis of apo-azurin folding: comparison between experiment and theory. *Biochemistry*, 2006, 45,6458-6466.

[8] Baker, D. A surprising simplicity to protein folding. *Nature*, 2000, 405, 39-42.

[9] Plaxco, KW; Simons, KT; Baker, D.Contact order, transition state placement and the refolding rates of single domainproteins.*J. Mol. Biol.*, 1998, 277, 985-994.

[10] Gromiha, MM; Selvaraj, S. Comparison between long-range interactions and contact order in determining the folding rate of two-state proteins: application of long-range order to folding rate prediction. *J. Mol. Biol.*, 2001,310, 27-32.

[11] Dixit, PD; Weikl, TR. A simple measure of native-state topology and chain connectivity predicts the folding rates of two-state proteins with and without crosslinks. *Proteins*, 2006, 64, 193-197.

[12] Orengo, CA; Jones, DT; Thornton, JM. Protein superfamilies and domain superfolds, *Nature*, 1994, 372, 631-634.

[13] Alexander, PA; Rozak, DA; Orban, J; Bryan, PN. Directed evolution of highly homologous proteins with different folds by phage display: Implications for the protein folding code. *Biochemistry*,2005, 44, 14045-14054.

[14] He, Y; Yeh, DC; Alexander, P; Bryan, PN. Solution NMR structures of IgG binding domains with artificially evolved high levels of sequence identity but different folds. *Biochemistry*, 2005, 44, 14055-14061.

[15] Alexander, PA; He, Y; Chen, Y;Orban, J; Bryan, PN.The design and characterization of two proteins with 88% sequence identity but different structure and function, *Proc. Natl. Acad. Sci. USA*, 2007, 104, 11963-11968.

[16] He, Y; Chen, Y; Alexander, PA; Bryan, PN;Orban, J.NMR structures of two designed proteins with high sequence identity but different fold and function, *Proc. Natl. Acad. Sci. USA*, 2008, 105, 14412-14417.

[17] Gunasekaran, K;Eyles, SJ;Hagler, AT;Gierasch, LM. Keeping it in the family: Folding studies of related proteins. *Curr. Opin. Struct. Biol.*, 2002, 11, 83-93.

[18] Kikuchi, T; Némethy, G; Scheraga, HA. Prediction of the location of structural domains in globular proteins. *J. Protein Chem.*, 1988,7, 427-471.

[19] Kikuchi, T.Contact maps derived from the statistics of average distances between residues in proteins. Application to the prediction of structures and active sites of proteins and peptides. In: Pandalai SG. (ed). *Recent research developments in protein engineering*. Research Signpost, Kerala, India, 2002, 1-48.

[20] Nishikawa, K; Ooi, T; Isogai, Y; Saito N. Tertiary structure of proteins. I. Representation and computation of the conformations. *J. Phys. Soc. Jpn.*, 1972, 32, 1331-1337.

[21] Phillips, DC. The development of crystallographic enzymology. In: Goodwin TW(ed.) *British Biochemistry Past and Present, Biochem.* Soc. Symp. No. 30,Academic Press, London, 1970, 11-28.

[22] Kikuchi, T. Inter-Cα atomic potentials derived from the statistics of average interresidue distances in proteins: Application to bovine pancreatic trypsin inhibitor. *J Comput. Chem.*, 1996, 17, 226-237.

[23] Kikuchi, T. Analysis of 3D structural differences in the IgGbinding domains based on the interresidue average distance statistics.*Amino Acids*, 2008, 35, 541-549.

[24] Kikuchi, T. Inter-Cα atomic potentials derived from the statistics of average interresidue distances in proteins: Application to bovine pancreatic trypsin inhibitor. *J Comput. Chem.*, 1996, 17,226-237.

[25] Metropolis, N; Rosenbluth, A; W.,Rosenbluth, MN; Teller, AH; Teller E. Equation of state calculations by fast computing machines. *J. Chem. Phys., 1953,21*,1087-1092.

[26] Daggett, V; Fersht, AR. Transition states in protein folding. In: R. Pain, (ed.) *Mechanisms of Protein Folding*, 2nd edition, Oxford University Press, Oxford, 2000, 175-211.

[27] Ichimaru, T; Kikuchi, T. Analysis of the differences in the folding kinetics of structurally homologous proteins based on predictions of the gross features of residue contacts. *Proteins*,2003, 51, 515-530.

[28] Burns, LL; Dalessio, PM;Ropson, IJ. Folding mechanism of three structurally similar β–sheet proteins. *Proteins*, 1998, 33, 107-118.

[29] Dalessio, PM; Ropson, IJ. β-sheet proteins with nearly identical structures have different folding intermediates. *Biochemistry*, 2000, 39, 860-871.

[30] Burns, LL; Ropson, IJ. Folding of intracellular retinol and retinoic acid binding proteins. *Proteins*, 2001, 43, 292-302.

[31] Liu, ZP; Riao, J; Gierasch, LM. Equilibrium folding studies of cellular retinoic acid binding protein, a predominantly β–sheet protein. *Biochemistry*, 1994, 33, 134-142.

[32] Kim, K; Cistola, DP; Frieden, C. Intestinal fatty acid binding protein: The structure and stability of a helix-less variant. *Biochemistry*, 1996, 35, 7553-7558.

[33] Nakajima, S;Álvarez-Salgado, E; Kikuchi, T; Arredondo-Peter, R.Prediction of folding pathway and kinetics among plant hemoglobins by using an average distance map method.*Proteins*, 2005, 61, 500-506.

[34] Jennings, PA; Wright, PE. Formation of a molten globule intermediate early in the kinetic folding pathway of apomyoglobin. *Science*, 1993, 262, 892-896.

[35] Cavagnero, S; Dyson, HJ; Wright, PE. Effect of H helix destabilizing mutations on the kinetic and equilibrium folding of apomyoglobin. *J. Mol. Biol.*, 1999, 285, 269-282.

[36] Nishimura, C; Prytulla, S; Dyson, HJ; Wright, PE. Conservation of folding pathways in evolutionarily distant globin sequences. *Nature Struct. Biol.*, 2000, 7, 679-686.

[37] Nakajima, S; Kikuchi, T. Analysis of the Differences in the folding mechanisms of c-type lysozymes based on contact maps constructed with interresidue average distances. *J. Mol. Model.*, 2007, 13, 587-594.

[38] Hooke, SD; Radford, SE; Dobson, CM. The refolding of human lysozyme: a comparison with the structurally homologous hen lysozyme. *Biochemistry*, 1994, 33, 5867-5876.

[39] Forge, V; Wijesinha, RT; Balbach, J; Brew, K; Robinson, CV; Redfield, C; Dobson, CM. Rapid collapse and slow structural reorganisation

during the refolding of bovine α-lactalbumin. *J. Mol. Biol.*, 1999, 288, 673-688.

[40] Sato, S; Religa, TL; Daggett, V; Fersht, AR. Testing protein-folding simulations by experiment: B domain of protein *A. Proc. Natl. Acad. Sci.* USA 101, 2004, 6952-6956.

[41] Sato, S; Religa, TL; Fersht, AR.Φ-Analysis of the folding of the B domain of protein a using multiple optical probes. *J. Mol. Biol.*, 2006,360, 850-864.

[42] Sato; S, Fersht, AR. Searching for multiple folding pathways of a nearly symmetrical protein: Temperature dependent Φ-value analysis of the b domain of protein A. *J. Mol. Biol.*, 2007, 372, 254-267.

[43] McCallister, EL; Alm, E; Baker, D. Critical role of β-hairpin formation in protein G folding. *Nature Struct. Biol.*, 2000, 7, 669-673.

In: Advances in Proteomics Research
Editors: Ya Li Huang et al. pp. 63-109
ISBN: 978-1-61942-227-8

Chapter 3

MODELLING OF PROTEIN FOLDING AND PREDICTION OF RATE BASED ON NUCLEATION MECHANISM

Oxana V. Galzitskaya*
Institute of Protein Research, RussianAcademy of Sciences,
Pushchino, Moscow Region, Russian Federation, Russia.

ABSTRACT

The problem of protein self-organization is one of the most important problems of molecular biology nowadays. Despite the recent success in the understanding of general principles of protein folding, details of this process are yet to be elucidated. Moreover, the prediction of protein folding rates has its own practical value due to the fact that aggregation directly depends on the rate of protein folding. The time of folding and transition state ensembles for 67 proteins with known experimental data at the point of thermodynamic equilibrium between unfolded and native state have been calculated using a Monte Carlo method and Dynamic programming one where each residue is considered to be either folded as in the native state or completely disordered. The times of folding for 67 proteins which reach the native state within a limit of 10^8 Monte Carlo steps are in a good correlation with experimentally measured folding time at mid-transition point (the correlation coefficient is -0.82). A lower

* Corresponding author: E-mail: ogalzit@vega.protres.ru

correlation was obtained if to use Dynamic programming approach (the correlation coefficient is -0.72). The capillarity model allows us to predict the folding rate at the same level of correlation as by Monte-Carlo simulations. The calculated model entropy capacity (conformational entropy per residue divided by the average contact energy per residue) for 67 proteins correlates by about 78% with the experimentally measured folding rate at the mid-transition point. Theoretical consideration of a capillarity model for the process of protein folding demonstrates that the difference in the folding rate for proteins sharing more ball-like and less ball-like folds is the result of differences in the conformational entropy due to a larger surface of the boundary between folded and unfolded phases in the transition state for proteins with more ball-like fold.

INTRODUCTION

The problem of protein folding is one of the important and actual problems in biophysics. Besides of its fundamental significance the understanding of the mechanism of protein folding is of great importance for many practical tasks such as development of drugs and design of *de novo* artificial proteins with given properties (Jiang et al., 2008; Röthlisberger et al., 2008). Violation of proteins folding *in vivo*, and often concomitant process of their aggregation in many cases evoke diseases (Chiti et al., 1999; Fändrich et al., 2001).

Today theoretical and experimental investigations of the mechanism of self-organization of globular proteins result in qualitative understanding of protein folding (Thirumalai, 1995; Gutin et al., 1996; Finkelstein and Badretdinov, 1997; Plaxco et al.,1998; Jackson, 1998; Koga and Takada, 2001; Finkelstein and Galzitskaya, 2004). However, until now the details of the protein folding process is not yet known. Not numerous models of protein folding (Muñoz and Eaton, 1999; Galzitskaya and Finkelstein, 1999; Ivankov and Finkelstein, 2001; Alm et al., 2002; Garbuzynskiy et al., 2004; Galzitskaya, 2010) allow us to describe more or less correctly only the folding of not large one-domain globular proteins (less than 200 amino acid residues).

The time of folding of different proteins varies in many orders, from microseconds to seconds and even hours. Small proteins usually fold quickly and without intermediates of folding (i.e. the process occurs in one stage, "one-stage" kinetics is observed). Larger proteins fold slower, and under folding metastable intermediates are often observed (i.e. the process of folding occurs in many stages, "multi-state" kinetics is observed) (Jackson, 1998).

One of the first analytical theories of folding of one-domain globular proteins was that of Finkelstein and Badretdinov (1997). In the framework of this theory developed on the base of a nucleation mechanism, it has been obtained that the rate of protein folding at the point of mid-transition depends on the value of border between two phases at the transition state, and loops protruding from the folded part of the protein create additional surface tension decreasing the process of protein folding. This implies that since the border between two phases depends for a ball-like globule on the number of amino-acid residues in the protein chain as $L^{2/3}$, then the rate of protein folding should depend on the number of amino-acid residues in protein L in the same way:

$$\ln k_{mt} \sim -L^{2/3} \tag{1}$$

where $\ln k_{mt}$ is the logarithm of protein folding rate at the point of thermodynamic equilibrium of two states of the protein, the native and the denatured ones. However, the detected correlation between $\ln k_{mt}$ and $L^{2/3}$ does not reach a unity (see Table 1). This makes us take into account other factors which can additionally affect protein folding rate as well as the length of the protein chain.

Simultaneously, another analytical estimation of the dependence of the protein folding rate on the protein chain size has been suggested on conditions that the native state is more stable than the unfolded one (Thirumalai, 1995):

$$\ln k_f^w \sim -L^{1/2} \tag{2}$$

Where $\ln k_f^w$ is the logarithm of the protein folding rate in water. At that the correlation coefficient for a set of 69 proteins was 0.74 (Naganathan and Muñoz, 2005).

In computer experiments on folding of model protein chains using a cubic lattice (Gutin et al., 1996) it has been obtained that when the stability of native state is maximal the natural logarithm of rate should depend on the size of the protein chain as

$$\ln k_f^w \sim -\ln L \tag{3}$$

and correlation coefficient is 0.78 for the set of 69 proteins (Naganathan and Muñoz, 2005).

In a number of computer experiments it has been shown that (Koga and Takada, 2001) the rate of folding of model proteins on the lattice with simple potentials depends on the protein size as. This is in good agreement with dependences found by both Finkelstein and Thirumalai (Thirumalai, 1995; Finkelstein and Badretdinov, 1997).

Despite the different view of dependences of the rate of folding on the length of protein chain, all analytical theories are similar in that, as intuitively seems, that time of protein folding should growth with increasing of length of protein chain, it growths slower than exp(*L*).

In 2003 year it was demonstrated that the size of protein in the first place determines the rate of folding of multi-state proteins (Galzitskaya et al., 2003), their correlation coefficient is -0.80 for the dependence $\ln k_f^w \sim -L^P$ when $0 \leq P \leq 1$, at the same time for one-stage proteins (having chains of about an equal size) the correlation has not been detected (correlation coefficient is –0.07 (Galzitskaya et al., 2003)). It should be noted that the case $P = 0$ corresponds to the dependence $\ln k_f^w \sim -\ln L$, so $L^P = \exp(P \ln L) \approx 1 + P \ln L$ under $P \to 0$.

Thus, both from analytical theories and as from computer experiments that resolved the Levinthal's paradox it was conluded that the size of protein is one –and the only one – of the defining factors in the description of protein folding rate. Such a dependence helps to understand the reason for the difference in folding rates of proteins with essentially distinct sizes, but can not explain why proteins of about equal sizes often fold with essentially different rates.

From the point view of prediction of folding rate, all suggested dependences of folding rates on the number of residues in protein chain about equally agree with the observed protein folding rates: the correlation coefficient is about 70% (see Table 1).

Besides the size of protein, there are more factors which can additionally affect the protein folding rate. Thus, from the nucleation mechanism of folding it follows that the topology of transition state – path of protein chain in space – should be the same as that of the native structure (Fersht, 1997). This means that the larger is the number of contacts in protein between residues which are far along the chain the more probable it is that the protein could not avoid the loops protruding from the native-like part of protein in the transition state, and the folding will be slower. Just this is observed under comparison with experiment: for proteins of about equal size, the logarithm of folding rate is decreasing with the growth of contact order (*CO*), which is equal to the average distance (in amino acid residues) along the chain between atoms that are in contact in the native structure normalized on the number of amino acid residues in protein chain (Plaxco et al., 1998). However, topology itself can not explain the difference in the folding rates for some proteins with one and the same topology (pathway of protein chain in the space) (SH3-domains, cold-shock proteins, domains of fibronectin, and proteins with ferredoxine-like fold) (Guijarro et al., 1998; Plaxco et al., 1998; Perl et al., 1998; van Nuland et al., 1998; Zerovnik et al., 1998).

Table 1. Correlation coefficients between logarithms of folding rates in water and in mid-transition and structural parameters as connected with size of protein and no (*CO*)

parameter	$\ln k_f$, s^{-1} 84 proteins	$\ln k_f^{multi}$, s^{-1} 26 proteins	$\ln k_f^{two}$, s^{-1} 58 proteins
L	-0.65±0.06	-0.78±0.08	-0.42±0.11
$L^{1/2}$	-0.70±0.06	-0.81±0.07	-0.50±0.10
$L^{2/3}$	-0.69±0.06	-0.80±0.07	-0.47±0.10
$\ln L$	-0.71±0.05	-0.82±0.06	-0.55±0.09
AbsCO	-0.77±0.04	-0.78±0.08	-0.71±0.06
CO	-0.01±0.11	0.25±0.18	-0.41±0.11
parameter	$\ln k_f^{mt}$, s^{-1} 84 proteins	$\ln k_f^{mt\ multi}$, s^{-1} 26 proteins	$\ln k_f^{mt\ two}$, s^{-1} 58 proteins
L	-0.64±0.06	-0.58±0.08	-0.61±0.11
$L^{1/2}$	-0.73±0.05	-0.61±0.12	-0.71±0.06
$L^{2/3}$	-0.69±0.06	-0.60±0.13	-0.67±0.07
$\ln L$	-0.77±0.04	-0.64±0.12	-0.76±0.06
AbsCO	-0.77±0.04	-0.65±0.11	-0.78±0.05
CO	0.00±0.11	0.01±0.20	-0.17±0.13

Since *CO* does not depend on the protein size then it is not possible to predict the folding rates of all proteins by using this parameter. Integration of *CO* and the number of amino acid resides in proteins in one equation gives "absolute contact order" $AbsCO = CO{*}L$, including the influence of topology and size of protein. This parameter predicts better the protein folding rates than $CO$and$L^{2/3}$ separetely (Ivankov et al., 2003).

There is one more consequence of Finkelstein-Badretdinov's theory about the influence of the protein shape on its folding rate which has been established in (Galzitskaya et al., 2008°a,b; Ivankov et al., 2009). Namely, under equal conditions a ball-like protein independent of the pathway of folding can not avoid the large square of border between phases. But an oblong-like protein has a possability to choose such a pathway of folding in which the protein folding goes through the small square of border, and consequently through a less high barrier. Therefore, more ball-like proteins should fold slower. In (Galzitskaya et al., 2008°a,b; Ivankov et al., 2009) it has been shown that proteins of classα/β, on average, are more "ball-like" than proteins with another type of packing of secondary structure.

Also it has been shown that α/β-proteins, again on average, fold slower than proteins from other classes of about the same size. We explained this as foolows: under equal conditions for more ball-like proteins which are α/β-proteins, the surface border of phases in the transition state is larger and consequently the folding is slower.

Since the prediction of folding rate is in itself valuable, many parameters for prediction of folding rate have been proposed during recent years (Galzitskaya et al., 2003; Ivankov et al., 2003; Punta and Rost, 2005; Ivankov and Finkelstein, 2004; Zhou and Zhou, 2002; Gong et al., 2003; Capriotti and Casadio, 2007; Gromiha and Selvaraj, 2001; Gromiha et al., 2006; Ma et al., 2007). Some of them are modifications of *CO* (Ivankov et al., 2003; Zhou and Zhou, 2002; Zhou and Zhou, 2002), in others the prediction of folding rate is realized using secondary structure (Ivankov and Finkelstein, 2004; Gong et al., 2003) and number of contacts in the native structure (Makarov et al., 2002). Besides, search for the dependences has been done by bioinformatics methods (Gromiha et al., 2006; Ma et al., 2007; Gromiha, 2005). It has been revealed that there is different dependence of folding rate on the amino acid composition (Ma et al., 2007) and physicochemical properties of amino acids of proteins (Gromiha et al., 2006; Gromiha, 2005) for proteins with one-stage and multi-stage kinetics of folding in water. However, the bioinformatics methods cannot give a physical explanation of the obtained results.

The above rather contradictory data demonstrate that the theory of protein folding requires further development and subsequent search for factors affecting the rate of folding. In this work the process of protein folding of separate protein molecules and structural properties connected with the folding has been investigated. The statistical analysis has been made for the dependence of rate of folding on the size of protein and the number of stages in this process.

One of important questions in molecular biology is what determines folding pathways: native structure or protein sequence. There are many proteins that have similar structures but very different sequences, and a relevant question is whether such proteins have similar or different folding mechanisms. To explain the differences in folding rates of various proteins, the theory of protein folding rate should be developed further.

The capillarity model (Finkelstein and Badretdinov, 1997; Wolynes, 1997) gave rise to the hypothesis that protein folding rates are determined by the average "entropy capacity" (the entropy capacity for the given protein structure is defined as conformational entropy per residue divided by the average contact energy per residue, or model entropy capacity as the average number of degrees of freedom divided by the number of contacts per residue; thus, this value is, in a sense, reciprocal to the expected melting temperature) (Galzitskaya et al., 2000). It has been shown (Galzitskaya and Garbuzynskiy, 2006) that entropy capacity correlates with folding rates for alpha-helical proteins (correlation coefficient is 0.79) and proteins with mixed (α/β) secondary structure (correlation coefficient is 0.84).

Consideration of the compactness specifically addresses the issue of why some proteins fold more rapidly than others. Statistical analysis demonstrates that four main structural classes (Murzin et al., 1995) of proteins (all-α, all-β, α/β, $\alpha+\beta$) differ from one another in a statistically significant manner with respect to the number of rotatable angles φ, ψ, and χ and the average number of contacts per residue (Galzitskaya and Garbuzynskiy, 2006). On the whole, it has been shown that among proteins of the same size α/β proteins have, on average, a greater number of contacts per residue due to their more compact (more ball-like, since a ball is the most compact geometrical body: a ball has the minimal accessible surface area in comparison with other geometrical bodies of equal volumes) structure, rather than to tighter packing (Galzitskaya et al., 2008a).

From previous works, it is possible to suggest a relationship between the number of contacts and folding rates. For 75 proteins for which both folding rates and tertiary structures are known, α-helical proteins have on average the fastest folding kinetics and the smallest number of contacts per residue (they are less compact than others), whereas α/β proteins have on average the slowest folding kinetics and the largest number of contacts (they are more compact than others) (Galzitskaya et al., 2008a). An explanation is that the expected surface of the boundary between folded and unfolded phases in the transition state (Galzitskaya et al., 2001) for a more ball-like protein is larger than for an oblong-like protein. Thus, the fact that α/β proteins are more ball-like explains both the more average number of contacts per residue (Galzitskaya et al., 2008a) and the slower folding kinetics.

The progress in the protein folding rate prediction is due to the analysis of multidimensional networks of the protein folding-unfolding trajectories done by various algorithms (Galzitskaya and Finkelstein, 1999; Alm and Baker, 1999). All these approaches (Galzitskaya and Finkelstein, 1999; Alm and Baker, 1999;Muñoz and Eaton, 1999) use different approximations and algorithms, consider only the attractive native interactions (the "Gō model", Taketomi et al., 1975) to reduce the energy frustrations and heterogeneity of interactions, and model the trade-off between the formation of attractive interactions and the loss of conformational entropy during protein folding. These works also simulate unfolding of known 3D protein structures rather than their folding, but the unfolding is considered close to the mid-transition point, where folding and unfolding pathways coincide according to the detailed balance principle. Under these "near-equilibrium" conditions, all single-domain proteins demonstrate two-state (i.e., "all-or-none") transitions both in thermodynamics (Privalov, 1979) and kinetics (Fersht, 1995; 1997). This means that at the mid-transition all semi-folded and misfolded globules are unstable relative to both native and unfolded states of protein chain, and this allows us to take into account only the pathways going from the native to the unfolded state and to neglect those leading to misfolded globules, stabilized by non-native interactions.

Calculation of protein folding in such model bases on the method of dynamic programming (Galzitskaya and Finkelstein, 1999), or by Monte Carlo method (Galzitskaya et al., 2000; Galzitskaya et al., 2005), or by solution of kinetic equations (Ivankov and Finkelstein, 2001). Correlation coefficient (without adjustable parameters) between experimentally investigated folding rates and calculated for 45 proteins and peptides is 0.78 (Ivankov and Finkelstein, 2001), for 17 proteins with well studied folding nucleus is 0.73 (Garbuzynskiy et al., 2004).

Under analysis of similar model in water the calculated folding rates correlate with experimental data at the level of 0.67 for the set 37 proteins (Alm et al., 2002).

Table 2. Methods for calculation of protein folding rates with known tree dimensional structures based on the nucleation mechanism

Method	Condition of modeling	Number of proteins	Correlation coefficient	reference
Diffusion equations on the one-dimension profile	water	22	0.87	Munoz and Eaton, 1999
Recursive search deep into	water	39	0.67	Almetal., 2002
Dynamic programming	mid-transition	17	0.73	Garbuzynskiy et al., 2004
Monte Carlo	mid-transition	10	0.70	Galzitskaya et al., 2005
Kinetic equations	mid-transition	45	0.78	Ivankov and Finkelstein, 2001

In this work the attention has been done to the folding of separate protein molecules and their structural properties connected with the process of protein folding. We predict folding time for 67 proteins with known experimental data, and compare the predicted things with experimental ones. We model the folding process by means of a relatively simple theoretical approach, and use two methods (Monte Carlo simulations and Dynamic Programming) to investigate free-energy landscapes of protein folding, and an entropy capacity derived from the capillarity model for the prediction of folding rate for 67 proteins.

Consideration of the entropy capacity specifically addresses the issue of why some proteins fold more rapidly than others. Statistical analysis demonstrates that four main structural classes of proteins (all-α, all-β, α/β, $\alpha+\beta$) differ from one another in a statistically significant manner with respect to the number of rotatable angles φ, ψ, and χ and the average number of contacts per residue. These parameters are able to explain the vast range of experimentally observed folding rates. The obtained result suggests that structural and sequence properties are important determinants of the folding rate.

RESULTS

Comparison of Different Parameters Describing the Shape of Protein Globules (Compactness) for Two-State and Multi-State Folders

Recently, we have found that in order to predict protein folding rates, any parameter should correlate well with the protein chain length (Ivankov et al., 2009). As a very illustrative example of this was observed with relative contact order (the normalized parameter, which has poor correlation with the logarithm of protein folding rates, see Table 1) and absolute contact order, which includes both the size of protein and the average length of loops and correlates well with the logarithm of protein folding rates (Ivankov et al., 2003; Ivankov et al., 2009).

On average, the folding of multi-state proteins is slower than that of two-state ones. At the same time, slow folding proteins are more ball-like (compact) than fast folding ones (Galzitskaya et al., 2008b). Thus, we suggest here protein compactness as a predictor of the protein folding type. This is naturally to expect since almost all known experimentally studied α/β proteins exhibit multi-state kinetics.

We have calculated the compactness, radius of cross-section and radius of gyration for each protein (see section Materials and http://phys.protres.ru/resources/compact.html).

Dependences of normalized radius of gyration, radius of gyration, radius of cross-section on the logarithm of the folding rate in water for multi-state and two-state folders are presented in Figure 1. Coefficient correlation for radius of gyration and radius of cross-section are -0.57 and -0.74, respectively. But coefficient correlation for normalized radius of gyration is small, is -0.33. This only underlined the above mentioned fact.

One can see that multi-state proteins have more spherical shape than two-state folders. The dependence of normalized radius of gyration demonstrates that, on average, two-state folders have more elongated shape than multi-state folders.

Table 3. Correlation coefficients between logarithms of folding rates in water and structural parameters as connected with size of protein and no

parameter	$\ln k_f$, s^{-1} 84 proteins	$\ln k_f^{multi}$, s^{-1} 26 proteins	$\ln k_f^{two}$, s^{-1} 58 proteins
V/S	-0.74 ± 0.05	-0.77 ± 0.08	-0.59 ± 0.09
ln(V/S)	-0.74 ± 0.05	-0.78 ± 0.08	-0.61 ± 0.08
*S/S**	-0.33 ± 0.10	-0.48 ± 0.15	-0.19 ± 0.13
*Rg/Rg**	0.23 ± 0.10	-0.01 ± 0.20	0.20 ± 0.13
Rg	-0.57 ± 0.07	-0.73 ± 0.09	-0.37 ± 0.11
ln(L)	-0.71 ± 0.05	-0.82 ± 0.06	-0.55 ± 0.09
$L^{2/3}$	-0.69 ± 0.06	-0.80 ± 0.07	-0.47 ± 0.10

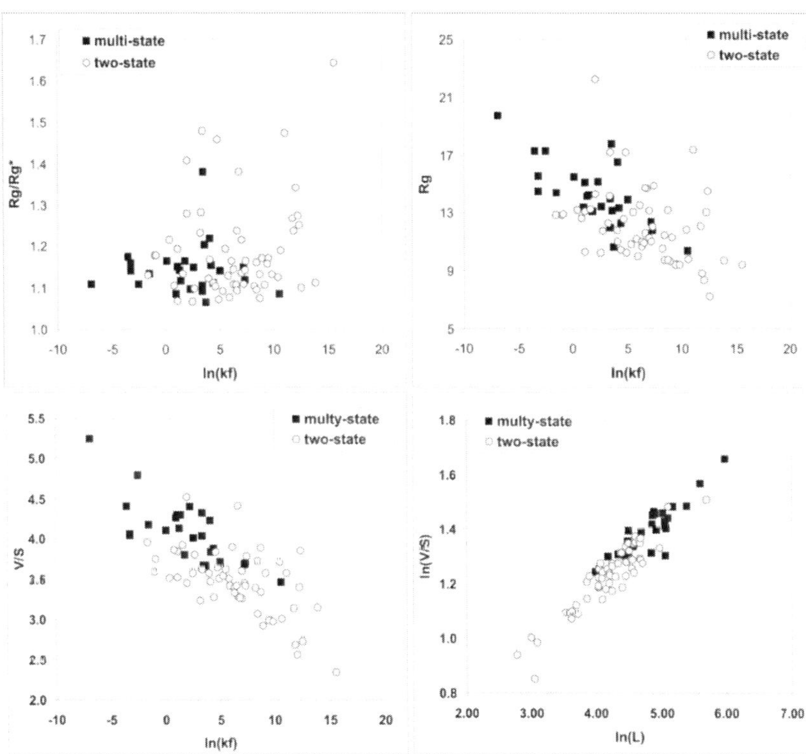

Figure 1. Dependence of normalized radius of gyration (a), radius of gyration (b), and radius of cross-section (c) on the logarithm of the folding rate in water for multi-state and two-state folders. (d) Dependence of logarithm of radius of cross-section on the logarithm of the number of amino acid residues in protein.

To exclude the influence of length, we analyzed the folding rate data, compactness, radius of cross-section, and radius of gyration within a given size range where the average size of proteins is nearly the same. To that end, we divided the set of our proteins into groups according to their size. Thus, we take into account the number of residues in protein structures. We obtained two groups where the number of proteins is sufficient for statistics (the ranges are 50-100 and 101-151). For every group we averaged the compactness, radius of cross-section, normalized radius of gyration and the folding rate logarithms in order to compare them for each size range (see Materials and Methods).

We have found that multi-state proteins indeed are more ball-like than proteins with two-state kinetics as judged by all considered characteristics of shape. This trend persists in both size ranges in which the number of proteins is sufficient for statistics. Thus, the observed difference in compactness is not a consequence of differences in size distribution between two classes of proteins.

Table 4. Average values of normalized radius of gyration, *compactness*, radius of cross-section, and logarithms of folding rates in-water for two- and multi-state folding proteins

Folding kinetics	Two-state		Multi-state	
Size range, residues	50—100	101—151	50—100	101—151
Number of proteins	36 proteins	7 proteins	9 proteins	8 proteins
Normalized radius of gyration, R_g/R_g*	1.18 ± 0.01		1.13 ± 0.01	
	1.16 ± 0.01	1.30 ± 0.06	1.13 ± 0.01	1.13 ± 0.01
Compactness, S_{ASA}/S^*_{ASA}	1.51 ± 0.01		1.48 ± 0.01	
	1.50 ± 0.01	1.60 ± 0.03	1.45 ± 0.02	1.52 ± 0.03
Radius of cross-section, V_{ASA}/S_{ASA}	3.57 ± 0.03		3.93 ± 0.05	
	3.54 ± 0.03	3.76 ± 0.05	3.75 ± 0.05	4.14 ± 0.07
$ln(k_f)$ in water	5.31 ± 0.47		3.45 ± 0.60	
	4.98 ± 0.57	7.03 ± 1.50	5.12 ± 0.90	1.58 ± 0.84

For proteins with studied folding kinetics, compactness and radius of cross-section depend on protein length in the manner expected from the analysis of 3769 protein domains (Ivankov et al., 2009). For the normalized radius of gyration one could expect that for 101-151 window size it will be slightly higher than for 50-100 window size. For two-state proteins the difference in Table 4 accords with this expectation, while for multi-state proteins the normalized radius of gyration is independent on the protein length, which is important.

Is the Protein Folding Rate Dependent on the Number of Folding Stages?

The results of comparison of average folding rates from the Table 4 are rather surprising. The only expected observation is that average folding rate for multi-state proteins from 101-151 size range is less than all others average values. One unexpected correspondence is that in the size range of 50-100 residues two-state folding is not faster than multi-state one. Next, for two-state proteins folding of larger proteins (101-151 residues) is faster than that of smaller ones (50-100 residues). The general opinion is that multi-state folders should demonstrate slower folding kinetics and, thus, the introduction of an intermediate should decrease the folding rate (probably, this opinion arose due to multi-state proteins are slower folders since they are bigger). Our analysis shows that this is not true for proteins of 50-100 residues long. However, in the size range of 101-151 residues multi-state proteins do fold slower, but this is not due to the differences in their length (we consider the same-length proteins). So, we suggest another explanation, namely, the slower folding for multi-state proteins of the same length can be explained by their more ball-like structure that requires more time for the burst phase and following packing of the 3D structure in the main phase, so the expected surface of the boundary between folded and unfolded phases in the transition state for a more ball-like protein is larger than that for a oblong-like protein (see Table 5) (Galzitskaya et al., 2008a,b).

There is an interesting example of the folding of the largest protein with two-state kinetics: Variable surface antigen VlsE (pdb entry 1L8W) is less ball-like than protein with a similar number of amino acid residues which exhibit multi-state kinetics (Tryptophan synthase α subunit, pdb entry 1QOP, see Tables 1 and 2 at the http://phys.protres.ru/ resources/compact.html). Despite of the fact that in the case of the correlation between contact order and folding rates, the correlation has a clear explanation in terms of the entropy cost of the size of loops and/or the ordering of residues between the contacting residues, contact order can not explain the behavior of this protein (Ivankov et al., 2009). VlsE does not obey contact-order correlation.

Table 5. Example of comparison two large proteins with geometrical bodies

PDB entry 1l8w, 341 residues, two-state protein Rg_{1l8w}=21.53 Å	$Rg = \sqrt{\frac{1}{2}r^2 + \frac{1}{12}l^2}$, l=4.5r
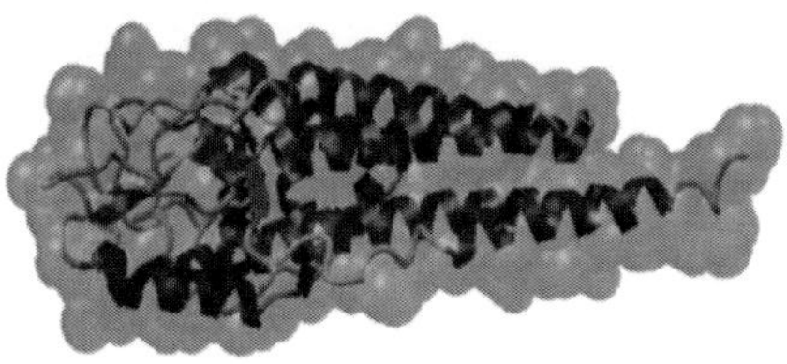	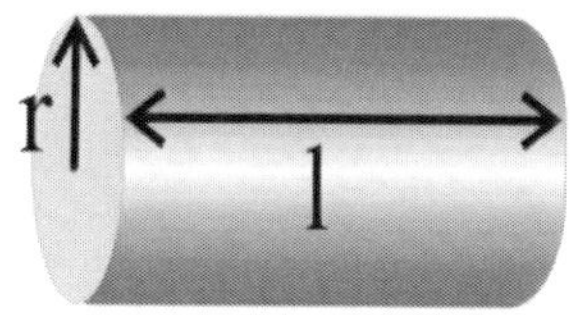
PDB entry 1qop, 396 residues, multi-state protein Rg_{1qop}=17.20 Å	$Rg = \sqrt{\frac{3}{5}R^2}$, R=1.5r
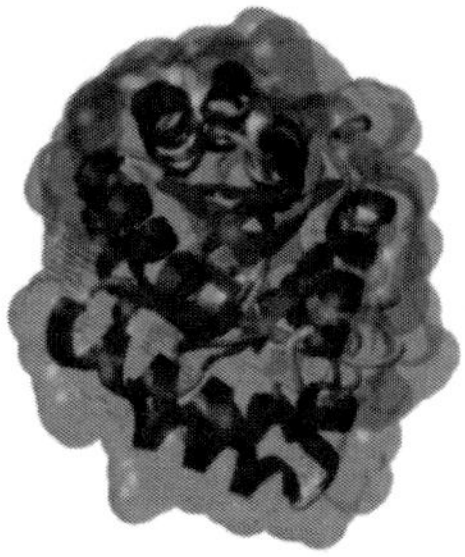	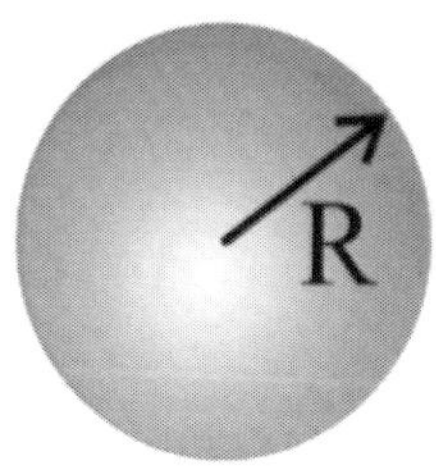
$\frac{Rg_{1l8w}}{Rg_{1qop}} = 1.25$	$\frac{Rg_{cylinder}}{Rg_{ball}} = 1.27$

From our analysis we can conclude that the barrier height for folding of large proteins is defined by size of surface of the boundary between folded and unfolded phases in the transition state (see Table 5).

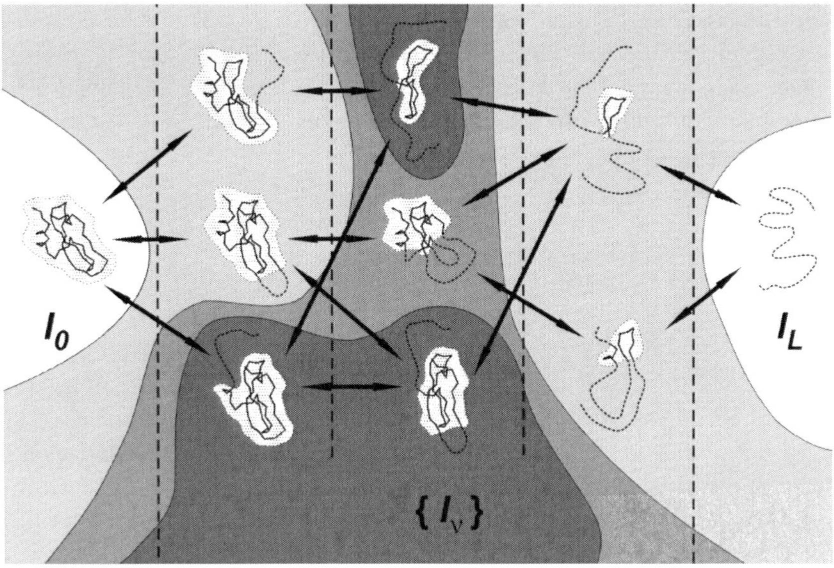

Figure 2. A sketch of the network of pathways of sequential unfolding (and folding) of native 3D protein structure (I0). IL is the coil where all L links of the protein chain are disordered. In each of the many intermediates of the type Iv, v chain links (shown in the dashed line) are unfolded, while the other L-v links keep their native positions and conformations (they are shown as the solid line against the background of a dotted cloud denoting the globular part of the intermediate). The central structure in the lower line exemplifies a microstate with v unfolded links forming one closed unfolded loop and one unfolded tail; the central structure in the central line exemplifies a microstate where v unfolded links form two closed unfolded loops. The networks used in computations are much larger than the one shown in the sketch: they include millions of semi-folded microstates.

Monte-Carlo Simulations of Protein Folding

To construct a theoretical pathway of protein folding, we did Monte Carlo simulations for 67 proteins (Galzitskaya et al., 2005; Galzitskaya, 2010). We performed travelling from the unfolded state to the native 3D structure without misfolding to other compact states. In our model, the folding pathways are treated as sequential insertion of residues from the unfolded state to their native positions according to the 3D native structure or removal of residues from the native position to the coil, respectively (Figure 2).

The removed (inserted) residues are assumed to loose (gain) all the non-bonded interactions and gain (loose) the coil entropy except that spent to close the disordered loops protruding from the remaining globule (Galzitskaya and Finkelstein, 1999). The general assumption of this model is that the residues remaining in the globule keep their native position and that the unfolded regions do not fold to another, non-native globule. Thus, we neglect non-native interactions that make our model similar to that of Gō(Taketomi et al., 1975).

Estimation of Free Energy

Our model considers the native structure I_0, the unfolded state I_L and an ensemble of intermediate microstates I_ν consisting of a native-like part and of ν unfolded chain links (ν=0 for I_0, ν=L for I_L, L being the total number of the chain links, and ν=1, …, L-1 for the semi-folded intermediates with ν disordered links). The model uses a simple free energy estimate (Galzitskaya and Finkelstein, 1999) of each microstate I:

$$F(I) = \varepsilon \times n_I^{nb} - T[\eta_I \times \sigma + \sum_{loops \in I} S_{loop}]. \quad (1)$$

n_I^{nb} is the number of native atom-atom contacts in the native-like part of I (n_I^{nb} does not include contacts of neighbor residues, also existing in the coil); ε is the energy of one contact; η_I is the number of residues in the unfolded part of I; T is the temperature; σ is the entropy difference between the coil and the native state of a residue (we take σ=2.3R according to Privalov (Privalov, 1979), R being the gas constant). The sum Σ is taken over all closed unfolded loops (see legend to Figure 2) protruding from the native-like part of I.

At the point of equilibrium between the native state I_0 and the coil I_L, we have $F(I_0)$=$F(I_L)$, i.e., the contact energy ε (which is influenced by the solvent) and the temperature$T$ are connected (at the mid-transition) by equation

$$\varepsilon = -TN\sigma / n_0^{nb} \quad (2)$$

where n_0^{nb} is the number of contacts in the native structure and N is the total number of the protein chain residues. It follows from equations (1) and (2) that the $F(I)/T$ values (which only determine the transition state, see equation (4) below) do not depend on temperature, provided that the solvent composition corresponds to the mid-transition at this temperature.

The entropy spent to close a disordered loop between the still fixed residues k and l is estimated (Finkelstein and Badretdinov, 1997) as

$$S_{loop} = -{}^5/_2 R \ln|k - l| - {}^3/_2 R\, (r^2_{kl} - a^2) / (2Aa|k - l|); \qquad (3)$$

here r_{kl} is the distance between the C_α atoms of residues k and l, a = 3.8Å is the distance between the neighbor C_α atoms in the chain, and A is the persistence length for a polypeptide (according to Flory (Flory, 1969), we take A = 20Å). The term $-{}^5/_2 R \ln|k - l|$ is the main in equation (3); the coefficient $-{}^5/_2$ (rather than Flory's value $-{}^3/_2$) follows from the condition that a loop cannot penetrate inside the globule (Finkelstein and Badretdinov, 1997).

We consider our model as an approximation of the protein folding process, rather than a detailed description of the chain motions. Thereby our model of folding is a trade-off between the configurational entropy loss and the gain of attractive interactions. The model takes into account the topology of the native state.

Investigation of Folding Kinetics

We calculated how long a given protein chain folds to its known native structure, starting from unfolded chain by Monte Carlo (MC) simulation using the Metropolis scheme (Metropolis et al., 1953) at point of mid-transition. The kinematic scheme of elementary movements includes removal of a residue from the native position to the coil or insertion of a residue from the coil to the native position (Galzitskaya and Finkelstein, 1998). Thus, we did a travelling from the unfolded state to the native 3D structure without misfolding to other compact states.

An elementary MC step was done as follows. We randomly chose a residue (namely, we generated a random number between 1 and L, where L being here the total number of residues; thus, a link was one residue-long). If the chosen residue had been already fixed in the native position, we tried to unfold it. If the chosen residue was in the coil, we tried to fix it according to its native position. Then we computed the free energy difference, ΔF, between new and previous intermediate structures. The MC step leads to the new structure with a probability w, which is equal to $exp(-\Delta F/RT)$, if $\Delta F>0$, or to 1, if $\Delta F\leq 0$. Thus, if $\Delta F\leq 0$, the MC step always leads to the new structure. If

$\Delta F>0$, w is compared with a random number ξ ($0<\xi<1$; ξ is generated according to the uniform distribution) if $w>\xi$, the transition is accepted; if $w\leq\xi$, it is rejected and the previous state is preserved.

To estimate the characteristic first passage time, $t_{1/2}$, we performed 50 MC runs for every protein (Galzitskaya and Finkelstein, 1998). For every set of values, $t_{1/2}$ was determined as the number of MC steps required to complete 50% of MC runs (25 of 50 runs). Each individual run was started from the completely unfolded structure, and was completed when the molecule became completely folded. In the limit of 10^8 MC steps, we could calculate the time of folding for 67 proteins from 84 investigated ones (Ivankov et al., 2009) (the rest 17 proteins could not fold during this number of steps). Figure 3 presents the typical MC Gō kinetics for three proteins (activation domain of procarboxypeptidase, spliceosomal protein, and ribosomal protein). One can see (in Figure 3a) that the protein chain stays near the unfolded state for a long time (in this case, for 277 000 of MC steps), then very quickly (compared to the first period of time) folds (the period of time of overcoming by protein chain of folding transition state barrier is 1000 of MC steps), then spends some time near folded state (the fraction of folded residues is near 90% for this protein) and finally comes to the completely folded state.

It should be noted that some almost folded structures have free energies not much higher compared to that of the completely folded structure (thus, even if each residue can be only in one of two states – folded and unfolded – there is a basin of native states rather than a single completely folded state). The same (in a less extent though) concerns also to the basin of the unfolded structures (however, it is definitely an ensemble because unfolded residues have more than one conformation by definition). The "almost folded" structures which are rather stable are usually those ones where one or several residues are still unfolded (these are usually those residues which form a small number of contacts in the completely folded structure). The brightest cases comprise NMR structures that have long tails forming virtually no contacts in the native structures. Thus, it is not a miracle that they "prefer" to be unfolded. Moreover, in some cases some almost folded structures have lower free energy compared to the completely folded one (see Figure 3d).

Figure 4 represents the typical MC kinetics for one of the 67 proteins (Chemotactic protein, CheY). In CheY (Figure 4), the *N*-terminal part of the molecule (residues 1-86) folds first (during 20% of the time of barrier crossing) forming an intermediate state which exists for quite a long time (see Figure 4) before the *C*-terminus folds. After that, the *C*-terminus folds, and the native state is complete. This behavior (the *N*-terminal part folds first) is roughly the same for all individual folding trajectories; however, there are some differences in the order of folding of individual elements of secondary structure. Such a scenario of protein folding has been suggested from the experimental study for this protein (Muñoz et al., 1994).

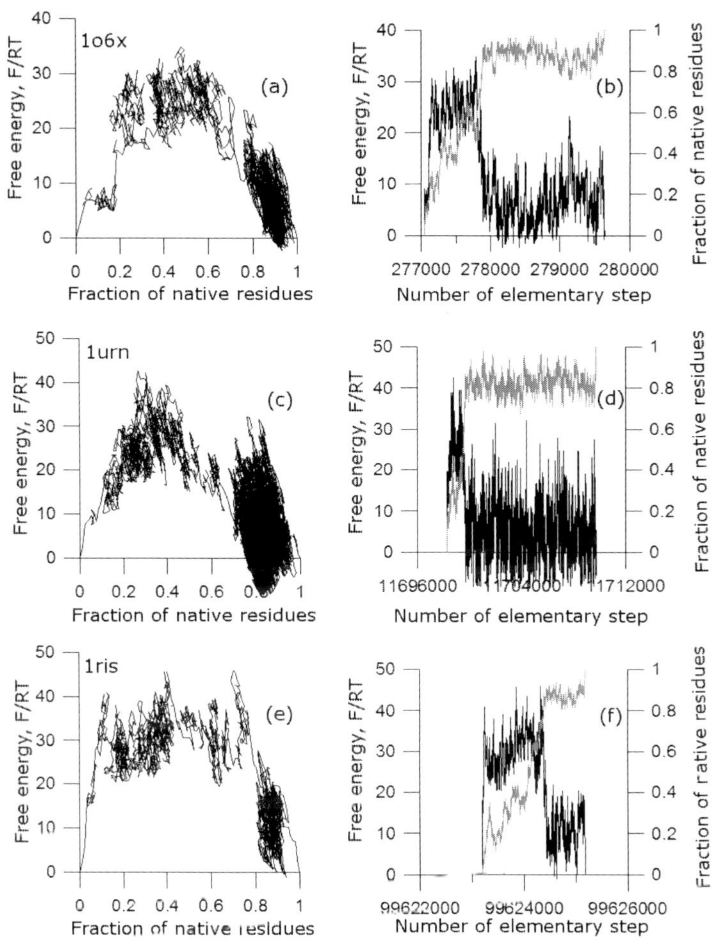

Figure 3. (a,c,e) Dependences of free energy on the fraction of amino acid residues fixed in the native position for one of the folding trajectories for proteins with a ferredoxin-like fold. (b,d,f) The same fragment of the same folding trajectory. Black curve is the dependence of free energy on time. Gray curve is the dependence of the number of native amino acid residues on time.

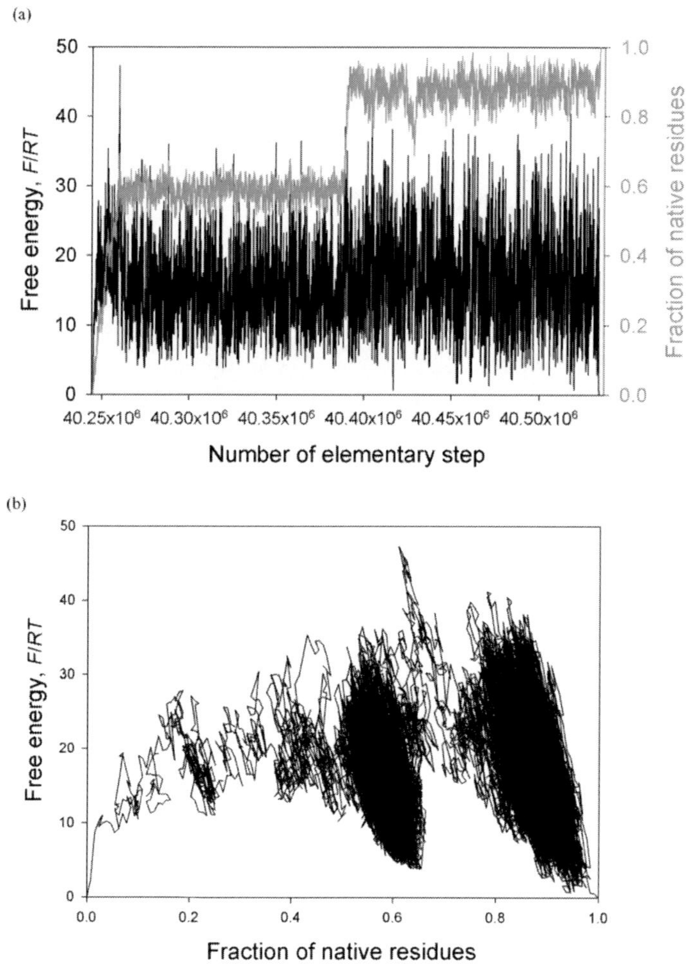

Figure 4. (a) A fragment of one of the folding trajectories for CheY. Black curve shows the dependence of free energy on time. Gray curve shows the dependence of the number of native amino acid residues on time. (b) The dependence of free energy on the number of native amino acid residues for the same fragment of the same folding trajectory.

The computed (for mid-transition) characteristic first passage time, $t_{1/2}$, values for 67 proteins are given in Tables 7, 8 and 9. They are in good correlation with $\ln k_f^{mt}$: the correlation coefficient is -0.82±0.04 (see Figure 5). It should be noted here that proteins with two-state kinetics have a higher correlation coefficient (-0.83±0.04) than proteins with multi-state kinetics -0.68±0.13 (see Table 6).

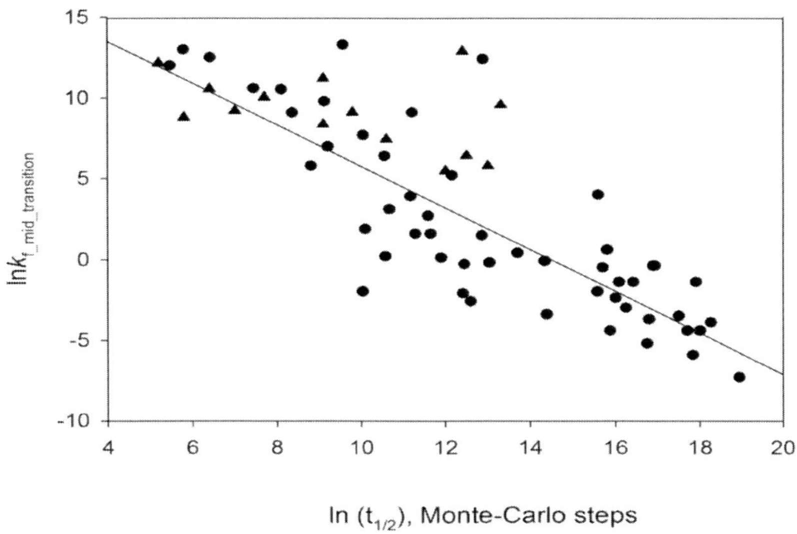

Figure 5. Correlation between the computed characteristic first passage time $t_{1/2}$ (the number of MC steps made until a half of molecules folds) and the experimentally measured folding rate at the mid-transition for 67 proteins, where the folding simulation has been completed within 10^8 MC steps. The time of simulation, $t_{1/2}$, is measured in MC steps. Both are represented in a logarithmic scale. The correlation coefficient is -0.82 for all proteins, -0.83 for two-state folders (circle) and for multi-state is -0.68 (triangle).

Table 6. Correlation coefficients between logarithms of folding rates in mid-transition and parameters connected with protein size

Parameters connected with protein size	$\ln k_{mt}$ *67 proteins*	$\ln k_{mt}^{multi}$ *16 proteins*	$\ln k_{mt}^{two}$ *51 proteins*
L	-0.69±0.06	-0.52±0.18	-0.72±0.07
ln(*L*)	-0.76±0.05	-0.60±0.16	-0.75±0.06
Radius of cross section, V/S,Å	-0.53±0.09	-0.49±0.19	-0.49±0.11
ln(*Entropy capacity*)	-0.78±0.05	-0.57±0.17	-0.78±0.05
ln($t_{1/2}$), MC steps	-0.82±0.04	-0.68±0.13	-0.83±0.04
F_{eff}	-0.72±0.06	-0.59±0.16	-0.73±0.07
F_{min}	-0.77±0.05	-0.57±0.17	-0.78±0.05

It is interesting to compare the correlation between the folding rate in the mid-transition with the length and different colors (*ln(L)*, $L^{2/3}$, $L^{1/2}$) of the length. From Table 6 one can see that *L* and *ln(L)* has a high correlation coefficient with folding rates at the mid-transition, especially for the proteins with two-state kinetics. Although, the dependence of the logarithm of folding rate proportional to *L* has Levinthal's estimation of folding time, it is not applicable for consideration. Such a good correlation means that there is a rather great scatter in the data, or the range of variation is too small.

At the same time the radius of cross-section has a worse correlation coefficient with the folding rate than the size of proteins for the considered set of proteins. But the protein size can not explain the difference in the folding rates for proteins of a similar size (or proteins sharing a similar fold, practically with a similar number of amino acid residues).

Table 7. Characteristics of proteins from class *a*

PDB entry	Protein (or domain) name, Number of amino acid residues in structure, Behavior	$\ln k_f^{mt}$	$\ln(k_f)$ in water	$\ln(t_{1/2})$ (MC steps)	$Ln(\nu/m)$	F_{eff}/RT	F_{min}/RT
1enh	Engrailed homeodomain, 54, multi	8.1	10.5	10.54	-1.33	6.96	12.16
2cro	Phage 434 cro protein, 65, multi	0.3	3.7	11.20	-1.52	8.4	13.53
1ayi	Colicin E7 immunity protein, 85, multi	2.8	7.2	12.15	-1.50	11.25	16.77
1a6n	Apomyoglobin, 151, multi	-1.4	1.1	17.47	-1.63	19.52	24.86
1l2y	Trp-cage protein, 20, two	13	12.5	5.79	-1.09	3.13	4.95
1vii	Villin headpeace subdomain, 36, two	10.6	9.4	7.44	-1.20	2.64	6.06
2pdd	Peripheral subunit-binding domain, 41, two	9.8	9.8	9.13	-1.30	4.93	9.52
1prb	GA module of albumin binding domain, 47, two	13.3	13.8	9.57	-1.41	6.47	11.06
1gv2	c-Myb-transforming protein, 47, two	3.1	8.7	10.67	-1.35	7.72	11.91
1ba5	TRF1 Myb domain, 49, two	1.6	5.9	11.29	-1.29	9.11	13.71
1fex	RAP1 Myb domain, 59, two	3.9	8.2	11.17	-1.41	4.86	10.57
1bdd	B-domain of staphylococcal proteinA, 60, two	5.8	11.7	8.81	-1.38	2.07	8.64
1jyg	Hypothetical protein encoded by the Yjbj gene from E.col, 69, twoi	6.4	9.1	10.56	-1.41	3.92	10.02
2a3d	α3D, 73, two	12.4	12.2	12.88	-1.39	11.69	16.25
1lmb	l-repressor, 80, two	5.2	10.4	12.16	-1.57	10.75	15.16

PDB entry	Protein (or domain) name, Number of amino acid residues in structure, Behavior	$\ln k_f^{mt}$	$\ln(k_f)$ in water	$\ln(t_{1/2})$ (MC steps)	$Ln(\nu/m)$	F_{eff}/RT	F_{min}/RT
1imq	Colicin E9 immunity protein, 85, two	-1.4	7.3	16.43	-1.60	10.18	14.94
1nti	Acyl-coenzyme A binding protein, 86, two	-0.3	7	12.45	-1.53	9.16	16.13
256b	Cytochrome b562, 106, two	-0.1	12.3	14.34	-1.58	11.35	15.48
1cun 1	16th domain of brain α – spectrin, 106, two	-2	4.8	15.57	-1.75	15.53	22.17
1cun 2	17th domain of brain α – spectrin, 107, two	-3.4	3.4	14.39	-1.51	14.86	21.46
1u5p	15th domain of brain α – spectrin, 110, two	4	11	15.59	-1.53	15.13	21.09

Table 8. Characteristics of proteins from class *b*

PDB entry	Protein (or domain) name, Number of amino acid residues in structure, Behavior	$\ln k_f^{mt}$	$\ln(k_f)$ in water	$\ln(t_{1/2})$ (MC steps)	$Ln(\nu/m)$	F_{eff}/RT	F_{min}/RT
1tit	Immunoglobulin domain of cardiac titin, 89, multi	-6.9	3.6	16.54	-1.54	16.21	21.45
1hng	C-terminal domain of the cell-surface receptor protein CD2, 95, multi	-3.5	1.8	13.68	-1.54	12.26	18.04
1eal	Ileal lipid binding protein, 127, multi	-2.8	1.3	18.02	-1.50	21.76	26.77
1ifc	Intestinal fatty acid binding protein, 131, multi	-2.8	3.4	17.45	-1.57	21.64	26.1
1opa	Cellular retinol binding protein II, 133, multi	-5	1.4	18.21	-1.55	21.21	24.91
beta	C-terminal β-hairpin of protein GB1, 16, two	12	12	5.47	-0.71	4.4	6.08
1pin	Pin WW domain, 34, two	9.1	9.5	8.36	-1.19	4.82	8.58
1e0l	Formin-binding protein, 37, two	9.1	10.6	11.21	-1.14	1.15	6.18
1e0m	Prototype WW domain, 37, two	7.7	8.9	10.05	-1.24	2.04	6.98

Table 8. (Continued).

PDB entry	Protein (or domain) name, Number of amino acid residues in structure, Behavior	$\ln k_f^{mt}$	$\ln(k_f)$ in water	$\ln(t_{1/2})$ (MC steps)	*Ln(ν/m)*	F_{eff}/RT	F_{min}/RT
1jmq	Yes kinase-associated protein, 40, two	7	8.4	9.21	-1.29	2.94	8.48
1rlq	Src SH3 domain, 56, two	0.4	4.4	13.70	-1.51	11.54	18.14
1shg	α-spectrin SH3 domain, 57, two	-3.7	1.1	16.80	-1.52	10.91	16.85
1avz	Fyn SH3 domain, 57, two	-2	4.9	10.05	-1.54	1.29	6.67
1jo8	Actin binding protein ABP1 SH3 domain, 58, two	-2.1	2.5	12.42	-1.56	10.04	15.27
1c9o	Cold shock protein B, 66, two	0.2	7.2	10.58	-1.48	5.54	10.72
1g6p	Cold shock protein B, 66, two	-2.6	6.3	12.60	-1.54	9.31	15.71
1csp	Cold shock protein B, 67, two	2.7	6.5	11.59	-1.51	4.8	10.49
1mjc	Cold shock protein A, 69, two	1.6	5.3	11.65	-1.59	6.699	13.49
1m9s	SH3-like domain of virulence protein internalin B, 76, two	0.1	4	11.90	-1.47	9.27	14.3
1ten	Third fibronectin type III repeat of tenascin, 89, two	-4.4	1.1	17.70	-1.60	18.69	23.198
1wit	18th module of muscle protein twitchin, 93, two	-5.9	0.4	17.83	-1.71	20.99	26.6
1fnf2	Tenth fibronectin type III domain of fibronectin, 94, two	-0.5	5.5	15.70	-1.70	14.3	20.18

Table 9. Characteristics of proteins from class *d*

PDB entry	Protein (or domain) name, Number of amino acid residues in structure, Behavior	$\ln k_f^{mt}$	$\ln(k_f)$ in water	$\ln(t_{1/2})$ (MC steps)	$Ln(\nu/m)$	F_{eff}/RT	F_{min}/RT
1ubq	Ubiquitin, 76, multi	-1.5	7.3	12.16	-1.49	9.87	14.45
1gxt	N-terminal domain of HypF, 88, multi	-0.8	4.4	17.03	-1.62	15.98	21.07
Suc1#	Cell-cycle regulatory protein p13suc1, 96, multi	-1	4.2	14.23	-1.47	13.65	19.30
1bni	Barnase, 108, multi	-4.3	2.6	18.50	-1.63	18.14	22.92
2vik	Villin 14T, N-terminal domain of villin, 126, multi	-1.6	5	16.10	-1.65	13.6	19.97
1t8j	BBA5 mini-protein, 22, two	12.5	11.8	6.42	-0.91	3.08	5.74
1divN	N-terminal domain from ribosomal protein L9, 56, two	1.9	6.6	10.10	-1.34	6.17	11.69
3gb1	B1 domain of streptococcal protein G, 56, two	-0.4	6.3	16.90	-1.47	9.00	15.33
2ptl	Immunoglobulin light chain-binding domain of protein L, 60, two	-1.4	4.1	17.90	-1.51	14.01	20.02
1c8c	Sso7d protein, 63, two	0.6	7	15.80	-1.36	8.97	15.2
2ci2	Chymotrypsin inhibitor 2, 64, two	-3.5	5.8	17.50	-1.48	10.22	17.00
1rfa	Ras-binding domain of C-raf-1, 78, two	-0.2	8.4	13.04	-1.55	11.92	16.30
1o6x	Activation domain of procarboxypeptidase A2, 81, two	1.5	6.8	12.86	-1.55	13.41	18.37
1poh	Histidine-containing phosphocarrier protein, 85, two	-3	2.7	16.26	-1.66	15.64	20.94
1divC	C-terminal domain from ribosomal protein L9, 92, two	-4.4	3.3	15.88	-1.55	17.43	22.93
1n88	Ribosomal protein L23	-2.4	2	16.00	-1.56	12.78	18.75

Table 9. (Continued).

PDB entry	Protein (or domain) name, Number of amino acid residues in structure, Behavior	$\ln k_f^{mt}$	$\ln(k_f)$ in water	$\ln(t_{1/2})$ (MC steps)	$Ln(v/m)$	F_{eff}/RT	F_{min}/RT
1urn	Spliceosomal protein U1A, 96, two	-0.4	4.6	16.94	-1.58	16.49	23.09
1ris	Ribosomal protein S6, 97, two	-3.9	6.1	18.25	-1.49	18.5	25.53
2acy	Common-type acylphosphatase, 98, two	-4.4	0.8	17.99	-1.63	18.73	24.83
1aps	Muscle acylphosphatase, 98, two	-7.3	-1.6	18.95	-1.64	19.76	25.39
1spr	Src SH2 domain, 103, two	-1.4	8.7	16.08	-1.59	15.57	21.87
1fkf	FK506 binding protein, 107, two	-5.2	1.6	16.76	-1.63	16.1	22.83

Dynamic Programming Method

A Simplified Description of a Network of Folding/Unfolding Pathways

In our model (Galzitskaya and Finkelstein, 1999) we consider a network of simplified stepwise unfolding pathways (see Figure 2), each step of which is the removal of one "chain link" (i.e., a chain fragment of one or a few residues) from the native protein 3D structure. The removed chain fragments are assumed to form a random coil; they lose all their non-bonded interactions and gain the coil entropy (except that spent to close the disordered loops protruding from the remaining globule). This reductive description of the unfolded chain is our first simplification. The next is the assumption that the chain residues remaining in the globule keep their native positions and conformations and that the unfolded regions do not fold into another, nonnative globule. Thus, we actually neglect nonnative interactions (cf. Taketomi et al., 1975). The last and main simplification is that we concentrate on the transition state (TS) and its free energy, i.e., on the stability (actually, the instability) of partly unfolded intermediates rather than on a detailed description of the chain motions.

To use Dynamic Programming in searching for the TS at a network of folding-unfolding pathways, we have, for computational reasons, to restrict this network by no more than 10^6–10^7 intermediates. Therefore we divide an N-residue protein chain into L~20–30 chain links (of $l=N/L$ residues each, except for the last link, which may include l or less residues), and use these links rather than residues as units of unfolding. To the same end, i.e., to restrict the number of semi-folded intermediates, we consider only the intermediates with no more than two closed disordered loops in the middle of the chain plus the N- and the C-terminal disordered tails. These four unfolded regions should be enough to describe unfolding of a protein up to $N \approx 100$ residues, since the estimated (Finkelstein and Badretdinov, 1997) number of coil regions in the folding nucleus is close to $N^{2/3}/6$.The above assumptions sharply decrease the time that is necessary for the calculations, while the links of lesser than $N/10 \approx 6$–10 residues limit the accuracy of our calculations only a little: these links are still much smaller than the expected size of a nucleus in the vicinity of mid-transition between the folded and unfolded phases (where the folded nucleus should include roughly $N/3$–$N/2$ residues (Finkelstein and Badretdinov, 1997)).

Thus, a network of protein folding/unfolding pathways on a free energy landscape is obtained. Further, on each of the pathways, we search (using a dynamic programming method) (Aho et al., 1976; Finkelstein and Roytberg, 1993) for a free-energy maximum (i.e., the transition state of this pathway; the part of the molecule which is structured in the transition state is a folding nucleus). Then, the free energies of all pathways are compared and the pathway with the minimum free energy of the transition state F_{min} is revealed (this is the optimal pathway since it has the lowest free energy barrier).

Considering all possible pathways, we thus obtain the ensemble of transition states (each of which possesses its own free energy) and the ensemble of folding nuclei. The effective height of the free energy barrier was calculated as

$$F_{eff} = -RT \ln \sum_{I^{\#}} \exp\left(-F_I^{\#} / RT\right) \qquad (4)$$

where $F_I^{\#}$ is the free energy of a single transition state, and the summation is over all transition states.

Estimation of Protein Folding Rate from Calculations of Free Energy Barrier

To use dynamic programming in searching for the TS at a network of folding-unfolding pathways, we have, for computational reasons, to restrict this network by no more than ~10^6 intermediates. Therefore, we divide an *N*-residue protein chain into *L*~20–30 chain links and use a limited number of loops. Using the Monte Carlo (MC) simulation of folding, we, in principle, can avoid these simplifications.

Since the folding rate k_f should be proportional to exp($-F^{\#}/RT$), and since our model allows us to calculate the transition state free energy$F^{\#}$ (see eq. 4), we can estimate a correlation of computed $F^{\#}/RT$ values with experimentally obtained folding rates k_f (or rather, ln(k_f)). The correlation coefficient is -0.72 between the computed (for mid-transition, see above) $F^{\#}/RT$ values and ln($k_{f\_at\_mid\text{-}transition}$) (see Figure 6).

At the same time, the calculated minimal values of free energy barrier correlate somewhat better with the logarithm of experimentally measured folding times at the point of thermodynamic equilibrium: the correlation coefficient for all 67 proteins is -0.77 (see Table 6). On the other hand, the values of free energy barriers correlate somewhat worse with the logarithm of experimentally measured time of folding in water, far from the point of thermodynamic equilibrium: in this case the correlation coefficient of the theory and experiment is -0.66 for all 67 considering proteins. The decrease of the correlation in the last case is not surprising since the calculated values of free energy barriers correspond to the point of thermodynamic equilibrium.

Influence of the Average Conformational Entropy and the Average Energy of Residue in Protein on the Protein Folding Rate

First-order phase transitions proceed by a nucleation mechanism in which a small droplet of the ordered phase is formed within the metastable disordered phase (Lifshits and Pitaevskii, 1991). A similar mechanism could apply to the folding of a protein with the ordered phase identified with the native state and the disordered state identified with the unfolded phase (Pande et al., 1998). A number of recent experiments and theoretical studies suggest that a crucial step of folding is the formation of a native-like folding nucleus (Matouschek et al., 1989; Matouschek et al., 1990; Fersht et al., 1992; Abkevich et al., 1994; Finkelstein and Badretdinov, 1997; Finkelstein and Galzitskaya, 2004). The nucleation barrier is intrinsic for the folding process, since each protein first has to form its nucleus (Fersht, 1995; Fersht, 1997).

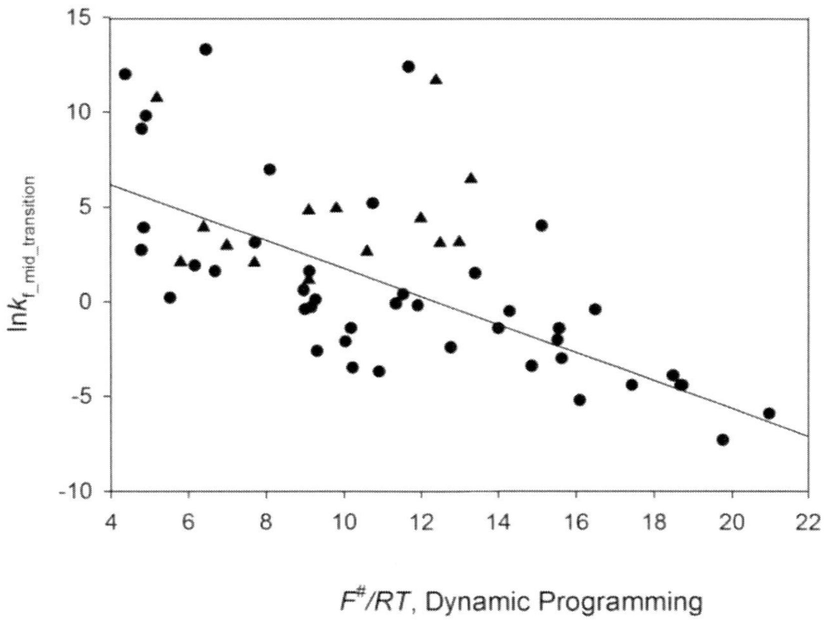

Figure 6. Correlation between the computed transition state free energyF#/RT and the mid-transition folding rate (measured in sec-1 and represented in a logarithmic scale) for all 67 investigated wild-type proteins. The correlation coefficient is -0.72 for all proteins, -0.73 for two-state folders (circle) and for multi-state is -0.59 (triangle).

The formation of a sufficient number of interactions between amino acid residues is necessary to compensate for a loss of the conformational entropy during the protein folding process. Therefore, structural uniqueness of the native state is a result of the balance between the conformational entropy and the energy of interactions between residues. Taking this phenomenon into account, the entropy capacity for a given protein chain with a chosen topology has been suggested (Galzitskaya et al., 2000). This parameter characterizes the relation between the conformational entropy and energy of residue-residue interactions. The estimation of the influence of the average conformational entropy (in consideration per residue of protein chain) and the average energy of residue on the protein folding rate is possible considering the consequences from the capillarity model of protein folding (Wolynes,1997; Finkelstein and Badretdinov, 1997).

$$G_N = N\varepsilon - \mu N^{2/3}\varepsilon \tag{5}$$

is the free energy of the native state;

$$G_0 = -TNs \tag{6}$$

is the free energy of the unfolded state;

$$G_n = n\varepsilon - \mu n^{2/3}\varepsilon - T(N-n)s \tag{7}$$

is the free energy of the intermediate state with n fixed residues in the native topology. Here, ε is the average contact energy per residue; $\mu n^{2/3}$ takes into account the surface residues having less interactions than the internal ones, where μ= 1.5 for a ball-like body (and $\mu$is larger for a not ball-like body (Finkelstein and Badretdinov, 1997)); s is the average conformational entropy per residue for an unfolded chain, and T is the temperature.

$$\Delta G_n = G_n - G_0 = n\varepsilon - \mu n^{2/3}\varepsilon + Tns \tag{8}$$

is the free energy difference between intermediate and unfolded states. We can simplify this expression using $\xi = -\varepsilon/RT > 0$and $\sigma = s/R > 0$. Then we have:

$$g_n = \Delta G_n / RT = -n\xi + \mu n^{2/3}\xi + n\sigma \tag{9}$$

The transition state on this pathway is $g^{\#} = \max\{g_n\}$. To find the transition state (the maximum) we take the derivative of equation (9) with respect to n: $n_0 = (\frac{2}{3}\times\frac{\mu}{1-\sigma/\xi})^3$. If we substitute the value of n_0 in equation (9) and introduce an "entropy capacity" $C = \sigma/\xi$ (Galzitskaya et al., 2000) ($0 < C < 1$) then we obtain the equation

$$g^{\#}(C) = \frac{4}{27}\times\frac{\mu^3\sigma}{C(1-C)^2} \tag{10}$$

To answer the question about changing of the free energy barrier with two major parameters, ξ and σ, let us write the changing of the free energy barrier in partial derivatives in ξ and σ:

$$dg^{\#} = g^{\#} \times \frac{1}{(1-\frac{\sigma}{\xi})}\left[(2\frac{\sigma}{\xi})\frac{d\sigma}{\sigma} + (1-3\frac{\sigma}{\xi})\frac{d\xi}{\xi}\right] \qquad (11)$$

At the point of equilibrium we have $G_N - G_0 = 0$, that is,

$$-N(\xi-\sigma) + \mu N^{2/3}\xi = 0 \qquad (12)$$

and $\sigma/\xi = 1 - \mu N^{-1/3}$. Putting this equation in (10) and neglecting $\mu N^{-1/3}$ (which is not large in comparison with 1 at large N) we obtain:

$$dg^{\#} = (\frac{g^{\#}}{\mu}N^{1/3}) \times \left[2\frac{d\sigma}{\sigma} - 2\frac{d\xi}{\xi}\right] = (2\frac{g^{\#}}{\mu}N^{1/3}) \times \frac{\xi}{\sigma}d\frac{\sigma}{\xi} \qquad (13)$$

Introducing the entropy capacity $C = \sigma/\xi$ we obtain the dependence of the changing of free-energy barrier on the changing of entropy capacity at an equal meaning of N:

$$dg^{\#} = (2\frac{g^{\#}}{\mu}N^{1/3}) \times d\ln C \text{ or} \qquad (14)$$

$$d\ln g^{\#} = (2\frac{N^{1/3}}{\mu}) \times d\ln C \qquad (15)$$

One of the main determinants of the protein folding rate is the number of degrees of freedom that are to be fixed during the rate-limiting step of folding. Therefore, the difference in the folding rate for proteins sharing the ball-like and oblong-like fold is the result of differences in the conformational entropy due to a larger surface of the boundary between folded and unfolded phases in the transition state for protein with a ball-like fold (see eqs. 13-15, μ is larger for a not ball-like body which causes diminishing of the free energy barrier). Moreover, the unfolded closed loops protruding from the folded part (the nucleus) create an additional surface tension (Ivankov et al., 2009; Galzitskaya, 2010).

Statistical Analysis of Average Conformational Entropy and Average Number of Contacts Per Residue for Different Classes of Proteins

Now we are interested only in the dependence of the change of the free-energy barrier on $dg^{\#}$ the change of value C, which depends on the properties of amino-acid residues in protein (see equation 15). Since the value of conformational entropy is proportional to the number of degrees of freedom (i.e. the number of rotatable angles φ, ψ, and χ) and the value of energy per residue proportional to the number of atom-atom (or residue-residue) contacts in protein, then the entropy capacity is proportional to the relation of the above values: $C \approx const \times C_{\text{mod}}$ where $C_{\text{mod}} = \nu/m$ with m being the number of residue-residue contacts in the native structure (two residues were considered in contact with each other if any atom-atom pairs were at a distance of less than 8Å, the contacts between adjacent residues were not taken into account), and ν being the number of rotatable angles φ, ψ, and χ (see Table 11). The model entropy capacity has been calculated for 67 proteins with known experimental data for the folding rate and for which the Monte-Carlo simulations has been done for comparison of two methods for prediction of protein folding rate (Galzitskaya, 2010) (see Tables 7-9). Figure 7 demonstrates that the logarithm of entropy capacity correlates by about 78% with the logarithm of protein folding rate in the mid-transition.

Table 10. Correlation coefficients between logarithms of folding rates in mid-transition and parameters connected with protein size and shape for three protein classes (*a*, *b*, *d*)

	$\ln k_{mt}$ *67 proteins*	$\ln k_{mt}^{a}$ *21 proteins*	$\ln k_{mt}^{b}$ *22 proteins*	$\ln k_{mt}^{d}$ *22 proteins*
L	-0.69±0.06	-0.70±0.11	-0.76±0.09	-0.72±0.10
$Ln(L)$	-0.76±0.05	-0.73±0.10	-0.85±0.06	-0.82±0.07
$L^{1/2}$	-0.73±0.06	-0.72±0.11	-0.82±0.07	-0.77±0.09
$L^{2/3}$	-0.72±0.06	-0.72±0.11	-0.80±0.08	-0.75±0.09
AbsCO	-0.81±0.04	-0.76±0.09	-0.88±0.05	-0.74±0.10
RelativeCO	-0.12±0.12	0.37±0.19	0.44±0.17	-0.38±0.18
*Rg/Rg**	0.08±0.12	-0.34±0.19	0.41±0.18	0.32±0.19
Radius of cross-section, *V/S*	-0.53±0.09	-0.47±0.17	-0.55±0.15	-0.48±0.16
Ln(Entropy capacity)	0.78±0.05	0.74±0.10	0.85±0.06	0.86±0.06
$Ln(t_{1/2})$, MC steps	-0.82±0.04	-0.74±0.10	-0.83±0.07	-0.84±0.06
$Ln(F_{eff}/RT)$	-0.72±0.06	-0.62±0.13	-0.74±0.09	-0.79±0.09
$Ln(F_{min}/RT)$	-0.77±0.05	-0.69±0.12	-0.80±0.08	-0.84±0.07

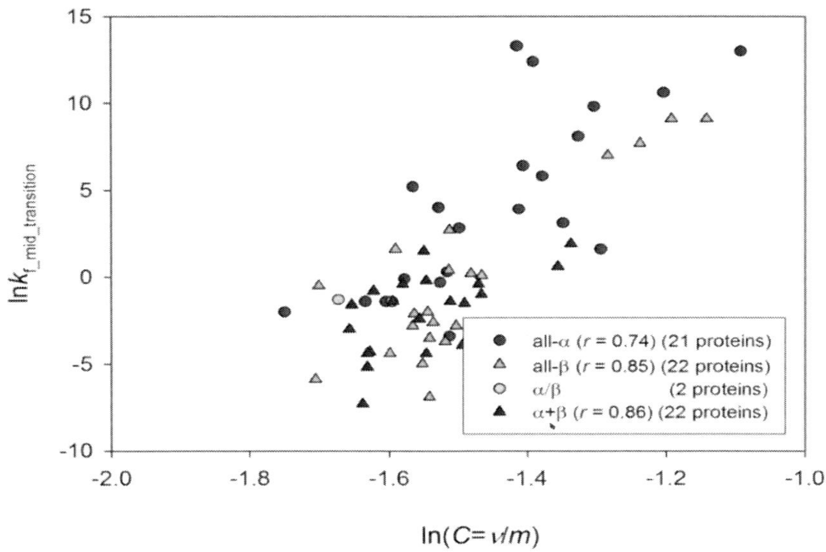

Figure 7. Correlation between the computed model entropy capacity and the experimentally measured folding rate at the mid-transition for 67 proteins. Both are represented in a logarithmic scale. The correlation coefficient is 0.78±0.05.

It should be noted that entropy capacity correlates with folding rate in mid-transition practically at the same level as the first passage times obtained from Monte Carlo simulations (82%, see Table 10) (Galzitskaya, 2010). The capillarity model allows us to predict the folding rate at the same level of correlation as by Monte Carlo simulations but without time consuming calculations required for large proteins. The correlation between the logarithm of the first passage times in Monte Carlo simulations and the logarithm of folding rates for separate classes of proteins is sufficiently high: –0.74 for class *a*, –0.83 for class *b*, –0.84 for class *d* (see Table 10, and http://phys.protres.ru/resources/compact.html, the correlation for class *c* is absent so only two proteins are included in the set of 67 proteins).

We compare the correlation between folding rates and a set of structural parameters for 67 proteins: contact order, length and the different colors of length (see Table 10). It is worth to underline here, that the correlation between folding rates and such structural parameters as contact order is absent for all proteins. The correlation with the length reaches 70% as has been mentioned in the Introduction (see Table 1, for 84 proteins).

Table 11. Number of rotatable angles for amino acid residues of 20 types

Type of residue	ALA	ARG	ASN	ASP	CYS	GLN	GLU	GLY	HIS	ILE
Degrees of freedom	2	6	4	4	3	5	5	3*	4	4
Type of residue	LEU	LYS	MET	PHE	PRO	SER	THR	TRP	TYR	VAL
Degrees of freedom	4	6	5	4	1	3	3	4	4	3

*The set of conformations for the main chain of glycine is larger than that of other residues; this is taken into account by assigning three rather than two rotatable angles for glycine.

It is surprising that the correlation between the folding rate and the different colors of lengths (*ln(L)*, $L^{2/3}$, $L^{1/2}$) is high, which means that the size of the proteins is one of the important and determining parameters of protein folding (Galzitskaya et al., 2003; Ivankov et al., 2009) (see Table 10). But the protein size can not explain the difference in the folding rates for proteins of a similar size (or proteins sharing a similar fold, practically with a similar number of amino acid residues). All other considered parameters are used to explain the differences in protein folding for proteins with practically the same size. We demonstrate that the relation between the folding rate and entropy capacity has class-specific features. It is surprising that average structural properties give a high correlation with the folding rate in each structural class. At the same time the radius of the cross-section (*V/S*) has a worse correlation coefficient (-0.53) with the folding rate than the size of proteins for the considered set of proteins (-0.69).

Influence of Flexible Loops on the Rate of Protein Folding

Functional activity of a protein molecule depends on a subtle balance between its flexibility and rigidity. We have demonstrated that the difference in the folding rates for proteins displaying similar folding topologies with similar compactness of 3D structures can be explained by different rigidity of protein molecules: the more rigid proteins have faster kinetics (Galzitskaya, 2009). The FoldUnfold program has been used to find flexible regions in protein chains (Galzitskaya et al., 2006; Dovidchenko et al., 2008).

Comparison of proteins having similar native topologies is an important approach for elucidating fundamental aspects of the protein folding process.

We have compared compactness of homologous proteins. Unfortunately, there are no such examples for 101-151 residues proteins; all such groups belong to a protein size range from 50 to 100 residues.

An interesting example is the folding of cold shock proteins. The absence of correlation between the thermodynamic stability and folding rate, as observed for cold shock proteins, indicates that proteins with a more stable folded state do not necessarily fold faster. Cold shock proteins B are less compact (average compactness for three proteins is 1.50) than Cold shock proteins A (compactness is 1.43), and the folding of Cold shock proteins B is faster (Perl et al., 1998). The difference in the other parameters demonstrates the same trend (1.10 and 1.09 for the normalized radius of gyration and 3.40 and 3.54 for the radius of cross-section, for Cold shock proteins B and Cold shock protein A modules, respectively, see the web address, http://phys.protres.ru/resources/compact.html). However, among three Cold shock proteins B, the difference in compactness can not explain the small difference in folding rates. It should be noted that number of residues in flexible regions for Cold shock proteins B (1csp) is smaller (24 residues) than for Cold shock protein A (29 residues).

There are proteins displaying similar folding topologies with practically the same radius of gyration where the difference in the folding rates can be explained by rigidity of these proteins. These are muscle and common-type acylphosphatases (van Nuland et al., 1998) which are slow two-state folders (logarithms of their folding rate in water are -1.6 and 0.8, compactness is 1.44 and 1.48, respectively) and a fast multi-state folder HypF-N (the logarithm of the folding rate is 4.4 and compactness is 1.42). The authors of the original paper explain such a behavior by a different hydrophobic content of these proteins. In addition, it can be speculated that the observed differences can be explained by differences in the rigidity and flexibility of loops in these proteins. Indeed, fast folding HypF-N is the most rigid since it contains eight proline residues and, according to the FoldUnfold program, has the least number of residues in flexible regions (15 residues for HypF-N, 24 for common-type acylphosphatases and 27 for muscle acylphosphatases, see Table 12).

The slowest protein includes the largest number of residues belonging to the flexible regions. Our explanation does not contradict the above; so it has been shown that amino acids with small side chains tend to have greater backbone flexibility than those with large side chains which are mostly hydrophobic (Goodman et al., 2000).

Among four small three-helix bundle proteins, the engrailed-homeodomain is the fastest folder with three-state kinetics (logarithms of folding rates are 10.5, 8.7, 8.2 and 5.9 for En-H, C-Myb, hRAP1 and hTRF1, respectively, see Table 13). Normalized radii of gyration are the same (1.08, 1.07, 1.10 and 1.07 for En-H, C-Myb, hRAP1 and hTRF1, respectively); compactness is 1.41, 1.39, 1.47 and 1.40 for En-H, C-Myb, hRAP1 and hTRF1, respectively; radius of cross-section is 3.46, 3.34, 3.39 and 3.42 for En-H, C-Myb, hRAP1 and hTRF1, respectively. The faster folding of En-H can be also explained again by its rigidity. This protein has no flexible regions according to the FoldUnfold program in comparison with other proteins (C-Myb, hRAP1 and hTRF1) calculated by the FoldUnfod program (see Table 13).

Table 12. Parameters of compactness and characteristic time of folding from experiment and Monte Carlo simulations for proteins with ferredoxin-like fold

Name of protein Pdb code	3D structure with colored flexible regions	$\ln(k_f)$ in water/in mid-point	Mean packing density (flexible regions)	$t_{1/2}$ in MC steps (minimum number of MC steps)
HypF-N 1gxt V_{ASA} / S_{ASA} **3.88** S_{ASA} / S^*_{ASA} **1.42** *Rg*/*Rg** **1.11**	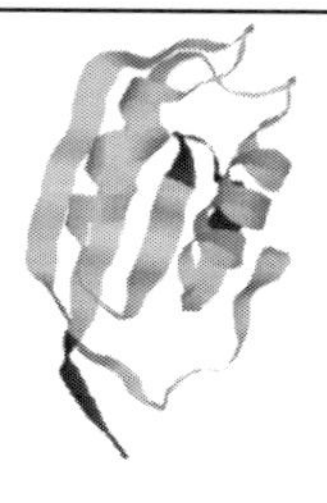	4.4/-0.9	21.22 15 residues 1-7 39-46	24,874,862 (471,786)
CT AcP 2acy V_{ASA} / S_{ASA} **3.87** S_{ASA} / S^*_{ASA} **1.48** *Rg*/*Rg** **1.11**	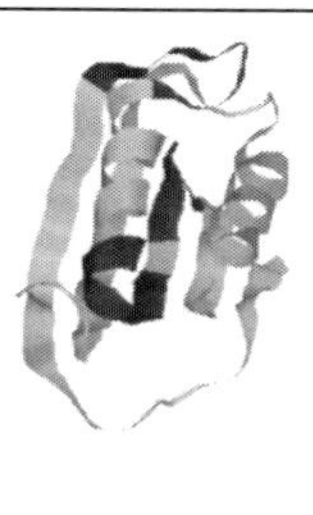	0.8/-4.4	20.77 24 residues 42-48 50-57 68-76	65,114,308 (912,270)

Name of protein Pdb code	3D structure with colored flexible regions	ln(kf) in water/in mid-point	Mean packing density (flexible regions)	t1/2 in MC steps (minimum number of MC steps)
mAcP 1aps V_{ASA} / S_{ASA} **3.96** S_{ASA} / S^{*}_{ASA} **1.44** *Rg/Rg** **1.13**	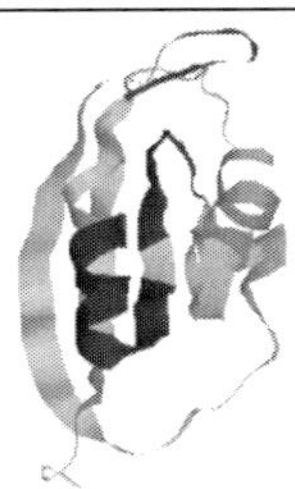	-1.6/-7.5	20.59 27 residues 42-48 50-60 68-76	169,227,106 (521,770)

Table 13. Parameters of compactness and characteristic time of folding from experiment and Monte Carlo simulations for proteins belonging to homeodomain-like superfamily

Name of protein Pdb code	3D structure with colored flexible regions	$\ln(k_f)$ in water/in mid-point	Mean packing density (flexible regions)	$t_{1/2}$ in MC steps (minimum number of MC steps)
En-H 1enh V_{ASA} / S_{ASA} **3.49** S_{ASA} / S^{*}_{ASA} **1.40** *Rg/Rg** **1.08**	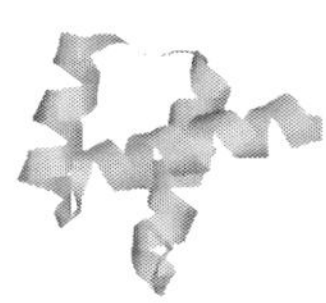	10.5/8.1	20.86 0 residues	37,828 (578)
C-Myb 1gv2 V_{ASA} / S_{ASA} **3.37** S_{ASA} / S^{*}_{ASA} **1.38** *Rg/Rg** **1.07**	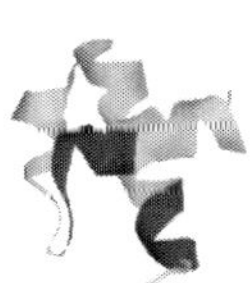	8.7/3.1	20.83 12 residues 5-9 32-38	43,161 (2841)

Table 13. (Continued).

Name of protein Pdb code	3D structure with colored flexible regions	$\ln(k_f)$ in water/in mid-point	Mean packing density (flexible regions)	$t_{1/2}$ in MC steps (minimum number of MC steps)
hRAP1 1fex V_{ASA} / S_{ASA} **3.42** S_{ASA} / S^*_{ASA} **1.45** *Rg*/*Rg** **1.10**	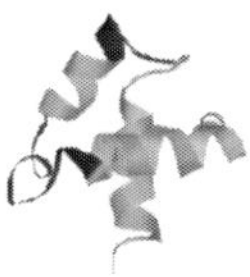	8.2/3.9	20.79 17 residues 19-30 37-41	71,215 (3091)
hTRF1 1ba5 V_{ASA} / S_{ASA} **3.45** S_{ASA} / S^*_{ASA} **1.39** *Rg*/*Rg** **1.07**	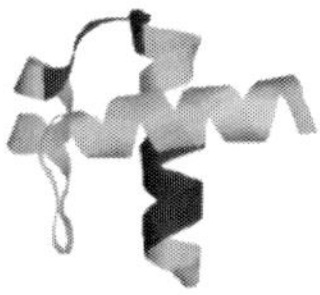	5.9/1.6	21.22 12 residues 10-15 21-26	79,791 (3887)

From the above examples we can conclude that the difference in the folding rates for proteins displaying similar folding topologies either can be explained by the differences in compactness or, for those with similar compactness, by different rigidity of protein molecules (different distribution of flexible regions in the protein chain in our case).

CONCLUSION

The presented model of protein folding is a rough approximation of the process. But it can describe a substantial point of the folding procedure. Consideration of models with native topology is an efficient way to explore global structural features of biological molecules and provide some information about the folding pathway both in theoretical models and in real proteins.

The presented theoretical simulations and the available experimental data for the rate of folding show the existence of agreement between them. In our theoretical modeling of protein folding the rate of achievement of the native state at the mid transition is limited by value of transition state barrier on the pathway from the unfolded to native state.

Considering the theoretical dependence of the folding rate between experimental data and number of Monte-Carlo steps, effective free energy barriers, and entropy capacities from nucleation mechanism we can predict the folding rate of proteins with unknown experimental data using the Monte Carlo Gō simulations, dynamic programming, and calculation of model entropy capacity. The obtained results may be useful in prediction of protein folding rate using only 3D protein structure.

Rapidly and slowly folding proteins have additional structural diversities that contribute to their differing folding rates. From our analysis we can conclude that the barrier height for folding of large proteins is defined by the size of the boundary between folded and unfolded phases in the transition state. This boundary is larger for a ball-like protein globule than for an oblong-like one. Theoretical consideration of the capillarity model for the process of protein folding demonstrates that the difference in the folding rate for proteins sharing more spherical and less spherical folds is the result of differences in the conformational entropy due to a larger surface of the boundary between folded and unfolded phases in the transition state for proteins with more a spherical fold. The entropy capacity follows from nucleation mechanism allows us to predict the folding rate at the same level of correlation as by Monte Carlo simulations.

MATERIALS AND METHODS

Database

We consider 84 proteins for which both folding rates and tertiary structures are known. Among them 26 proteins exhibit multi-state kinetics and 58 proteins exhibit two-state kinetics (see, http://phys.protres.ru/resources).

Calculation of Protein Structure Compactness

We have calculated the solvent-accessible surface area a S_{ASA} nd volume s V_{ASA} urrounded by this surface for each protein considered. We made these calculations with the program YASARA [http://yasara.org], using 1.4 Å as the radius of probe water molecule. To explore the protein shape, we used two parameters: V_{ASA} / S_{ASA} which we call radius of cross-section (for different geometric bodies of equal volumes, this ratio should be maximal for a ball) and S_{ASA} / S^{*}_{ASA} which Tsai and Nussinov called compactness (Tsai and Nussinov, 1997a,b) (i.e. the ratio of the accessible surface area of protein S_{ASA} to the surface area of sphere S^{*}_{ASA} of the same volume V_{ASA} as the protein; for the ball, this ratio is 1).

Molecular Protein Surface

In order to calculate normalized radius of gyration, we should estimate radius of gyration of an ideal ball from volume V_{mol} enclosed by the protein molecular surface (see eq. (19) below). The difference between the molecular surface and accessible surface is that ASA is a surface formed by the center of a probe molecule rolled over a protein molecule, while the molecular surface is a surface formed by the van der Waals sphere of a probe molecule rolled over a protein molecule. If the probe is water, the water molecule is modeled by a sphere of radius 1.4 Å. This means that the molecular surface is “thinner” than ASA and the “distance” between them is 1.4 Å. In fact, the molecular surface is obtained from the van der Waals surface if all crevices and interiors inaccessible for water are smoothed by means of the van der Waals surface of a water molecule. We accomplished the calculations of the molecular surface by YASARA [http://yasara.org], setting the radius of a probe molecule to be 1.4 Å [by the way, at http://www.yasara.org/AddEnv.jpg one can see the difference between molecular and accessible surfaces].

Radius of Gyration

If to consider atoms by points in 3D space, the radius of gyration R_g of a protein is calculated according to the following equation:

$$R_g^2 = \sum m_i (\mathbf{r}_i - \mathbf{R}_C)^2 / M \quad (16)$$

where m_i is the mass of *i-th* atom, $\mathbf{r}_i$ is its Cartesian coordinates, M is the mass of the protein, and $\mathbf{R}_C$ is the coordinate vector of the mass center of the protein calculated as follows:

$$\sum m_i (\mathbf{r}_i - \mathbf{R}_C) = 0 \tag{17}$$

Since protein structures often have no hydrogen atoms, then in eq. (16) we should take into account only non-hydrogen atoms, and M is the net mass of non-hydrogen atoms. In this case if the mass of all non-hydrogen atoms is taken approximately equal to each other, eq. (16) is simplified to the following:

$$R_g^2 \cong \sum_{i=1}^{N} (\mathbf{r}_i - \mathbf{R}_C)^2 \Big/ N \tag{18}$$

where N is the number of protein non-hydrogen atoms. The difference between R_g values calculated according to eqs. (16) and (18) is less than 0.1 Å.

For calculation of the normalized radius of gyration we computed the radius of gyration of an ideal ball with uniform density and the same volume as the considered protein according to the following equation:

$$R_g^{*2} = \frac{3}{5} R^2 = \frac{3}{5} \left(\frac{3V_{mol}}{4\pi} \right)^{2/3} \tag{19}$$

where V_{mol} is the volume enclosed inside the protein molecular surface. Note that the radii of gyration R_{gx}^*, R_{gy}^*, and R_{gz}^* of an ideal ball with uniform density corresponding to the rotations around Cartesian axes x, y, and z going through the mass center are calculated from the eq. $R_{gx}^{*2} = R_{gy}^{*2} = R_{gz}^{*2} = \frac{2}{5} R^2$. The factor 3/5 in the eq. (19) instead of 2/5 is due to the fact that there are many axes a protein can be rotated around; in this case radius of gyration "averaged" over all possible rotations is calculated according to the equation $R_g^{*2} = \frac{1}{2}\left(R_{gx}^{*2} + R_{gy}^{*2} + R_{gz}^{*2}\right)$, see ref. (Sivukhin, 1989).

ACKNOWLEDGMENTS

I am grateful to A.V. Finkelstein for discussion, and S.O. Garbuzynskiy, D.N. Ivankov, M.Yu. Lobanov, A.V. Glyakina, and N.S. Bogatyreva for their assistance in preparation of some figures and calculations. This work was supported by the programs "Molecular and Cellular Biology" (01200959110) and “Fundamental Sciences to Medicine”, by the Russian Foundation for Basic Research (08-04-00561), by the “Russian Science Support Foundation”, and by a grant from the Federal Agency for Science and Innovation (#02.740.11.0295).

REFERENCES

Abkevich, V. I., Gutin, A. M. and Shakhnovich, E. I. (1994). Specific nucleus as the transition state for protein folding: evidence from the lattice model. *Biochemistry*, *33*, 10026-10036.

Aho, A., Hopcroft, J. and Ullman, J. (1976). *The Design and Analysis of Computer Algorithms* (Addison-Wesley, Reading, MA).

Alm, E. and Baker, D. (1999). Prediction of protein-folding mechanisms from free-energy landscapes derived from native structures. *Proc. Natl Acad. Sci.*,USA,*96*, 11305-11310.

Alm, E., Morozov, A. V., Kortemme, T. and Baker, D. (2002). Simple physical models connect theory and experiment in protein folding kinetics. *J. Mol. Biol.*, *322*, 463-476.

Capriotti, E. and Casadio, R. (2007). K-Fold: a tool for the prediction of the folding kinetic order and rate. *Bioinformatics*, *23*, 385-386.

Chiti, F., Webster, P., Taddei, N., Clark, A., Stefani, M., Ramponi, G. and Dobson, C.M. (1999). Designing conditions for in vitro formation of amyloid protofilaments and fibrils. *Proc. Natl. Acad. Sci. USA*,*96*, 3590-3594.

Dovidchenko, N. V., Bogatyreva, N. S. and Galzitskaya, O. V. (2008). Prediction of loop regions in protein sequence.*J. Bioinform. Comput. Biol.*, *6*, 1035-1047.

Fändrich, M., Fletcher, M. A. andDobson, C. M. (2001). Amyloid fibrils from muscle myoglobin. *Nature*,*410*, 165-166.

Fersht, A. R. (1995). Characterizing transition states in protein folding: an essential step in the puzzle. *Curr. Opin. Struct. Biol.*, *5*, 79-84.

Fersht, A. R. (1997). Nucleation mechanisms in protein folding. *Curr. Opin. Struct. Biol.*, *7*, 3-9.

Fersht, A. R., Matouschek, A. and Serrano, L. (1992).*J. Mol. Biol.*,*224*, 771-782.

Finkelstein, A. V. andBadretdinov, A. Ya. (1997). Rate of protein folding near the point of thermodynamic equilibrium between the coil and the most stable chain fold. *Fold. Des.2*, 115-121.

Finkelstein, A. V. and Roytberg, M. A. (1993). Computation of biopolymers: a general approach to different problems. *Biosystems*, *30*, 1-19.

Finkelstein, A. V. and Galzitskaya, O. V. (2004). Physics of protein folding. *Phys. Life. Rev.*, *1*, 23-56 (2004).

Flory, P. J. (1969). *Statistical Mechanics of Chain Molecules* (Interscience, New York).

Galzitskaya O. V., Garbuzynskiy, S. O., Ivankov, D. N. and Finkelstein, A. V. (2003). Chain length is the main determinant of the folding rate for proteins with three-state folding kinetics. *Proteins*, *51*, 162-166.

Galzitskaya O. V., Ivankov, D. N. and Finkelstein, A. V. (2001). Folding nuclei in proteins. *FEBS Lett.489*, 113-118.

Galzitskaya O. V., Reifsnyder, D. C., Bogatyreva, N. C., Ivankov, D. N. and Garbuzynskiy, S. O. (2008a). More compact protein globules exhibit slower folding rates. *Proteins*,70,329-332.

Galzitskaya O. V., Garbuzynskiy S. O. and Finkelstein A. V. (2005). Theoretical study of protein folding: outlining folding nuclei and estimation of protein folding rates. *Journal ofPhysics*: *Condensed* Matter., *17*, S1539-S1551.

Galzitskaya, O. V. and Finkelstein, A. V. (1999). A theoretical search for folding/ unfolding nuclei in three-dimensional protein structures. *Proc. Natl Acad. Sci. USA*,*96*, 11299-11304.

Galzitskaya, O. V. and Garbuzynskiy, S. O. (2006). Entropy capacity determines protein folding. *Proteins*, *63*, 144-154.

Galzitskaya, O. V. Estimation of Protein Folding Rate from Monte-Carlo Simulations and Entropy Capacity.*Curr Protein Pept Sci.* in press.

Galzitskaya, O. V. (2009). Influence of flexible loops on the rate of protein folding. *Current Topics in Peptide and Protein Research*. *9*, 71-82.

Galzitskaya, O. V., Bogatyreva, N. S. and Ivankov, D. N. (2008b). Compactness Determines Protein Folding Type. *J. Bioinform. Comput. Biol.*, *6*, 667-680.

Galzitskaya, O. V. and Finkelstein, A. V. (1998). Folding rate dependence on the chain length of RNA-like heteropolymers. *Foldingand Design*, *3*, 69-78.

Galzitskaya, O. V., Garbuzynskiy, S. O. and Lobanov, M.Yu. (2006). FoldUnfold: Web Server for the Prediction of Disordered Regions in Protein Chain. *Bioinforamtics*, *22*, 2948-2949.

Galzitskaya, O. V., Surin, A. K. and Nakamura, H. (2000). Optimal Region of Average Side-Chain Entropy for Fast Protein Folding. *Protein Sci.*, *9*, 580-586.

Garbuzynskiy, S. O., Finkelstein, A. V. and Galzitskaya, O. V. (2004).Outlining folding nuclei in globular proteins. *J. Mol. Biol.*, *336*, 509-525.

Gong, H., Isom, D. G., Srinivasan, R. and Rose, G. D. (2003). Local secondary structure content predicts folding rates for simple, two-state proteins. *J. Mol. Biol.*, *327*, 1149-1154.

Goodman, J. L., Pagel, M. D. and Stone, M. J. (2000). Relationships between protein structure and dynamics from a database of NMR-derived backbone order parameters. *J. Mol. Biol.*, *295*, 963-978.

Gromiha, M. M. (2005). A statistical model for predicting protein folding rates from amino acid sequence with structural class information. *J. Chem. Inf. Model*, *45*, 494-501.

Gromiha, M. M. and Selvaraj, S. (2001). Comparison between long-range interactions and contact order in determining the folding rate of two-state proteins: application of long-range order to folding rate prediction. *J. Mol. Biol.*, *310*, 27-32.

Gromiha, M. M., Thangakani, A. M. and Selvaraj, S. (2006). FOLD-RATE: prediction of protein folding rates from amino acid sequence. *Nucl. Acids Res.*, *34*, W70-W74.

Guijarro, J. I., Morton, C. J., Plaxco, K. W., Campbell, I. D. and Dobson, C. M. (1998). Folding kinetics of the SH3 domain of PI3 kinase by real-time NMR combined with optical spectroscopy. *J. Mol. Biol.*, *276*, 657-667.

Gutin, A. M., Abkevich, V. I. and Shakhnovich, E. I. (1996). Chain length scaling of protein folding time. *Phys. Rev. Lett.*, *77*, 5433-5456.

Ivankov, D. N. and Finkelstein, A. V. (2004). Prediction of protein folding rates from the amino acid sequence-predicted secondary structure. *Proc. Natl. Acad. Sci.*, USA, *101*, 8942-8944.

Ivankov, D. N. andFinkelstein, A. V. (2001). Theoretical study of a landscape of protein folding-unfolding pathways. Folding rates at midtransition. *Biochemistry*,*40*, 9957-9961.

Ivankov, D. N., Bogatyreva, N. S., Lobanov, M. Yu. and Galzitskaya, O. V. (2009). Coupling between Properties of the Protein Shape and the Rate of Protein Folding. *PLoS ONE*, *4*, e6476.

Ivankov, D. N., Garbuzynskiy, S. O., Alm, E., Plaxco, K. W., Baker, D. and Finkelstein, A. V. (2003). Contact order revisited: influence of protein size on the folding rate. *Protein Sci.*, *12*, 2057-2062.

Jackson, S. E. (1998). How do small single-domain proteins fold? *Fold. Des.3*, R81-R91.

Jiang, L., Althoff, E. A., Clemente, F. R., Doyle, L., Röthlisberger, D., Zanghellini, A., Gallaher, J. L., Betker, J. L., Tanaka, F., Barbas, C. F. 3rd, Hilvert, D., Houk, K. N., Stoddard, B. L. and Baker, D. (2008) De novo computational design of retro-aldol enzymes. *Science,319*, 1387-1391.

Koga, N. and Takada, S. (2001). Roles of native topology and chain-length scaling in protein folding: a simulation study with a Go-like model. *J. Mol. Biol.*, *313*, 171-180.

Lifshits, E. M. and Pitaevskii, L. P. (1991). *Physical Kinetics.* Pergamon, Oxford, UK.

Ma, B. G., Chen, L. L. and Zhang, H. Y. (2007). What determines protein folding type? An investigation of intrinsic structural properties and its implications for understanding folding mechanisms. *J. Mol. Biol.*, *370*, 439-448.

Makarov D. E., Keller, C. A., Plaxco, K. W. and Metiu, H. (2002). How the folding rate constant of simple, single-domain proteins depends on the number of native contacts. *Proc. Natl. Acad. Sci. USA*, *99*, 3535-3539.

Matouschek, J. T., Kellis, Jr, Serrano, L. and Fersht, A. R. (1989). Mapping the transition state and pathway of protein folding by protein engineering, *Nature*, *340*, 122-126.

Matouschek, J. T., Kellis, Jr., Serrano, L., Bycroft, M. and Fersht, A. R. (1990). Transient folding intermediates characterized by protein engineering. *Nature*, *346*, 440-445.

Metropolis, N., Rosenbluth, A., Rosenbluth, M., Teller, A. and Teller, E. (1953). Folding kinetics of proteins and copolymers. *J. Chem. Phys.*, *96*, 768-780.

Muñoz, V. and Eaton, W. A. (1999). A simple model for calculating the kinetics of protein folding from three-dimensional structures. *Proc. Natl Acad. Sci. USA,96*, 11311-11316.

Muñoz, V., Lopez, E. M., Jager, M. and Serrano, L. (1994). Kinetic characterization of the chemotactic protein from Escherichia coli, CheY.

Kinetic analysis of the inverse hydrophobic effect. *Biochemistry, 33*, 5858-5866.

Murzin, A. G., Brenner, S. E., Hubbard T. and Chothia, C. (1995). SCOP: a structural classification of proteins database for the investigation of sequences and structures. *J. Mol. Biol., 247*, 536-540.

Naganathan, A. N. and Muñoz, V. (2005) Scaling of folding times with protein size. *J. Am. Chem. Soc., 127*, 480-481.

Pande, V. S., Grosberg, A. Yu., Tanaka, T. and Rokhsar, D. S. (1998 Pathways for protein folding: is a new view needed? *Curr. Opin. Struct. Biol., 8*, 68-79.

Perl, D., Welker, Ch., Schindler, Th., Schroder, K., Marahiel, M. A., Jaenicke, R. and Schmid, F. X. (1998). Conservation of rapid two-state folding in mesophilic, thermophilic and hyperthermophilic cold shock proteins. *Nature Struct. Biol., 5*, 229-235.

Plaxco, K. W., Guijarro, J. I. Morton, C. J. Pitkeathly, M., Campbell, I. D. and Dobson, C. M. (1998). The folding kinetics and thermodynamics of the Fyn-SH3 domain. *Biochemistry, 37*, 2529-2537.

Plaxco, K. W., Simons, K. W. and Baker, D. (1998) Contact order, transition state placement and the refolding rates of single domain proteins. *J. Mol. Biol., 277*, 985-994.

Privalov, P. L. (1979). Stability of proteins: small globular proteins. *Adv. Protein Chem.33*, 167-241.

Punta, M. and Rost, B. (2005). Protein folding rates estimated from contact predictions. *J. Mol. Biol., 348*, 507-512.

Röthlisberger, D., Khersonsky, O., Wollacott, A. M., Jiang, L., DeChancie, J., Betker, J., Gallaher, J. L., Althoff, E. A., Zanghellini, A., Dym, O., Albeck, S., Houk, K. N., Tawfik, D. S. and Baker, D. (2008). Kemp elimination catalysts by computational enzyme design. *Nature,453*, 190-195.

Sivukhin, D. V. (1989). *General course of physics*. 1.

Taketomi, H., Ueda, Y. and Gō, N. (1975). Studies on protein folding, unfolding and fluctuations by computer simulation. I. The effect of specific amino acid sequence represented by specific inter-unit interactions. *Int. J. Pept. Protein Res., 7*, 445-459.

Thirumalai, D. (1995). From minimal models to real proteins: time scales for protein folding kinetics. *Journal de Physique Orsay Fr.5*, 1457-1467.

Tsai, C. J. and Nussinov, R. (1997a). Hydrophobic folding units at protein-protein interfaces: implications to protein folding and to protein-protein association. *Protein Sci., 6*, 1426-1437.

Tsai, C. J. and Nussinov, R. (1997b) Hydrophobic folding units derived from dissimilar monomer structures and their interactions. *Protein Sci.*, *6*, 24-42.

van Nuland, N. A., Chiti, F., Taddei, N., Raugei, G., Ramponi G. and Dobson, C. M. (1998). Slow folding of muscle acylphosphatase in the absence of intermediates. *J. Mol. Biol.*, *283*, 883-891.

Wolynes, P. G. (1997). Folding funnels and energy landscapes of larger proteins within the capillarity approximation. *Proc. Natl Acad. Sci.,* USA, *94*, 6170-6175.

Zerovnik, E., Virden, R. Jerala, R. Turk V. and Waltho, J. P. (1998). On the mechanism of human stefin B folding: I. Comparison to homologous stefin A. Influence of pH and trifluoroethanol on the fast and slow folding phases," *Proteins*, *32*, 296-303.

Zhou, H. and Zhou, Y. (2002). Folding rate prediction using total contact distance. *Biophys. J.*, *82*, 458-463.

In: Advances in Proteomics Research
Editors: Ya Li Huang et al. pp. 111-158
ISBN: 978-1-61942-227-8

Chapter 4

STABILITY AND STABILIZATION OF PROTEINS: THE RIBONUCLEASEA EXAMPLE

Ulrich Arnold [1]
Martin-LutherUniversity, Institute of Biochemistry and Biotechnology, Halle, Germany.

ABSTRACT

Despite much progress in molecular biology, biophysics, and biochemistry, the mechanisms by which unfolded polypeptide chains gain their native conformation are not yet fully understood. Likewise, the network of forces that stabilize folded proteins and prevent them from unfolding elude a thorough accounting so far. Such an accounting is, however, necessary to engineer protein stability, which is often required for enzymes in technical applications.

The folding process of proteins starts with a hydrophobic collapse or local events at so-called 'nuclei' or 'initiation sites' and proceeds stepwise to the natively folded protein. The occurrence of rate-limiting steps often leads to the population of folding intermediates. In contrast to the successive protein folding process, protein *un*folding is highly cooperative. Due to the principle of microscopic reversibility, unfolding must be a progressive process as well, which is postulated to start at a

[1] E-mail address: ulrich.arnold@biochemtech.uni-halle.de

confined region—'unfolding region', 'critical region' or similar—of the tertiary structure of the native protein molecule.

The rate constants of the folding (k_f) and unfolding reaction (k_U), both of which determine the respective free energy of activation $\Delta G_f^\ddagger$ and $\Delta G_U^\ddagger$, provide information on the contribution of these reactions to the thermodynamic stability (Gibbs free energy $\Delta G = \Delta G_U^\ddagger - \Delta G_f^\ddagger$). The comparison of proteins with their chemically modified or, preferably, genetically engineered variants yields information on the involvement of specific residues in the folding or unfolding reaction.

RibonucleaseA (RNaseA) has been a model protein for half a century and is one of the most thoroughly studied examples concerning the protein folding problem. Whereas the folding reaction is complex due to proline isomerization reactions, the unfolding reaction can be described by a single-exponential reaction. Modifications by, *e.g.*, genetic engineering have revealed the importance of confined regions for the unfolding and refolding reaction, respectively.

Starting from basic principles of thermodynamics and kinetics, the effect of protein modifications on the stability and tools for protein stabilization are presented with special focus on work on RNase A.

INTRODUCTION

Despite their predominant role as nutrient, proteins (or more precisely: enzymes) have been exploited for processing materials—wine, bread, or cheese production, tanning of leather, *etc.*—for ages. In contrast to the early applications, where whole microorganisms were used, (non-purified) enzymes were used in, *e.g.*, bile soap. In 1833, Anselme Payen isolated an active substance from barley, which converted starch to dextrose ('diastase'), and in 1835, Theodor Schwann isolated a ferment from gastric juice ('pepsin'). In 1878, Friedrich Wilhelm Kühne created the term 'enzyme' (Greek: *en zyme* = from yeast) and in 1897, Eduard Buchner discovered that the fermentation of sugar to alcohol can be accomplished even with yeast cell extracts ('zymase'). However, it took time until 1926, when James B. Sumner crystallized urease [1] and postulated that enzymes are proteins (with the exception of ribozymes, whose existence was postulated in 1967 by Woese, Crick, and Orgel and which were discovered in the 1980s by Cech and Altman [2,3]).

The application of enzymes (such as proteases, lipases, amylases, and esterases) in laundry detergents, in food processing, in biofuel production, or in paper industry as well as for the production of bulk and fine chemicals, and pharmaceutics is, however, often restricted by their limited stability, as these technical *in vitro* conditions usually are not optimal with respect to the maintenance of the native protein structure. Despite a multitude of covalent and non-covalent bonds within protein structures, the thermodynamic stability ΔG, *i.e.*, the difference between the free energy of the folded and the unfolded state of proteins is rather small (20–60 kJ mol^{-1}) [4]. The structures of tens of thousands of proteins, protein variants or fragments, or protein•ligand complexes have been determined by X-ray crystallography or NMR spectroscopy and innumerable experiments revealed hydrogen bonds, hydrophobic interactions, ionic interactions, and van der Waals interactions as the main stabilizing forces of the native protein structure. In addition, cofactors, metal ions, or modifications like lipidation or glycosylation may contribute to the stability of proteins. The unfolded polypeptide chain is largely unstructured and, thus, possesses high conformational freedom (entropy). Consequently, it adopts a multitude of conformations so that the unfolded state is very heterogeneous. Upon folding, the polypeptide chain loses entropy, but this loss is over-compensated by enthalpic effects, which maintain the natively folded structure of the protein. Despite often crystal-like properties, also native proteins exhibit a certain degree of flexibility, which is necessary for, *e.g.*, ligand binding or catalysis. Consequently, also the native state represents an ensemble of various conformations in which, however, the energy barriers between the discrete conformations is usually marginal in comparison to the energy barrier between the folded and the unfolded state [5].

Nearly four decades ago, Anfinsen hypothesized that the "information dictating the native fold of protein domains is encoded in their amino acid sequence" [6]. This 'dogma' was, however, challenged, as numerous proteins show a comparable fold but have high sequence diversity[7]. In fact, proteins with as little as 1–2% sequence identity may still adopt the same native fold [8]. Thus, the 'fold code' is valid for amino acid sequence (1-D) patterns rather than for whole proteins. Nevertheless, 'fold-conserved information' is encoded in 2-D protein contact maps or 3-D protein structures [9]. Still, as the nascent polypeptide chain begins to fold *in vivo*—often by means of helper proteins like chaperones—before all information of the complete polypeptide chain is available, *in vivo* folding and *in vitro* folding are only contingently comparable.

Despite all the detailed knowledge on stabilizing forces, disulfide bond formation, and folding pathways, the interactions in the amino acid polymers are so diverse that they elude being fully understood and, more important, being systematically exploitable for tailoring protein attributes. However, the comparison of proteins from mesophilic sources with homologues from thermophilic counterparts revealed a number of obviously more general strategies to stabilize the native structure of proteins [4,10,11]:

(i) increase in the number of charged amino acid residues at the surface that form ion pairs
(ii) increase in the number of hydrogen bonds, particularly in loops and turns as well as at the termini of the polypeptide chain (fixation)
(iii) more complete packing of the hydrophobic core (cavity filling) and decrease of the number of solvent-exposed hydrophobic residues
(iv) strengthening of the interactions between subunits in oligomeric proteins and increase in the degree of oligomerization
(v) entropic destabilization of the unfolded polypeptide chain by introduction of disulfide bonds or proline residues and elimination of glycine residues
(vi) shortening of loops

The stabilization efficiency of these alterations of the protein structure is, however, context-dependent. Notwithstanding the advancements in predictions and rational design, the quest for more stable protein variants is mostly a matter of trial and error, which is facilitated by modeling studies, directed evolution and recombination approaches, and high-throughput screening methods.

THERMODYNAMIC STABILITY

The term 'stability' is used in rather different contexts, some of which are linked, including thermodynamic stability, kinetic stability, resistance against inactivation, resistance against proteolysis, resistance against aggregation, and reversibility of denaturation. The thermodynamic stability (or Gibbs free energy, ΔG) characterizes the difference between the free energy of the folded (N, native) and the unfolded (U) state of proteins (at constant pressure and temperature) and amounts for most proteins to 20–60 kJ mol^{-1} *in vitro*[4]. The value of ΔG can be determined experimentally by equilibrium unfolding experiments using temperature, pressure, or chemical denaturants as unfolding agents. (The determination of ΔG values is valid only for completely reversible unfolding reactions—otherwise only so-called 'apparent' values are obtained.) The concepts on how chemical denaturants induce the unfolding of polypeptide chains (by interacting with the polypeptide chain, which leads to the disturbance and disruption of the intramolecular interactions) were developed in particular by A. Schellman and co-workers[12]. The equations for the analysis of experimental data were developed and advanced by numerous groups [13-15]. Starting from

$$G = H - T \cdot S \tag{1}$$

where H is the enthalpy, T is the absolute temperature, and S is the entropy,

$$\Delta G = \Delta H - T \cdot \Delta S \tag{2}$$

is obtained, as only differences rather than absolute values can be measured. For chemical reactions such as

$$a\mathrm{A} + b\mathrm{B} \leftrightarrows c\mathrm{C} + d\mathrm{D} \tag{3}$$

with the reactants A–D and their respective concentration *a–d* the free energy of the system is the difference between the free energy of the products and the substrates. Thus

$$\Delta G = \Delta G^{\circ} - RT \ln \frac{[\mathrm{C}]^c [\mathrm{D}]^d}{[\mathrm{A}]^a [\mathrm{B}]^b} \tag{4}$$

where $\Delta G$is the free energy under standard conditions (25°C, 1 atm, concentration of reactants 1 M; for biochemical reactions: pH 7.0, *i.e.*, the concentration of H_3O^+ is not 1 M but 10^{-7} M, which is usually indicated by $\Delta G^{\circ\prime}$) and R is the gas constant. In equilibrium, the driving forces of the forward reaction are equal to those of the reverse reaction so that $\Delta G = 0$ and

$$\Delta G^{\circ} = -RT \ln K \tag{5}$$

with K being thc equilibrium constant of the reaction system (eq. 3 and 4). As under experimental conditions only systems in equilibrium are studied, the "o" superscript is omitted, the more so as it is often used to indicate the value of ΔG in the absence denaturant ("0 M denaturant"). Likewise, in biochemical literature, the prime (*vide supra*) is omitted as well, so that $\Delta G'$ is identified as ΔG.

The unfolding of small proteins (Figure 1) can often be well described by a two-state model

$$\mathrm{N} \leftrightarrows \mathrm{U} \qquad (6)$$

where N and U symbolize energetically clearly distinct states, which are the macroscopic sum of numerous microscopically different but energetically similar states [5]. The occurrence of folding intermediates is generally not in contradiction to the two-state model, as those intermediates are usually thermodynamically unstable so that they are not populated under equilibrium conditions. Criteria for a valid treatment of experimental data according to the two-state model were already established by Lumry *et al.*[16] and apply mostly to the congruence of signal changes of various optical probes (far- and near-UV circular dichroism, fluorescence spectroscopy, absorption) as a function of the denaturant concentration.

Data obtained from thermal unfolding of proteins can be treated according to Pace *et al.*[15] as follows

$$y = \frac{(y_\mathrm{N}^0 + m_\mathrm{N} \cdot T) - (y_\mathrm{U}^0 + m_\mathrm{U} T)\exp\left[\left(\frac{\Delta H_\mathrm{m}}{RT}\right)\left(\frac{T - T_\mathrm{m}}{\mathrm{T_m}}\right)\right]}{1 + \exp\left[\left(\frac{\Delta H_\mathrm{m}}{RT}\right)\left(\frac{T - T_\mathrm{m}}{\mathrm{T_m}}\right)\right]} \qquad (7)$$

where y is the measured signal, y_N^0 and y_D^0 are the (extrapolated) signals of the native and unfolded protein, respectively, m_N and m_U are the slopes of the linear signal changes in the pre- and posttransition regions of the curve, T_m is the temperature at the transition midpoint, and ΔH_m is the enthalpy at T_m (van't Hoff enthalpy, which can be determined alternatively from the slope of the van't Hoff plot ln*K* *vs.* 1/T). By means of the Gibbs-Helmholtz equation

$$\Delta G = \Delta H_\mathrm{m}(1 - T/T_\mathrm{m}) - \Delta C_\mathrm{p}\left[(T_\mathrm{m} - T) + T\ln(T/T_\mathrm{m})\right] \qquad (8)$$

where ΔC_p is the difference in molar heat capacity between the folded and the unfolded protein, ΔG can be calculated at any temperature (by calculation of f_N-values, *i.e.*, the fraction of native protein (Figure 1 right) from the experimentally determined transition curve (Figure 1 left), ΔG can be calculated alternatively by means of eq. 5). The value of ΔC_p can be obtained from differential scanning calorimetry (DSC) experiments or from transition curves by chemical denaturants at different temperatures [17] and can be roughly estimated to 50 J mol^{-1} K^{-1} per amino acid residue [18]. The congruence of ΔH determined by DSC (ΔH_{cal}) and ΔH_m is also sufficient to qualify an unfolding reaction as a two-state process [19].

The ΔG*vs.*T curve (Figure 2) evinces a clear curvature indicating not only heat unfolding but also cold unfolding of proteins. The comparison of the ΔG*vs.*T curves of a model protein and a more stable variant reveals that T_m and/or ΔG can be affected by changes in T_m and/or ΔH_m and/or ΔC_p (eq. 8).

As, however, thermal unfolding of proteins is often accompanied by aggregation and the determination of ΔG from such curved functions is problematic, $\Delta G^{(H_2O)}$ (ΔG in the absence of denaturant) is often determined from chemically induced transition curves. From the linear dependence of ΔG on the concentration of denaturant ([D]), $\Delta G^{(H_2O)}$ is calculated by the linear extrapolation method (linear free energy model [20]). However, in some cases the denaturant interacts specifically with the protein leading to deviations from the linearity [12,21,22]. Data obtained from chemically induced transition curves (Figure 1 left) can be treated according to Santoro und Bolen [13] with the modification by Clarke and Fersht [14]:

$$y = \frac{(y_N^0 + m_N[D]) + (y_U^0 + m_U[D])\exp(\frac{-m_{\Delta G}([D]_{0.5} - [D])}{RT})}{1 + \exp(\frac{-m_{\Delta G}([D]_{0.5} - [D])}{RT})} \qquad (9)$$

The slope $m_{\Delta G}$, which is proportional to the change in the solvent accessible surface area between the folded and unfolded protein [23], indicates the dependence of ΔG on [D], $\Delta G^{[D]}$ is ΔG at the respective concentration of denaturant, and $[D]_{0.5}$ corresponds to the concentration of denaturant at the turning point of the transition curve, *i.e.*, where [U] = [N].

As, however, the determination of ΔG requires complete reversibility of the respective processes, which is usually not the case for *in vivo* systems, and the polypeptide chain starts to fold during biosynthesis, *i.e.*, not from the completely synthesized but unfolded state, thermodynamic considerations have to be treated with caution when *in vivo* processes are analyzed [24]. Moreover, 'molecular crowding', *i.e.*, the high concentration of molecules within living cells (up to 400 mg mL^{-1}), and the presence of small-molecule osmolytes can significantly affect protein stability and folding/unfolding processes [25,26].

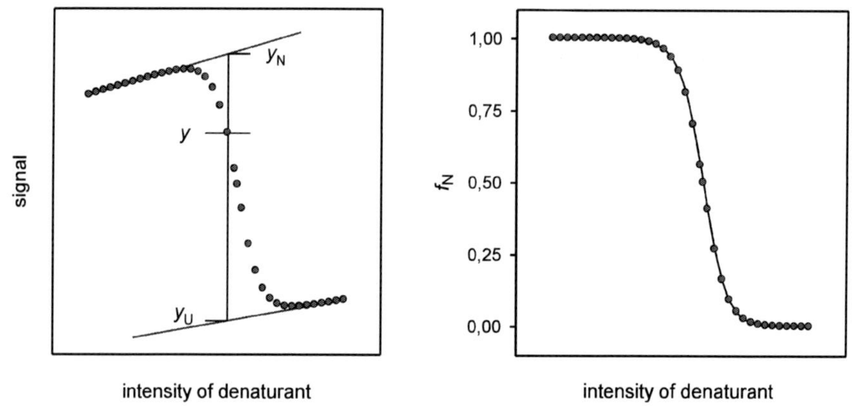

Figure 1. Unfolding of a protein according to a two-state model. Left: Change in signal intensity (y) as a function of temperature, pressure, or concentration of a chemical denaturant. y_N and y_U correspond to the extrapolated signal under the respective conditions. Right: Fraction of native protein (f_N) as a function of temperature, pressure, or concentration of a chemical denaturant, from which the equilibrium constant K can be calculated ($K = [U]/[N] = (1 - f_N)/f_N$).

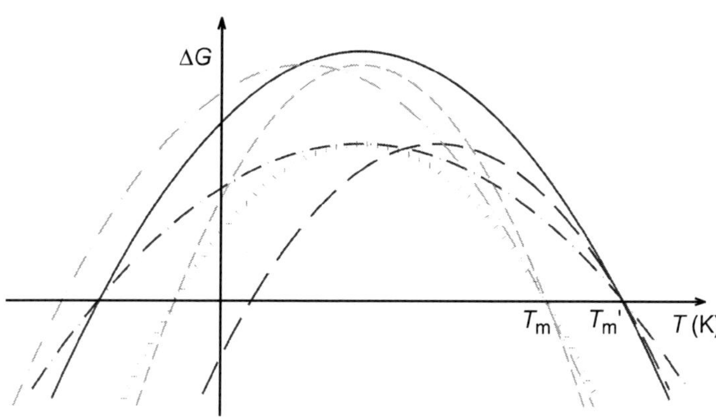

Figure 2. Gibbs free energy (ΔG) as a function of temperature. The stability of a protein (dotted red line) can be increased by a decrease in ΔC_p and/or an increase in ΔH_m and/or in T_m (T_m', blue). Possibly, the temperature of maximum stability is shifted (a sole increase in T_m causes the cold denaturation to set on at higher temperatures; adapted from [10]).

KINETIC STABILITY

A value $\Delta G < 0$ is no guarantee that the equilibrium state will be reached at a measurable rate. The reaction velocity depends on the height of the energy barrier between the native and the unfolded state (Figure 3) so that thermodynamically unstable proteins can be kinetically stable and *vice versa* [27]. While the relative homogeneity of the native state usually results in single-exponential unfolding kinetics (an exception, for instance, is the staphylococcal nuclease, which exhibits parallel unfolding pathways due to an X_{aa}–Pro isomerization reaction in the native state [28,29]), the heterogeneity of the polypeptide chain in the unfolded state often results in multiple, parallel folding pathways to the native state. The energy landscape between U and N becomes even more rugged by the presence of intermediates [30], *i.e.*, partially folded states (I, Figure 3). Consequently, also the transition state is an *ensemble* of (mostly similar) structures [31], which in most cases largely resemble the native state of the protein. While in the process of protein folding intermediates are frequently populated, the rate-limiting step in unfolding is the N→TS reaction (Figure 3) so that unfolding intermediates are rarely detected. Nevertheless, the principle of microscopic reversibility postulates that the same intermediates occur in both directions [32].

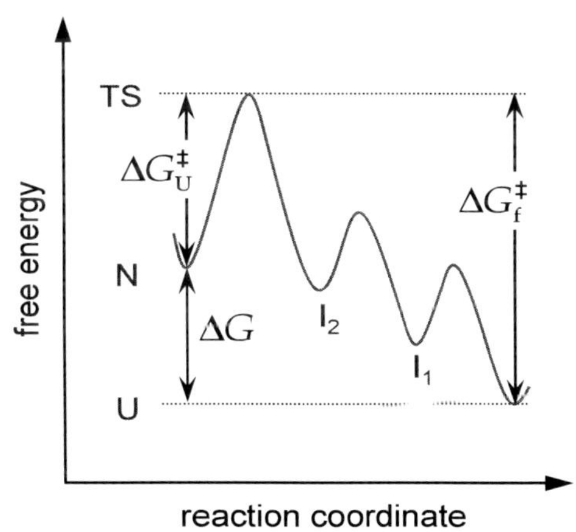

Figure 3. Free energy profile of a protein under denaturing conditions. Despite the presence of intermediates (I1 , I2), a monophasic unfolding kinetics is usually observed as the rate-limiting step is the N→TS reaction. The intermediates will possibly be populated and, thus, be detectable in the refolding reaction resulting in multiphasic folding kinetics.

The reaction velocity and, thus, the reaction rate constant k (k_U for the unfolding reaction, k_f for the folding reaction) depends inversely proportionally on the energy difference between the initial state and the transition state (TS; Figure 3), *i.e.*, the activation free energy ($\Delta G^{\ddagger}$):

$$\frac{k}{T} = \frac{\kappa k_B}{h} \exp\left(\frac{-\Delta G^{\ddagger}}{RT}\right) \text{and } \ln\frac{k}{T} = \ln\frac{\kappa k_B}{h} + \Delta S^{\ddagger}/R - \Delta H^{\ddagger}/(RT) \qquad (10)$$

where k_B is Boltzmann's constant, h is Planck's constant, and κ is the transmission coefficient, which indicates the probability of TS to react forward to the final state rather than back to the initial state ($0 \leq \kappa \leq 1$; http://goldbook.iupac.org/; note that the interactions in protein folding results from a 'diffusion' within the polypeptide chain, not in the—theoretic—gas phase [23]). For two-state folders [33], k_f [U] = k_U [N] applies and, thus, not only K = [U]/[N] but $K = k_U/k_f$[23,34]. As $\Delta G^{\ddagger}$ like ΔG depends linearly on the concentration of denaturant (eq. 11; [12] and references therein), k_U and k_f change linearly as a function of the concentration of denaturant in the semi-logarithmic presentation.

$$\Delta G^{\ddagger[D]} = \Delta G^{\ddagger(H2O)} + m^{\ddagger}[D] \qquad (11)$$

$$\ln k^{[D]} = \ln k^{(H2O)} + m^{\ddagger}[D]/(RT) \qquad (12)$$

where $m^{\ddagger}$ is the slope representing the change in solvent accessible surface area between the initial state and TS [21,31] and $k^{[D]}$ and $k^{(H2O)}$ are the rate constants at the respective concentration of denaturant and in the absence of denaturant, respectively. The plot of the experimentally observable rate constant k_{obs} as a function of the concentration of denaturant ($\ln k_{obs}$ *vs.* [D]) yields a so-called chevron plot, which for a two-state folder exhibits linear folding and unfolding branches (Figure 4).

The comparison of kinetic and thermodynamic data is another possibility to verify a two-state transition of a protein [34]: $\Delta G = \Delta G_U^{\ddagger} - \Delta G_f^{\ddagger}$ and $m_{\Delta G} = m_U^{\ddagger} - m_f^{\ddagger}$, whereas discrepancies indicate the occurrence of intermediates. The population of intermediates often results in a multiphasic folding behavior or kinks in the (folding) branch(es) of the chevron plots ('roll over' [35]). Such intermediates often accumulate during refolding experiments under native-like conditions. They can occur either on the pathway from U to

N ('on-pathway') or they can be linked to U only ('off-pathway') [23]. Moreover, if the energy barriers between the different species within the unfolded state are too high, the interconversion between the different unfolded species becomes slower than conformational folding resulting in parallel folding pathways and, thus, in non-linear chevron plots [36]. A common reason for parallel folding pathways and rate-limiting steps are isomerization reactions of X_{aa}–Pro peptide bonds[37] due to the high energy barrier (about 80 kJ mol^{-1}) for the isomerization reaction. The *cis/trans* ratio of X_{aa}–non-Pro peptide bonds is about 1:1000 in model peptides, and only about 0.03% of X_{aa}–non-Pro peptide bonds were found to be in *cis* conformation in proteins so that here isomerization reactions only rarely affect the conformational folding. In contrast, the *cis/trans* ratio of X_{aa}–Pro peptide bonds is roughly 1:5 in model peptides and about 5.2% of the X_{aa}–Pro peptide bonds were found to be in *cis* conformation in proteins [38-41]. The rate constant for *trans*→*cis* isomerization reactions is about 0,01 s^{-1} at 25°C thus possibly delaying conformational folding as k_f values are often of similar magnitude [42]. Due to the *cis* conformation of the X_{aa}–Pro peptide bond, *cis*-Pro residues are often found in turns between β-strands. Still, a substitution of Pro by, *e.g.*, Ala not necessarily results in a loss of the *cis* conformation of the respective peptide bond but usually in a loss of conformational stability for the protein [43]. On the other hand, a stabilization of the *cis* conformation of the X_{aa}–Pro peptide bond in the unfolded state by structural mimics results in a stabilization of the respective peptides or proteins [44-47]. According to Levitt [48], the isomerization of X_{aa}–Pro peptide bonds either does not influence the conformational folding (type I, for instance Pro13 of the bovine pancreatic trypsin inhibitor BPTI), or influences the rate of the conformational folding but does not limit it (type II, for instance Pro2 und Pro9 in BPTI or Pro114 in RNase A), or limits the rate of the conformational folding (type III, for instance Pro8 in BPTI or Pro93 in RNase A). The rate constant of the isomerization reaction of X_{aa}–Pro peptide bonds does not depend on the concentration of denaturant but strongly depends on the temperature due to the high activation energy. Moreover, X_{aa}–Pro isomerization reactions can be accelerated by acids or by peptidyl prolyl *cis/trans* isomerases (PPIases [49,50]).

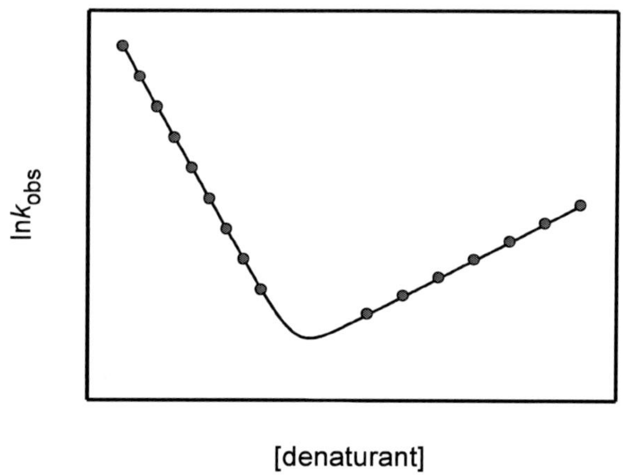

Figure 4. Schematic presentation of lnkobs as a function of the concentration of denaturant (chevron plot). The folding and unfolding branches are linear for 'two-state folders' and kobs corresponds to kU or kf under the respective extreme conditions.

Double-jump experiments are an efficient method to characterize the accumulation and stability of intermediates. In the respective 'interrupted folding experiments', unfolded protein is subjected to refolding conditions and unfolded again after defined intervals (D→N→D [51]). From the amplitudes of the signal change in the respective unfolding reactions, conclusions regarding on-pathway intermediates or parallel refolding pathways can be drawn. Furthermore, the rate constants of the unfolding reactions yield information on the stability of the intermediate(s) [51]. Of course, double-jump experiments can also be carried out by a brief unfolding of protein followed by its refolding (N→D→N). By this means, unfolding intermediates or slow isomerization reactions subsequent to the conformational unfolding can be detected [37].

In contrast to the linear dependence of lnk_{obs} on the concentration of denaturant, the respective temperature-dependent plots (ln(k/T) *vs.* 1/T; Eyring plot) exhibit curvatures due to the differences in the molar heat capacities of N, TS, and U. While the curvature for ln(k_U/T) *vs.* 1/T is often only marginal, ln(k_f/T) *vs.* 1/T is considerably curved [30,31,52] resulting in two intersection points of the ln(k_U/T) *vs.* 1/T and ln(k_f/T) *vs.* 1/T curves, which correspond to the T_m values of cold and heat denaturation [30,52].

MECHANISTIC ASPECTS OF PROTEIN UNFOLDING AND PROTEIN STABILIZATION

As the unfolding reaction starts from a rather homogeneous native state both *in vitro* and *in vivo*, *in vitro* unfolding experiments should reflect the situation *in vivo* fairly well. Nevertheless, molecular crowding within living cells often causes a stabilization of the native state by a decrease of k_U and an increase in k_f [25,26]. *In vitro* folding experiments, however, usually start from a full-length and unfolded polypeptide chain (and possibly with reduced disulfide bonds [53]), which clearly deviates from *in vivo* conditions, where folding starts within the nascent polypeptide chain [24]. In particular, the unfolded polypeptide chain is strongly prone to irreversible consecutive reactions*in vivo* like aggregation (which can be prevented by chaperones) and proteolysis (Figure 5). Moreover, chemical modifications *etc.* may become crucial *in vitro*, for instance in technical applications, where biocatalysts are requested to operate in an environment quite different from its natural habitat [24]. Owing to these irreversible consecutive reactions, the difference in ΔG between N and TS ($\Delta G_U^{\ddagger}$) is pivotal to maintaining the native, *i.e.*, biologically active form, of a protein as a destabilization of U increases k_f and, thus, promotes the refolding reaction to N but likewise promotes irreversible consecutive reactions (by lowering the activation free energy for the irreversible reaction $\Delta G_i^{\ddagger}$; Figure 5).

Consequently, the elucidation of protein unfolding processes has gained increasing interest. As, however, the transition state (ensemble) is usually structurally still close to the native state [21] and the N→TS reaction usually is the rate-limiting step, the (locally confined) structural changes that initiate global unfolding are difficult to detect. Due to the principle of microscopic reversibility, however, the characterization of *folding* intermediates yields also information on the unfolding pathway of the respective protein. Note that this principle is valid for the back and forth reaction under the *same* experimental conditions only. Unfolding studies are, however, usually carried out under denaturing conditions whereas folding studies are carried out under native conditions so that the free energy levels of N, TS, and U (and all intermediates I) differ, which can lead to different, not comparable pathways.

The finding that amino acid residue replacements (mutations) in the interior of a protein ('core') often predominantly affect the folding reaction [54] whereas mutations on the surface of the protein molecule predominantly affect the unfolding reaction [10,55] is consistent with the hydrophobic collapse protein folding hypothesis. Here, the hydrophobic residues of the later core collapse initially followed by the arrangement of the 'outer shell residues', which later form the surface of the protein molecule. In reverse, the process of unfolding should consequently start at confined regions of the protein's surface, and indeed numerous studies provide evidence for the existence of suchlike regions, which were termed 'unfolding region' [56-58], 'weak point' [59], 'critical region' [60], 'unfolding nucleation site' [61], or similar.

To test whether or not an amino acid residue is in a native-like structural environment in the transition state and, thus, is involved in the first step(s) of the unfolding or rather of the folding reaction, Fersht and co-workers developed the Φ-value analysis approach ($\Delta\Delta G_f^{\ddagger} / \Delta\Delta G$ [62,63]). Here, the effect of an amino acid residue substitution is analyzed with respect to its influence on the thermodynamic stability and folding rate: $\Phi_f = 0$ indicates that the native interactions around this residue are poorly formed in TS, whereas $\Phi_f = 1$ indicates a native structural environment. This approach of comparing kinetic and thermodynamic data can, of course, be used for the unfolding reaction as well ($\Phi_U = \Delta\Delta G_U^{\ddagger} / \Delta\Delta G$ [47,64-66]). The Φ-value analysis resembles the Tanford β-value analysis ($\beta_T = m_f / m_{\Delta G}$, [67]), which compares the slopes of the curves in the chevron plot and the transition curve (for most two-state folders this value is 0,6–0,9 indicating the contiguousness of N and TS, [21]). However, while the β_T-value characterizes the protein globally, Φ_U- and Φ_f-values yield information regarding confined regions within the protein structure[31]. Limitations for the applicability of the Φ-value approach have been elaborated elsewhere [63].

Several distinctive features of proteins from thermophilic hosts have been outlined above and other strategies have evolved or have been conceived by researchers to stabilize the folded protein structure, such as the conjugation of proteins with lipids, nucleotides, metal ions, or carbohydrate moieties [68-71], the formation of isopeptide bonds[72], or—for technical applications—the conjugation with polyethylene glycol[73], dextrans [74], or carbohydrates[70,75], the introduction of cross-links [76-79], or the immobilization on carrier supports [58,80,81]. Moreover, 'medium engineering', that is, the addition of stabilizing substances, such as salts, polyols, or organic solvents [82-85], can also be applied to favor the native conformation of the protein.

Even though it is clear from the experimental data that most of these effects concern the surface residues of the respective proteins and the effects of stabilization in the sense of the 'unfolding region hypothesis' have been described mathematically [56,58,80], the results do not provide a conclusive answer to the question: Which regions of the surface of a protein are likely candidates for an unfolding region? Secondary structure elements such as α-helices or β-sheets are rather stable entities, but the interconnecting peptide segments—loops—often lack regular interactions. The resulting flexibility enables these loop segments to bind ligands or to serve themselves as substrate for phosphorylation or proteolytic cleavage, but also generates points of (local) instability. Loops between helices are often rather long and flexible but do not contribute considerably to the stability of the respective protein. In contrast, loops connecting helices and sheets were found to be of significant importance for unfolding processes and, thus, for global stability [86,87]. 'Loop' does not necessarily mean 'random coil' or 'disordered' as particular helix-sheet loops can form so-called Ω-loops [88] if the ends of the loop segment come into contact in the tertiary structure so that a network of (non-regular) interactions can be formed [89]. The decreased number of regular interactions qualifies such regions as likely candidates for 'unfolding regions' [65,90].

Unfortunately, flexible regions of proteins often elude or can complicate a characterization by X-ray crystallography or NMR spectroscopy. In contrast, proteolysis is an excellent method to localize flexible regions within native proteins, as the cleavage by proteases requires the flexibility of the substrate to interact efficiently with the enzyme [90-95]. Thus, the analysis of proteolytic fragments yields information on the localization of flexible regions and the kinetics of peptide bond cleavage yield information on the degree of flexibility (the loop's 'opening rate' [95]). Moreover, changes in the fragment pattern and proteolysis kinetics in dependence on the experimental conditions reveal structural changes [91,93,94,96-101]. A clear limitation of the proteolysis approach, however, is the substrate specificity of the respective protease, which possibly excludes parts of the target protein from being analyzed. In contrast, from a vast amount of data, NMR spectroscopy can provide information residue-by-residue, as long as the H–D exchange rates are of measurable magnitude. Also, nonspecific photolabeling may provide a more detailed figure on solvent-exposed regions, but the information is not site-specific as only the sum of, *e.g.*, labeled Tyr *vs.* nonlabeled Tyr can be determined [102].

The analysis of thermal unfolding processes by conventional spectroscopic methods is restricted by technical limitations making them rather rare [103,104]. Extreme temperature jumps, where the signal amplitude between the initial and final state is large, are hard to accomplish precisely, whereas under conditions where only small temperature differences have to be covered, the signal amplitude becomes too small. As proteases withdraw the unfolded protein from the equilibrium by degradation, the signal amplitude always amounts to 100% so that even processes with marginal spectroscopic signal amplitudes, that is, under native-like or marginally denaturing conditions, can be monitored precisely. In general, proteolysis is a comparably simple but sophisticated method to analyze unfolding processes both with respect to the position of the structural changes [90,93,97,100,105] and to the kinetics [65,66,98,106-110].

For proteases that are able to degrade a natively folded protein, the rate constant of proteolysis (k_p) increases linearly with the protease concentration ([P]). In contrast, k_p*vs.* [P] yields hyperbolic characteristics if the protease requires the unfolding of the substrate protein prior to degradation[106].

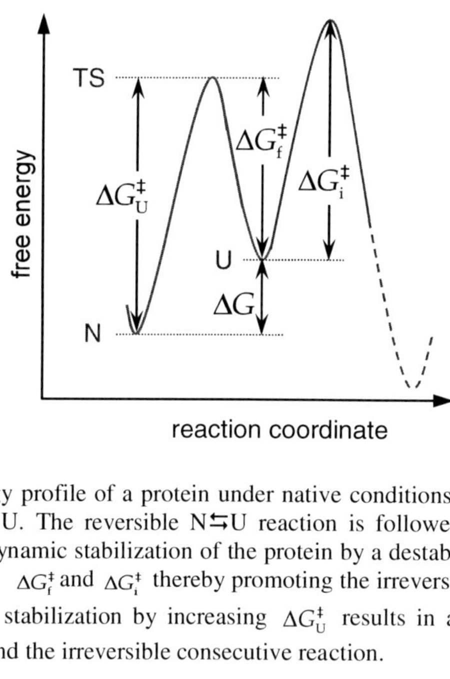

Figure 5. Free energy profile of a protein under native conditions with an irreversible process coupled to U. The reversible N⇆U reaction is followed by an irreversible reaction. A thermodynamic stabilization of the protein by a destabilization of U results in both a decrease in $\Delta G^{\ddagger}_{f}$ and $\Delta G^{\ddagger}_{i}$ thereby promoting the irreversible reaction as well. On the other hand, stabilization by increasing $\Delta G^{\ddagger}_{U}$ results in a suppression of the unfolding reaction and the irreversible consecutive reaction.

From the reaction scheme in eq. 13, Imoto *et al.* [107] developed eq. 14, by which k_U can be determined from proteolysis experiments under conditions where [U] and [U–P] are still small (that is under native-like or marginally denaturing conditions) so that $v = k_p$ [N] and [P] = $[P]_0$:

$$N \underset{k_f}{\overset{k_U}{\rightleftharpoons}} U \underset{k_b}{\overset{k_a[P]}{\rightleftharpoons}} U\text{–}P \xrightarrow{k_c} \textbf{protease + fragments} \qquad (13)$$

$$k_p = \frac{k_U [P]_0}{B + [P]_0} \text{ with } B = (k_b + k_c)\, k_f / (k_a\, k_c) \qquad (14)$$

This approach has been successfully used for the determination of k_U for lysozyme, RNase A, and β-lactoglobulin [107], the peroxidase from *Coprinus cinereus*[108], and numerous RNase A variants [65,109,111].

THE RIBONUCLEASEA EXAMPLE

RNase A (Figure 6) is probably one of the best characterized proteins (reviewed in [112,113]). Its remarkable career as a model began in the 1950s, when the American slaughterhouse and meatpacking company Armour and Co. (Chicago, IL) supplied researchers all over the world free of charge with RNase A. This protein was purified from bovine pancreas (under rather drastic conditions: solubilization of dried pancreas with acidic acetone, extraction with ether, and boiling [114] or by 0.25 N sulfuric acid at 5°C followed by incubation at pH 3.0, at 95–100°C [115,116]) where its abundance had been described already in 1920 by Jones [117]. The reversibility of its thermal unfolding [118] rendered RNase A a suitable model protein for numerous studies, many of which became a landmark [112,113]. RNase A was not only the third protein whose amino acid sequence was determined [119,120] and the fifth protein whose crystal structure was solved [121] but it served among others as a model for

- studies on the protein stability and folding problem (Nobel price for chemistry, Christian B. Anfinsen in 1972; 'folding code')
- studies on chemistry and catalysis (Nobel price for chemistry, Stanford Moore and William H. Stein in 1972)
- the chemistry of protein synthesis (Nobel price for chemistry, Robert B. Merrifield in 1984)
- the development of techniques (NMR spectroscopy[122], H–D exchange NMR spectroscopy to follow protein folding processes [123], intein-mediated protein ligation [124])

- studies on the evolutionary relationship of proteins (RNase A superfamily [125,126])
- studies on 'domain swapping' [127], by which RNase A forms multiple oligomers with novel biological properties [128]
- the development of protein-based therapeutics[129-131]

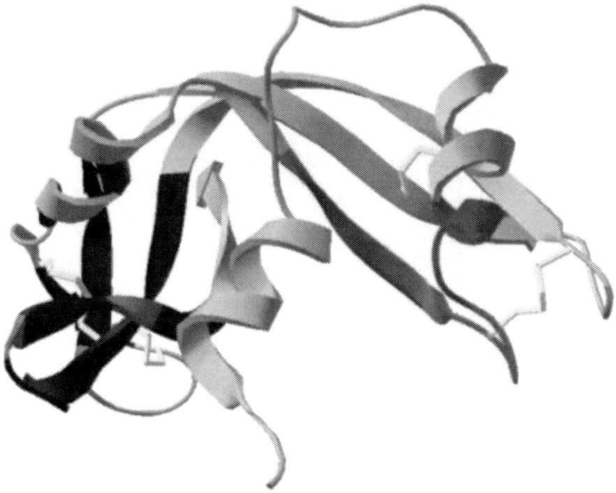

Figure 6. Tertiary structure of ribonuclease A. The model was taken from the Brookhaven Protein Data Bank (7rsa) and drawn using the program PDB Viewer. The proposed unfolding region (red), the proposed chain folding initiation site (blue), the proline residues (cis conformation—green, trans conformation—purple), and disulfide bonds (yellow) are indicated. See text for details.

Thermodynamic Stability of RNaseA

RNaseA is a small, monomeric protein of 124 amino acid residues[120]. With ΔG of $\approx$40 kJ mol^{-1}[65,132] and a T_m value of $\approx$64°C at pH 8.0 [47,66,133,134], RNaseA is a moderately stable protein. Its unfolding by chemical denaturants such as guanidine hydrochloride (GdnHCl) or urea is reversible [132], as is its thermal unfolding under mildly acidic conditions [133]. Its thermal unfolding at neutral pH, however, is not completely reversible [135] due to aggregation and chemical modification. Moreover, numerous other denaturants have been applied such as trifluorethanol [136], sodium dodecyl sulfate [137], lithium salts[138], trichloro acetic acid[139], or pressure [140].

The unfolding of RNaseA can be well described by a two-state transition (eq. 7 and 9) and also the coincidence of ΔH_{cal} and ΔH_m[141] indicates the validity of a two-state unfolding process under equilibrium conditions. Early studies employing proteolysis[96,105], NMR spectroscopy (to follow the signal change of the His-C2 atoms[142]), laser Raman spectroscopy[143], or the non-specific labeling of exposed amino acid residues[102] seemed to diverge and led to a hypothesis on a thermally induced stepwise unfolding of RNase A [144]. Despite marginal local variations, however, no thermodynamically stable intermediates have been characterized so that for the unfolding of RNase A—like for most small, single-domain proteins—a two-state assumption is justified.

Modifications of the protein structure of RNase A in order to study and to increase the (thermodynamic) stability will be outlined below. However, two homologues should be mentioned here: a naturally occurring form of RNase A, which is *N*-glycosylated at Asn34 (RNase B [145]) and onconase (or ranpirnase), a homologue from the Northern leopard frog *Rana* pipiens[146]. RNase B possesses the same amino acid sequence as RNase A but is more stable by 1.5°C ($\Delta\Delta G \approx +3$ kJ mol^{-1}[98,109,147,148]).

Despite a carbohydrate moiety of $GlcNAc_2Man_{(5-9)}$[149], the entire stabilizing effect is caused by the first GlcNAc unit attached to Asn34, as determined from partially deglycosylated RNase B derivatives[109]. This result is supported by the analysis of the crystal structure, which indicates a hydrogen bond between the first GlcNAc unit and the side chain of Lys37 [150].

The other homologue, onconase, and RNase A possess the same overall tertiary structure, the bilobal, kidney-shaped structure of the members of the RNase A superfamily, but share only 28% amino acid sequence identity [146]. As for the differences, onconase possesses, for instance, an extended hydrophobic cluster and a disulfide bond, which tethers the C-terminus to the protein body. Interestingly, onconase surpasses RNase A by almost 30°C in T_m[151,152], 1.4 M in $[GdnHCl]_{1/2}$, and 20 kJ mol^{-1} in ΔG[152].

Folding of RNaseA

The reversibility of the unfolding of RNase A enabled the comprehensive and detailed study of its folding and unfolding processes, for which mostly temperature and GdnHCl were applied. Moreover, Anfinsen *et al.* had shown that RNase A, which had been unfolded by urea and whose disulfide bonds had even been reduced by mercaptoethanol, folds spontaneously to yield active protein after removal of urea and mercaptoethanol by dialysis[153]. This finding had resulted in the 'folding code' concept, which postulates that the information for the formation of the native tertiary structure is encoded in the amino acid sequence [6].

After Tsong *et al.*[154] had shown that both the thermally induced folding and unfolding reactions of RNase A were biphasic processes, Garel and Baldwin were able to prove parallel folding pathways from the unfolded to the native protein [155]. According to the fast and slow refolding reactions, the distinct unfolded species were termed U_f and U_S, respectively. However, U_S is not homogeneous but consists of a minor (even slower folding) species (U_S^I) and a major species (U_S^{II}[156]). Isomerization reactions of X_{aa}–Pro peptide bonds (*vide supra*) were postulated to be responsible for the occurrence of the slow folding phases [37]. In fact, under native-like conditions the folding rate constant of U_S was found to be independent of the concentration of chemical denaturants but showed strong temperature dependence[157]. Moreover, it was increased by low pH[158] or by addition of a PPIase [159]. As all these findings coincide with the characteristics of X_{aa}–Pro peptide bond isomerization reactions, the folding of U_S^{II} was considered as being limited by one or more such processes.

Double-jump experiments (D→N→D) proved that the X_{aa}–Pro isomerization reaction(s) occurred after the conformational folding, which leads to the population of a native-like intermediate (I_N[160]). While the catalytic activity[156] and the UV spectroscopic properties of I_N are indistinguishable from those of native RNase A [160], I_N contains (at least one) X_{aa}–Pro peptide bond(s) in its/their non-native conformation [160], which leads to a different fluorescence behavior [161].

The subsequent studies accumulated much knowledge on the folding behavior of RNase A as well as on the populated intermediates I_1 and I_N[156,161-165] leading to the following scheme (the percentages indicate the amplitudes of the respective folding phases):

$$\begin{array}{l} U_f \rightarrow 20\% \\ U_s^{II} \rightarrow I_1 \rightarrow I_N \rightarrow U70\% \\ U_s^{I} \rightarrow (I_N?) \rightarrow N10\% \end{array} \qquad (15)$$

In contrast to these parallel folding pathways, the conformational unfolding of RNase A is a monophasic process [166,167], which is followed by X_{aa}–Pro isomerization reactions in the unfolded state (eq. 16 [155,157,168,169]). However, indications for a 'dry molten globule', where the polypeptide backbone conformation equals that of native RNase A but where the side chain of several amino acid residue can rotate freely, have been described [170].

$$N \rightarrow U_f \rightarrow U_f + U_s^{II} + U_s^{I} \tag{16}$$

As native RNase A contains two *cis*- (Pro93 and Pro114) und two *trans*-prolines (Pro42 and Pro117 [171]), further studies focused on the elucidation of the contribution of the X_{aa}–Pro isomerization reactions to the folding behavior of RNase A. While for the folding of both U_s^{II} and U_s^{I} X_{aa}–Pro isomerization reactions could be proven, U_f (amplitude about 20%, eq. 15) folds without rate-limiting X_{aa}–Pro isomerization reactions. Due to the *cis/trans* ratio of roughly 1:5 for X_{aa}–Pro peptide bonds in unstructured peptides[38,41], however, only about 4% of all unfolded RNase A molecules should possess all four X_{aa}–Pro peptide bonds in their native conformation. In fact, by applying specific reaction conditions (pH 3.0, 1.5 M GdnHCl) the refolding of U_f was found to become biphasic: a very fast phase (for the unfolded species U_{vf}, which constitutes about 4% of the total unfolded protein) and the fast phase (for U_f, which was suggested to possess Pro114 in *trans* conformation [172]). Moreover, a 'medium-refolding species' U_m was detected and postulated to consist of two species with either non-native *trans*-Pro93 or non-native *trans*-Pro114 plus non-native *cis*-Pro117 [173]. The fraction of U_m was estimated to about 4% [174].

With RNase A variants, which were generated by genetic engineering, the contribution of the individual proline residues to the folding behavior of RNase A could be probed in more detail [43,175-179]. The substitution of Pro by Ala revealed (indirectly, by elimination of 'proline phases') that *trans*-Pro42 does not affect the conformational folding and also *trans*-Pro117 has only little influence. In contrast, the *trans*→*cis* isomerization reaction of Pro114 and even more pronounced of Pro93 were shown to cause the complex folding behavior of RNase A [174-176].

By expressed protein ligation [180] or 'intein-mediated protein ligation' [124] (both of which base on the native chemical ligation [181]) it was possible to replace *cis*-Pro114 by a chemically modified proline residue—5',5'-dimethylproline (dmP)—which no longer can isomerize to the *trans* conformation [45]. In fact, dmP114-RNase A was found to be more stable by

ΔT_m = +3°C and $\Delta\Delta G$ = +6 kJ mol^{-1}, which was caused by a six-fold faster refolding reaction [47,111]. By this means, the involvement of a X_{aa}–Pro isomerization reaction was proven directly for the first time.

The exchange rate constants of the individual amide protons have been determined under a variety of experimental conditions, from which the respective ΔG values were calculated [182-184]. As expected from the involvement of the individual amino acid residues in elements of secondary structures [171,183], the exchange rates strongly differ from residue to residue. Even though it has been shown for several proteins that the most slowly exchanging residues belong to the 'folding core' [185,186], *i.e.* that they form the first contacts during the folding reaction ('chain folding initiation sites' CFIS [174,187]), this correlation did not prove to be valid for other proteins [188,189]. For RNase A, residues 106–118 (including *cis*-Pro114) had been suggested as CFIS from contact maps [187]. At least partial experimental support for this hypothesis was provided by hydrogen exchange measurements during the refolding of RNase A: Val47, His48, Val54, Val63, His72, Tyr73, Ile81, Cys84, Lys98, Ile106, Val108, Val116, Val118, and His119 became protected first during the refolding of RNase A (forming the intermediate I_1[190]; the intermediate I_Φ, which was described for the refolding of U_{vf}, *i.e.*, the unfolded RNase A species with all X_{aa}–Pro peptide bonds in their native conformation, is structurally comparable but much less stable [191]). By comparison of this protection pattern with the exchange kinetics in native RNase A, Neira *et al.* suggested a modified distribution of CFIS residues: Val54, Val57, Lys62–Ala64, Cys72–Ser75, Ile106–Cys110, and Val116–His119 [183] (Figure 6).

Val116 and Val118 show, however, a faster exchange than expected from global unfolding in low concentrations of urea[184], as does His119 in low concentrations of GdnHCl [182]. Locally confined, marginal structural changes were detected [182-184] or concluded from modeling studies [192] before the onset of the global unfolding, which concern, most of all, the termini of secondary structure elements. With increasing temperature a considerable increase in the exchange rate constants of selected amide protons was detectable, which was assigned to a 'fraying' of the termini of the secondary structure elements due to the general increase in the mobility. Limited proteolysis studies identified the Ω-loop including the C-terminus of helix II and the first β-strand (residues Met30–Phe46, Figure 6) as unfolding region of RNase A [65,90,93]. Stelea *et al.* concluded from DSC, CD, and FTIR studies "that the pretransitional changes ... are determined by the unwinding of the C terminus of helix II correlated with the modification of β-strand 43–49" [135], which coincides with the suggested unfolding region. In ostensible contrast, Kiefhaber and Baldwin [166] concluded from the analysis of the exchange rates of 49 amide protons "that a single rate-limiting step in unfolding breaks the entire network of peptide hydrogen bonds and causes the overall unfolding of ribonuclease A" and also Noronha *et al.* showed that thermal unfolding of RNase A followed by tyrosine fluorescence proceeds as "a single unfolding event" [167]. The faster H–D exchange for several residues, some of which interestingly are again located in the proposed unfolding region of RNase A, was explained by additional small fluctuations (EX2 mechanism [193]). As the disruption of interactions within the unfolding region does not necessarily result in an unfolding intermediate but rather *initiates* the global unfolding, 'unfolding region' and 'single rate-limiting step' are not mutually exclusive.

Apparent deviations from the two-state unfolding behavior were also detected by following the unfolding of RNase A by NMR (C2-His signals [194]) or laser Raman spectroscopy [143] or by proteolysis [96,100,110,136,195], but whether they arise from a general (but regionally varying) increase in 'local breathing' due to an increase in temperature (or denaturant concentration) or from a *state* different from the native state (N_I^*[196], N' [192]) remains a matter of discussion.

Despite the increase in ΔG, the folding of the above-mentioned glycosylated homologue RNase B is not changed in comparison to RNase A with respect to both the occurrence of the kinetic phases and their rate constants and amplitudes [197]. The unfolding reaction is, however, decelerated ($\Delta\Delta G_U^{\ddagger} = +3\ \mathrm{kJ\ mol^{-1}}$, determined by the limited proteolysis approach [98]) and the resulting Φ_U–value (≈ 1) reveals a stabilization of N as reason for the increase in ΔG. Again, the stabilizing effect was the same for all partially deglycosylated RNase B derivatives[109]. The stabilization mode by the carbohydrate moiety, which is attached to Asn34, is in full accordance with the concept of the unfolding region.

Also the unfolding of onconase, the other homologue mentioned above, is considerably decelerated [152,198]. The folding behavior of onconase, however, is different from that of RNase A [198,199], which is caused by a different disulfide bond pattern and the lack of *cis*-prolines. In the folding of onconase, a X_{aa}–Pro *cis*→*trans* isomerization reaction occurs in the unfolded state before the protein folds to its native state *via* on on-pathway intermediate [199]. This intermediate, which requires the presence of the C-terminal disulfide bond [200], is nevertheless comparable to I_1 in the refolding of RNase A [199].

Stabilization of RNase A

Numerous attempts have been made to stabilize RNase A and/or to characterize the contribution of single amino acid residues to the stability or folding of RNase A (Table 1) as well as to its biological activity. The interior of the RNase A molecule consisting of two hydrophobic clusters is tightly packed [201,202] and four disulfide bonds tether the small, 124 amino acid residues protein [171] (Figure 6). Thus, chances seem to be rather limited for a considerable stabilization and, in fact, most modifications led to a decrease in stability. In most cases, thermodynamic stability parameters (T_m and/or ΔG) have been determined, which alone do not provide a comprehensive characterization of the respective (de)stabilizing effects. As outlined above, the contribution of an individual amino acid residue to the unfolding or folding reaction can be estimated from Φ_U- ($\Delta\Delta G^{\ddagger}_{U} / \Delta\Delta G$) and/or Φ_f-values (), if the $\Delta\Delta G^{\ddagger}_{U} / \Delta\Delta G$ kinetics of the unfolding or refolding reaction has been followed in addition to equilibrium measurements.

The strongest stabilization of RNase A was achieved by the introduction of an extrinsic cross-link between Lys7 and Lys41 (1,5-difluoro-2,4-dinitrobenzene [203]). Thereby, T_m increased by 25°C [77] and ΔG by 12.5 kJ mol^{-1}[204], which was almost exclusively caused by a deceleration of the unfolding reaction ($\Delta\Delta G^{\ddagger}_{U} \approx$ +11 kJ mol^{-1}, $\Phi_U =$ 0.9 [204]). Another successful cross-linking approach used thiolation of a number of lysine residues with *N*-acetylhomocysteine thiolactone followed by cross-linking either by oxidation or by reaction with bifunctional cross-linking reagents[205]. By this means, several RNase A derivatives were generated that were more stable by about 10°C [78], but the effect was not assigned to the folding or unfolding reaction.

Many modifications by site-directed mutagenesis were designed to probe the contribution of individual amino acid residues to the catalytic [206] or cytotoxic activity [151,207], thermodynamic stability [65,133,140, 202,208,209], proteolytic resistance[210,211], and to the folding [65,66,104,175,176] or unfolding reaction [65,66] (Table 1). Most modifications resulted in a change in stability with Φ_U-values close to 1 (Φ_f-values close to 0 [65,66,169,204]).

Table 1. Contribution of individual amino acid residues of RNase A to its stability and folding behavior

Amino acid residue	Effect of substitution / references
Glu2	essential for stabilizing helix I by ionic interaction with Arg10 [216]
Ala4	A4C/V118C: ΔT_m = +5°C [66,213,214], $\Delta\Delta G$ = +7 kJ mol^{-1}, $\Delta\Delta G_U^{\ddagger}$ = +6 kJ mol^{-1}, Φ_U = 0.8 [66]
Lys7	K7A/R10A: ΔT_m = –4°C [217], K7A: no impact on stability [218], cross-link to Lys41: ΔT_m = +25°C [77] and $\Delta\Delta G$ = +12 kJ mol^{-1}, $\Delta\Delta G_U^{\ddagger} \approx$ +11 kJ mol^{-1}, Φ_U = 0.9 [204]
Phe8	F8L: ΔT_m = –14°C, $\Delta\Delta G$ = –17 kJ mol^{-1}[202]
Arg10	K7A/R10A: ΔT_m = –4°C [217], R10A: ΔT_m = –3°C [218], R10C/R33C: ΔT_m = –9°C, $\Delta\Delta G$ = –10 kJ mol^{-1}, $\Delta\Delta G_U^{\ddagger}$ = –6 kJ mol^{-1}, Φ_U = 0.6 [66]
His12	H12A/H119A: ΔT_m = –9°C (Klink and Raines in [219])
Met13	M13A: ΔT_m = –10°C, $\Delta\Delta G$ = –12 kJ mol^{-1}[202]
Ala19	A19P and A19P/Q28L: ΔT_m = –2°C [220]
Ala20	A20P and A20P/S21P: no impact on stability [65] (but hindrance of proteolysis by subtilisin and proteinase K [210,211])
Ser21	S21L, S21P, and A20P/S21P: no impact on stability [65] (but hindrance of proteolysis by subtilisin, proteinase K, and elastase [210,211])
Tyr25	Y25F: ΔT_m = –6°C, $\Delta\Delta G$ = –8 kJ mol^{-1}, faster unfolding, slower refolding [221]
Cys26	C26A/C84A:ΔT_m = –38°C [133]
Gln28	Q28A: no impact on stability [202]
Met30 ‡	M30C/N44C: ΔT_m = –19°C, $\Delta\Delta G$ = –21 kJ mol^{-1}, $\Delta\Delta G_U^{\ddagger}$ = –12 kJ mol^{-1}, Φ_U = 0.6 [66], M30A:ΔT_m = –10°C, $\Delta\Delta G$ = –12 kJ mol^{-1}[202]
Lys31 ‡	A19P/Q28L/K31C/S32C: no effect on T_m (but dimerization like bovine seminal RNase [220]), K31A/R33S: $\Delta\Delta G$ = –10 kJ mol^{-1}, $\Delta\Delta G_U^{\ddagger}$ = –13 kJ mol^{-1}, $\Phi_U \approx$ 1 [65]
Ser32 ‡	A19P/Q28L/K31C/S32C: no effect on T_m (but dimerization like bovine seminal RNase [220])
Arg33 ‡	K31A/R33S: $\Delta\Delta G$ = –10 kJ mol^{-1}, $\Delta\Delta G_U^{\ddagger}$ = –13 kJ mol^{-1}, $\Phi_U \approx$ 1 [65], R10C/R33C: ΔT_m = –9°C, $\Delta\Delta G$ = –10 kJ mol^{-1}, $\Delta\Delta G_U^{\ddagger}$ = –6 kJ mol^{-1}, Φ_U = 0.6 [66]
Asn34 ‡	first GlcNAc entity of the carbohydrate moiety of RNase B causes ΔT_m = +2°C, $\Delta\Delta G$ = +3 kJ mol^{-1}, $\Delta\Delta G_U^{\ddagger}$ = +3 kJ mol^{-1}, Φ_U = 1.0 [98,109], N34D: no effect on T_m[65]
Leu35 ‡	L35A or L35S: $\Delta\Delta G$ = –10 or –15 kJ mol^{-1}, $\Delta\Delta G_U^{\ddagger}$ = –6 or –10 kJ mol^{-1}, Φ_U = 0.6 [65]
Lys37	K37A: no effect on T_m[222]
Asp38	D38A: no effect on T_m[222], D38R: ΔT_m = –4°C [151], D83R/R39D: ΔT_m = –4°C [207]

Table 1. (Continued).

Amino acid residue	Effect of substitution / references
Arg39	D83R/R39D: ΔT_m = –4°C [207]
Cys40 ‡	C40A/C95A: ΔT_m = –21°C [133]
Lys41 ‡	K41R/G88R: no effect on T_m (but strong decrease of activity [218]), cross-link to Lys7: ΔT_m = +25°C [77] and $\Delta\Delta G$ = +12 kJ mol^{-1}, $\Delta\Delta G^{\ddagger}_{U} \approx$ +11 kJ mol^{-1}, Φ_U = 0.9 [204]
Pro42 ‡ *trans*	P42A: almost no effect on T_m and folding behavior [176]
Val43 ‡	V43C/R85C: ΔT_m = +2°C, $\Delta\Delta G$ = +3 to +7 kJ mol^{-1}, $\Delta\Delta G^{\ddagger}_{U}$ = +4 kJ mol^{-1}, Φ_U = 0.6 to > 1 [66], V43A: ΔT_m = +3°C, $\Delta\Delta G$ = +4 kJ mol^{-1}[202]
Asn44 ‡	M30C/N44C: ΔT_m = –19°C, $\Delta\Delta G$ = –21 kJ mol^{-1}, $\Delta\Delta G^{\ddagger}_{U}$ = –12 kJ mol^{-1}, Φ_U = 0.6 [66]
Thr45 ‡	T45G: ΔT_m = –10°C [223]
Phe46 ‡	F46Y: $\Delta\Delta G^{\ddagger}_{U}$ = –7 kJ mol^{-1}, Φ_U = 0.6 [65], F46L, V, E, K, or A: $\Delta\Delta G$ = –10 to –28 kJ mol^{-1} (and decrease of activity [65,208,209]), ΔT_m up to –26°C (F46K [208]), $\Delta\Delta G^{\ddagger}_{f}$ = +3 to +5 kJ mol^{-1}, Φ_f = 0.2 [209]
Val47	V47A: ΔT_m = –13°C, $\Delta\Delta G$ = –17 kJ mol^{-1}, V47G: ΔT_m = –27°C, $\Delta\Delta G$ = –32 kJ mol^{-1}[140]
Glu49	E49R/D53R: ΔT_m = –10°C [224]
Leu51	L51A: no impact on stability [202]
Asp53	E49R/D53R: ΔT_m = –10°C [224], D53A: ΔT_m = +5°C, $\Delta\Delta G$ = +7 kJ mol^{-1}[202]
Val54 ★	V54I, L, A, or G: ΔT_m = –3 to –19°C, $\Delta\Delta G$ = –6 to –22 kJ mol^{-1}[140]
Val57 ★	V57I, L, A, or G: ΔT_m = –1 to –20°C, $\Delta\Delta G$ = –6 to –25 kJ mol^{-1}[140]
Cys58	C58A/C110A: ΔT_m = –38°C [133]
Val63 ★	V63A or V63G: ΔT_m = –7 or –12°C, $\Delta\Delta G$ = –10 or –16 kJ mol^{-1}[140]
Ala64 ★	A64G: ΔT_m = –3°C, $\Delta\Delta G$ = –3 kJ mol^{-1}[140]
Cys65 ★	C65A/C72A: ΔT_m = –19°C [133]
Lys66	K66A:ΔT_m = –2°C [217]
Asn67	N67D: no effect on T_m but N67(iso)D:ΔT_m = –6°C, $\Delta\Delta G$ = –7 kJ mol^{-1}[225], N67R:ΔT_m = –7°C [207]
Cys72 ★	C65A/C72A: ΔT_m = –19°C [133]
Tyr73 ★	Y73A:ΔT_m = –8°C, $\Delta\Delta G$ = –11 kJ mol^{-1}[202]
Thr78	T78C/H105C: ΔT_m = –8°C or $\Delta\Delta G$ = –20 kJ mol^{-1}[214]
Met79	M79L: $\Delta\Delta G$ = –3 kJ mol^{-1} (J. Köditz, personal communication;$\Phi_U \approx$ 1, U. Arnold, unpublished data), M79A:ΔT_m = –8°C, $\Delta\Delta G$ = –8 kJ mol^{-1}[202]
Ile81	I81V, A or G: ΔT_m = –1 to –17°C, $\Delta\Delta G$ = –3 to –22 kJ mol^{-1}[140]
Asp83	D83A: ΔT_m = –4°C [223], D83E: ΔT_m = +5°C, $\Delta\Delta G$ = +6 kJ mol^{-1}, $\Delta\Delta G^{\ddagger}_{U} \approx$ 5 kJ mol^{-1}, Φ_U = 0.8 (U. Arnold, unpublished data)
Cys84	C26A/C84A:ΔT_m = –38°C [133]

Amino acid residue	Effect of substitution / references
Arg85	R85A: no effect on T_m[222], V43C/R85C: ΔT_m = +2°C, $\Delta\Delta G$ = +3 to +7 kJ mol^{-1}, $\Delta\Delta G_U^\ddagger$ = +4 kJ mol^{-1}, Φ_U = 0.6 to > 1 [66]
Thr87	T87A: no impact on stability [202]
Gly88	G88R: ΔT_m = −4°C, G88D no effect on T_m (but significantly reduced affinity to the RNase inhibitor[151])
Tyr92	Y92F: no impact on stability or folding behavior [221]
Pro93 *cis*	P93A: T_m−9°C, P93A/P114G:ΔT_m = −20°C [43], refolding of P93A still complex [175], P93A: ΔT_m = −11°C, k_U increases twofold, no U_f detectable [176], P93G: *trans* peptide bond ΔT_m = −6°C [177], P93A: *cis* peptide bond [178]
Cys95	C40A/C95A: ΔT_m = −21°C [133]
Tyr97	Y97F: ΔT_m = −5°C, $\Delta\Delta G$ = −12 kJ mol^{-1}, faster unfolding, slower refolding [221], Y97L or A: ΔT_m = −22 or −24°C [202]
Lys104	K104A: no effect on T_m[222]
His105	H105C/V124C: no effect on stability or folding [66]
Ile106 ⋆	I106V, L, or A: ΔT_m = −3 to −15°C, $\Delta\Delta G$ = −5 to −20 kJ mol^{-1}[140]
Ile107 ⋆	I107V, L, or A: ΔT_m = 0 to −10°C, $\Delta\Delta G$ = −5 to −13 kJ mol^{-1}[140], I107C/A122C: T_m−8°C, $\Delta\Delta G$ ≈−10 kJ mol^{-1}, $\Delta\Delta G_U^\ddagger$ ≈−8 kJ mol^{-1}, Φ_U = 0.8 [66]
Val108 ⋆	V108I, L, A or G: ΔT_m = 0 to −29°C, $\Delta\Delta G$ = −3 to −32 kJ mol^{-1}[140]
Ala109 ⋆	A109R: no effect on T_m[151], A109G: T_m−3°C, $\Delta\Delta G$ = −3 kJ mol^{-1}[140]
Cys110 ⋆	C58A/C110A: ΔT_m = −38°C [133]
Pro114 ⋆ *cis*	P114A and P114G: ΔT_m = −10°C, P93A/P114G:ΔT_m = −20°C [43], refolding without 'proline isomerization phase' [175], P114A: ΔT_m = −11°C, k_U increases twofold, changed proportions of U_f, U_S^I, and U_S^{II}[176], P114G: *trans* peptide bond [179], Pro114→5',5'-dimethylprolin: ΔT_m = +3°C, $\Delta\Delta G$ = +6 kJ mol^{-1}, $\Delta\Delta G_f^\ddagger$ = −6 kJ mol^{-1}, Φ_f = 1 [47,111]
Tyr115 ⋆	Y115F: $\Delta\Delta G$ = −10 kJ mol^{-1}[169], Y115W: ΔT_m = −3°C, $\Delta\Delta G$ = −3 kJ mol^{-1}, $\Delta\Delta G_U^\ddagger$ = −4 kJ mol^{-1}, Φ_U ≈ 1, Φ_f ≈ 0 [104]
Val116 ⋆	V116A or V116G: ΔT_m = −3 or −5°C, $\Delta\Delta G$ = −4 or −6 kJ mol^{-1}[140]
Pro117 ⋆ *trans*	P117A: ΔT_m = −7°C, k_U increases 1.5-fold, no U_S^I detectable [176], P117A: $\Delta\Delta G$ = −7 kJ mol^{-1}, k_U increases fourfold, $\Delta\Delta G_U^\ddagger$ = −3 kJ mol^{-1}, Φ_U ≈ 0.4 [169]
Val118 ⋆	A4C/V118C: ΔT_m = +5°C [66,213,214], $\Delta\Delta G$ = +7 kJ mol^{-1}, $\Delta\Delta G_U^\ddagger$ = +6 kJ mol^{-1}, Φ_U = 0.8 [66], V118A or V118G: ΔT_m = −6 or −11°C, $\Delta\Delta G$ = −9 or −13 kJ mol^{-1}[140]
His119 ⋆	H119A:ΔT_m = −2°C [206], H12A/H119A: ΔT_m = −9°C (Klink and Raines in [219])
Phe120	F120L, W, A, or G: ΔT_m = −1 to −20°C, $\Delta\Delta G$ = −1 to −20 kJ mol^{-1} (and decreased activity [226])

Table 1. (Continued).

Amino acid residue	Effect of substitution / references
Asp121	D121N and D121A:ΔT_m = −8°C [206], D121A: ΔT_m = −5°C, D121K ΔT_m = −8°C, ΔD121–V124: ΔT_m = −14°C (and strongly decreased activity [227])
Ala122	elimination of Ala122–Val124 ΔT_m = −6°C (and strongly impairs activity [227]), I107C/A122C ΔT_m = −8°C, $\Delta\Delta G \approx -10$ kJ mol⁻¹, $\Delta\Delta G_U^{\ddagger} \approx -8$ kJ mol⁻¹, $\Phi_U = 0.8$ [66]
Ser123	ΔS123–V124: ΔT_m = −4°C (and decreased activity [227])
Val124	ΔV124: ΔT_m = −3°C (and decreased activity [227]), k_U increases fivefold (U. Arnold, unpublished data), H105C/V124C: no effect on stability or folding [66]

‡ indicates residues in the proposed unfolding region ([65,90,93], ★ indicates residues in the proposed chain folding initiation site (CFIS [183,187]

Notably, even the modifications of CFIS-residues did not yield the expected Φ_f-values close to 1 [104,169,176]. This can be attributed to the multiple, parallel folding pathways, which result in different transition states, whereas the transition state of the unfolding reaction is rather homogenous. As, for instance, the amplitude of the folding of U_S^{II} is 0.6, the Φ_f-value for a respective amino acid residue in this folding pathway can be maximally 0.6. Moreover, the β_T-value of RNase A is only 0.62 meaning that RNase A is still unfolded to one third in the transition state of folding [212].

A sole exception from this consideration seems to be *cis*-Pro114 in the proposed CFIS of RNase A [187]. Here, a Φ_f-value of ≈ 1 (determined by investigation of the dmP114-RNase A variant [47,111]) revealed that isomerization to the native *cis* configuration is indispensible for the refolding of all unfolded RNase A species. The introduction of dmP114 resulted in an increase in ΔG by 6 kJ mol^{-1}[47,111].

An even more pronounced stabilization of RNase A was achieved by the introduction of an additional disulfide bond (A4C/V118C [66,213,214] or V43C/R85C [66]) or by point mutations (D53A [202] or D83E, U. Arnold, unpublished data) (Table 1). Despite being clearly localized distant from the unfolding region, D83E-RNase A is stabilized by a decrease in k_U (Φ_U = 0.8, Table 1) possibly due to a newly formed salt bridge between the γ-carboxyl group and the side chain of Arg85. Also, the introduction of the additional disulfide bond A4C/V118C led to a thermodynamic stabilization by a decrease in k_U (Φ_U = 0.8, Table 1), even though a CFIS-residue (Val118) is involved. Moreover, due to the chain entropy model, the introduction of a disulfide bond should increase k_f (due to an entropic destabilization of U [215]) rather than decrease k_U. Still, the covalent bond might tether the N-terminal helix I to the protein body, thereby stabilizing the native conformation and decelerating the unfolding reaction [66].

CONCLUSION

Despite its small size and an overall thermodynamic two-state unfolding behavior, RNase A shows a complex folding behavior. The conformational folding of RNase A, which starts from a heterogeneous mixture of unfolded conformers, is initiated by a restricted number of contacts (CFIS). Regardless of the isomerization state of the X_{aa}–Pro peptide bonds in the unfolded polypeptide chain, the initial contacts are obviously comparable (forming I_N and I_Φ). Subsequently to the formation of these initial contacts, which is accompanied by the formation of (parts of) certain secondary structure elements, the polypeptide chain is arranged to yield the native protein—potentially kinetically limited by a X_{aa}–Pro isomerization ($I_N \rightarrow N$). The heterogeneity of the unfolded state causes the existence of multiple, parallel folding pathways, which differ in the number as well as in the rate constants of the kinetic phases.

The conformational unfolding reaction, which starts from the homogeneous native state, is a global, single-step reaction in which the entire hydrogen bond network is lost. This process, which is initiated by the disruption of the interactions in the unfolding region—the Ω-loop from the C-terminus of α-helix II through the first β-strand (about residues Met30–Phe46)—and which is followed by the isomerization of the X_{aa}–Pro peptide bonds in unfolded RNase A, is overlapped by confined conformational changes in the native state ('breathing', 'fraying' of the termini of secondary structure elements). In contrast to the global unfolding, however, the extent of these confined processes and their increase with increasing temperature or denaturant concentrations strongly depends on local conditions and peculiarities: the intensity is much more pronounced in less ordered than in highly ordered regions (loops > turns or termini of secondary structure elements > center of secondary structure elements or hydrophobic core, Figure 7, see [110,184]).

The multiple but marginal and confined local changes, which are detectable in the pretransition region of the global unfolding by specific (local) probes, indicate an apparent deviation from the overall two-state unfolding behavior and explain, why not exclusively the stabilization of the unfolding region can lead to an efficient stabilization of the protein molecule.

In order to rationally exploit the multitude of possible approaches for protein stabilization, it is necessary to analyze the folding and unfolding processes of the respective target protein in the context with its tertiary structure and thermodynamic stability.

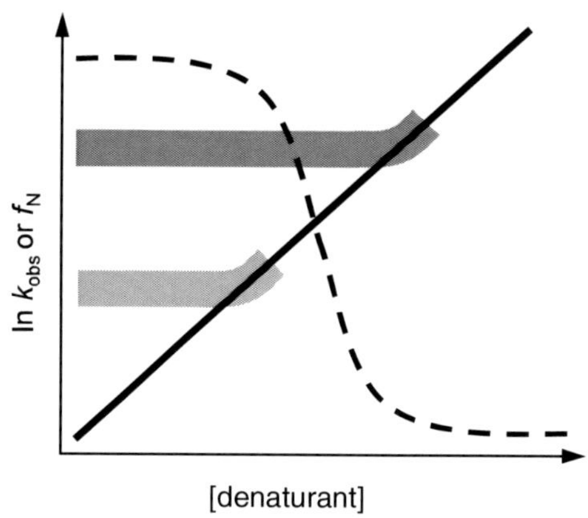

Figure 7. Schematic presentation of the unfolding rate constants of individual structural regions as a function of denaturant concentration. Core residues become exposed by global unfolding only (solid line). Residues at the termini of secondary structure elements or in turns become exposed by local unfolding events under native conditions (dark shaded area) but show a transition from accessibility in the native state (detectable by, e.g., H-D exchange via EX2 mechanism [193]) to accessibility by global unfolding (solid line, detectable by, e.g., H-D exchange via EX1 mechanism [193]). Residues in marginally structured regions or unstructured loops are highly exposed even under native conditions (light shaded area). Dashed line indicates the fraction of native protein (fN) at the respective concentration of denaturant.

REFERENCES

[1] Sumner, J. B. (1926). The isolation and crystallization of the enzyme urease: preliminary paper. *J. Biol. Chem.*, *69*, 435-441.

[2] Cech, T. R. (1990). Nobel lecture. Self-splicing and enzymatic activity of an intervening sequence RNA from Tetrahymena. *Biosci. Rep.*, *10*, 239-261.

[3] Altman, S. (1990). Nobel lecture. Enzymatic cleavage of RNA by RNA. *Biosci. Rep., 10*, 317-337.

[4] Richards, F. M. (1997). Protein stability: still an unsolved problem. *Cell. Mol. Life Sci., 53*, 790-802.

[5] Frauenfelder, H., Sligar, S. G. and Wolynes, P. G. (1991). The energy landscapes and motions of proteins. *Science, 254*, 1598-1603.

[6] Anfinsen, C. B. (1973). Principles that govern the folding of protein chains. *Science, 181*, 223-230.

[7] Govindarajan, S., Recabarren, R. and Goldstein, R. A. (1999). Estimating the total number of protein folds. *Proteins, 35*, 408-414.

[8] Mirny, L. A., Abkevich, V. I. and Shakhnovich, E. I. (1998). How evolution makes proteins fold quickly. *Proc. Natl. Acad. Sci. U. S. A., 95*, 4976-4981.

[9] Rackovsky, S. (1993). On the nature of the protein folding code. *Proc. Natl. Acad. Sci. U. S. A., 90*, 644-648.

[10] Vieille, C. and Zeikus, G. J. (2001). Hyperthermophilic enzymes: sources, uses, and molecular mechanisms for thermostability. *Microbiol. Mol. Biol. Rev., 65*, 1-43.

[11] Eijsink, V. G., Bjork, A., Gåseidnes, S., Sirevag, R., Synstad, B., van den Burg, B. and Vriend, G. (2004). Rational engineering of enzyme stability. *J. Biotechnol., 113*, 105-120.

[12] Schellman, J. A. (2002). Fifty years of solvent denaturation. *Biophys. Chem., 96*, 91-101.

[13] Santoro, M. M. and Bolen, D. W. (1988). Unfolding free energy changes determined by the linear extrapolation method. 1. Unfolding of phenylmethanesulfonyl alpha-chymotrypsin using different denaturants. *Biochemistry, 27*, 8063-8068.

[14] Clarke, J. and Fersht, A. R. (1993). Engineered disulfide bonds as probes of the folding pathway of barnase: increasing the stability of proteins against the rate of denaturation. *Biochemistry, 32*, 4322-4329.

[15] Pace, C. N., Hebert, E. J., Shaw, K. L., Schell, D., Both, V., Krajcikova, D., Sevcik, J., Wilson, K. S., Dauter, Z., Hartley, R. W. and Grimsley, G. R. (1998). Conformational stability and thermodynamics of folding of ribonucleases Sa, Sa2 and Sa3. *J. Mol. Biol., 279*, 271-286.

[16] Lumry, R. and Biltonen, R. (1966). Validity of the "two-state" hypothesis for conformational transitions of proteins. *Biopolymers, 4*, 917-944.

[17] Pace, C. N. and Laurents, D. V. (1989). A new method for determining the heat capacity change for protein folding. *Biochemistry*, *28*, 2520-2525.

[18] Makhatadze, G. I. and Privalov, P. L. (1990). Heat capacity of proteins. I. Partial molar heat capacity of individual amino acid residues in aqueous solution: hydration effect. *J. Mol. Biol.*, *213*, 375-384.

[19] Privalov, P. L. (1979). Stability of proteins: small globular proteins. *Adv. Protein Chem.*, *33*, 167-241.

[20] Greene, R. F., Jr. and Pace, C. N. (1974). Urea and guanidine hydrochloride denaturation of ribonuclease, lysozyme, alpha-chymotrypsin, and beta-lactoglobulin. *J. Biol. Chem.*, *249*, 5388-5393.

[21] Tanford, C. (1970). Protein denaturation. C. Theoretical models for the mechanism of denaturation. *Adv. Protein Chem.*, *24*, 1-95.

[22] Schellman, J. A. (1994). The thermodynamics of solvent exchange. *Biopolymers*, *34*, 1015-1026.

[23] Bieri, O. and Kiefhaber, T. (2000). Kinetic models in protein folding, in: ed. Pain, R. H., *Mechanisms of protein folding*, p. 34-64, New York, Oxford University Press Inc.

[24] Clark, P. L. (2004). Protein folding in the cell: reshaping the folding funnel. *Trends Biochem. Sci.*, *29*, 527-534.

[25] Cheung, M. S., Klimov, D. and Thirumalai, D. (2005). Molecular crowding enhances native state stability and refolding rates of globular proteins. *Proc. Natl. Acad. Sci. U. S. A.*, *102*, 4753-4758.

[26] Ebbinghaus, S., Dhar, A., McDonald, J. D. and Gruebele, M. (2010). Protein folding stability and dynamics imaged in a living cell. *Nat. Methods*, *7*, 319-323.

[27] Truhlar, S. M. and Agard, D. A. (2005). The folding landscape of an α-lytic protease variant reveals the role of a conserved β-hairpin in the development of kinetic stability. *Proteins*, *61*, 105-114.

[28] Evans, P. A., Dobson, C. M., Kautz, R. A., Hatfull, G. and Fox, R. O. (1987). Proline isomerism in staphylococcal nuclease characterized by NMR and site-directed mutagenesis. *Nature*, *329*, 266-268.

[29] Kuwajima, K., Okayama, N., Yamamoto, K., Ishihara, T. and Sugai, S. (1991). The Pro117 to glycine mutation of staphylococcal nuclease simplifies the unfolding-folding kinetics. *FEBS Lett.*, *290*, 135-138.

[30] Dill, K. A. and Chan, H. S. (1997). From Levinthal to pathways to funnels. *Nat. Struct. Biol.*, *4*, 10-19.

[31] Oliveberg, M., Tan, Y. J. and Fersht, A. R. (1995). Negative activation enthalpies in the kinetics of protein folding. *Proc. Natl. Acad. Sci. U. S. A.*, *92*, 8926-8929.

[32] Daggett, V. (2002). Molecular dynamics simulations of the protein unfolding/folding reaction. *Acc. Chem. Res.*, *35*, 422-429.

[33] Jackson, S. E. (1998). How do small single-domain proteins fold? *Fold. Des.*, *3*, R81-91.

[34] Jackson, S. E. and Fersht, A. R. (1991). Folding of chymotrypsin inhibitor 2. 1. Evidence for a two-state transition. *Biochemistry*, *30*, 10428-10435.

[35] Parker, M. J. and Marqusee, S. (1999). The cooperativity of burst phase reactions explored. *J. Mol. Biol.*, *293*, 1195-1210.

[36] Kiefhaber, T. and Schmid, F. X. (1992). Kinetic coupling between protein folding and prolyl isomerization. II. Folding of ribonuclease A and ribonuclease T1. *J. Mol. Biol.*, *224*, 231-240.

[37] Brandts, J. F., Halvorson, H. R. and Brennan, M. (1975). Consideration of the possibility that the slow step in protein denaturation reactions is due to cis-trans isomerism of proline residues. *Biochemistry*, *14*, 4953-4963.

[38] Grathwohl, C. and Wüthrich, K. (1981). NMR studies of the rates of proline *cis-trans* isomerization in oligopeptides. *Biopolymers*, *20*, 2623-2633.

[39] Stewart, D. E., Sarkar, A. and Wampler, J. E. (1990). Occurrence and role of *cis* peptide bonds in protein structures. *J. Mol. Biol.*, *214*, 253-260.

[40] Weiss, M. S., Jabs, A. and Hilgenfeld, R. (1998). Peptide bonds revisited. *Nat. Struct. Biol.*, *5*, 676.

[41] Reimer, U., Scherer, G., Drewello, M., Kruber, S., Schutkowski, M. and Fischer, G. (1998). Side-chain effects on peptidyl-prolyl cis/trans isomerisation. *J. Mol. Biol.*, *279*, 449-460.

[42] Balbach, J. and Schmid, F. X. (2000). Proline isomerization and its catalysis in protein folding, in: ed. Pain, R. H., *Mechanisms of protein folding*, p. 212-249, New York, Oxford University Press Inc.

[43] Schultz, D. A. and Baldwin, R. L. (1992). Cis proline mutants of ribonuclease A. I. Thermal stability. *Protein Sci.*, *1*, 910-916.

[44] Mutter, M., Wohr, T., Gioria, S. and Keller, M. (1999). Pseudo-prolines: induction of cis/trans-conformational interconversion by decreased transition state barriers. *Biopolymers*, *51*, 121-128.

[45] An, S. S. A., Cathy, C. C., Peng, J. L., Li, Y. J., Rothwarf, D. M., Welker, E., Thannhauser, T. W., Zhang, L. S., Tam, J. P. and Scheraga, H. A. (1999). Retention of the *cis* proline conformation in tripeptide fragments of bovine pancreatic ribonuclease A containing a non-natural proline analogue, 5,5-dimethylproline. *J. Am. Chem. Soc.*, *121*, 11558-11566.

[46] Renner, C., Alefelder, S., Bae, J. H., Budisa, N., Huber, R. and Moroder, L. (2001). Fluoroprolines as Tools for Protein Design and Engineering. *Angew. Chem. Int. Ed. Engl.*, *40*, 923-925.

[47] Arnold, U., Hinderaker, M. P., Köditz, J., Golbik, R., Ulbrich-Hofmann, R. and Raines, R. T. (2003). Protein prosthesis: a nonnatural residue accelerates folding and increases stability. *J. Am. Chem. Soc.*, *125*, 7500-7501.

[48] Levitt, M. (1981). Effect of proline residues on protein folding. *J. Mol. Biol.*, *145*, 251-263.

[49] Fischer, G., Bang, H. and Mech, C. (1984). [Determination of enzymatic catalysis for the cis-trans-isomerization of peptide binding in proline-containing peptides]. *Biomed. Biochim. Acta*, *43*, 1101-1111.

[50] Schiene, C. and Fischer, G. (2000). Enzymes that catalyse the restructuring of proteins. *Curr. Opin. Struct. Biol.*, *10*, 40-45.

[51] Schmid, F. X. (1983). Mechanism of folding of ribonuclease A. Slow refolding is a sequential reaction via structural intermediates. *Biochemistry*, *22*, 4690-4696.

[52] Chen, B. L., Baase, W. A. and Schellman, J. A. (1989). Low-temperature unfolding of a mutant of phage T4 lysozyme. 2. Kinetic investigations. *Biochemistry*, *28*, 691-699.

[53] Gahl, R. F. and Scheraga, H. A. (2009). Oxidative folding pathway of onconase, a ribonuclease homologue: insight into oxidative folding mechanisms from a study of two homologues. *Biochemistry*, *48*, 2740-2751.

[54] Shakhnovich, E., Abkevich, V. and Ptitsyn, O. (1996). Conserved residues and the mechanism of protein folding. *Nature*, *379*, 96-98.

[55] Collinet, B., Garcia, P., Minard, P. and Desmadril, M. (2001). Role of loops in the folding and stability of yeast phosphoglycerate kinase. *Eur. J. Biochem.*, *268*, 5107-5118.

[56] Schellenberger, A. and Ulbrich, R. (1989). Protein stabilization by blocking the native unfolding nucleus. *Biomed. Biochim. Acta*, *48*, 63-67.

[57] Ulbrich-Hofmann, R., Golbik, R. and Damerau, W. (1993). Fixation of the unfolding region - a hypothesis of enzyme stabilization, in: eds. van den Tweel, W. J. J., Harder, A., and Buitelaar, R. M., *Stability and stabilization of enzymes*, p. 497-504, Amsterdam, Elsevier.

[58] Ulbrich-Hofmann, R., Arnold, U. and Mansfeld, J. (1999). The concept of the unfolding region for approaching the mechanisms of enzyme stabilization. *J. Mol. Catal. B*, *7*, 125-131.

[59] Siddiqui, K. S., Rangarajan, M., Hartley, B. S., Kitmitto, A., Panico, M., Blench, I. P. and Morris, H. R. (1993). Arthrobacter D-xylose isomerase: partial proteolysis with thermolysin. *Biochem. J.*, *289*, 201-208.

[60] Eijsink, V. G., Veltman, O. R., Aukema, W., Vriend, G. and Venema, G. (1995). Structural determinants of the stability of thermolysin-like proteinases. *Nat. Struct. Biol.*, *2*, 374-379.

[61] Gåseidnes, S., Synstad, B., Jia, X., Kjellesvik, H., Vriend, G. and Eijsink, V. G. (2003). Stabilization of a chitinase from Serratia marcescens by Gly→Ala and Xxx→Pro mutations. *Protein Eng.*, *16*, 841-846.

[62] Fersht, A. R., Matouschek, A. and Serrano, L. (1992). The folding of an enzyme. I. Theory of protein engineering analysis of stability and pathway of protein folding. *J. Mol. Biol.*, *224*, 771-782.

[63] Fersht, A. R. and Sato, S. (2004). Phi-value analysis and the nature of protein-folding transition states. *Proc. Natl. Acad. Sci. U. S. A.*, *101*, 7976-7981.

[64] Matouschek, A., Kellis, J. T., Jr., Serrano, L. and Fersht, A. R. (1989). Mapping the transition state and pathway of protein folding by protein engineering. *Nature*, *340*, 122-126.

[65] Köditz, J., Ulbrich-Hofmann, R. and Arnold, U. (2004). Probing the unfolding region of ribonuclease A by site-directed mutagenesis. *Eur. J. Biochem.*, *271*, 4147-4156.

[66] Pecher, P. and Arnold, U. (2009). The effect of additional disulfide bonds on the stability and folding of ribonuclease A. *Biophys. Chem.*, *141*, 21-28.

[67] Fersht, A. R. (1999). Kinetics of protein folding - a guide to enzyme catalysis and protein folding, in, *Structure and mechanism in protein science*, p. 540-572, NewYork, W. H. Freeman and Company.

[68] Krebs, H., Rudolph, R. and Jaenicke, R. (1979). Influence of coenzyme on the refolding and reassociation in vitro of glyceraldehyde-3-phosphate dehydrogenase from yeast. *Eur. J. Biochem.*, *100*, 359-364.

[69] Relimpio, A., Iriarte, A., Chlebowski, J. F. and Martinez-Carrion, M. (1981). Differential scanning calorimetry of cytoplasmic aspartate transaminase. *J. Biol. Chem.*, *256*, 4478-4488.

[70] Pantoliano, M. W. (1992). Proteins designed for challenging environments and catalysis in organic solvents. *Curr. Opin. Struct. Biol.*, *2*, 559-568.

[71] Shareghi, B. and Moosavi-Movahedi, A. A. (1996). Kinetics and thermodynamics studies on the interaction of D-amino acid oxidase and sodium*n*-dodecyl sulphate in the presence and absence of flavin adenine dinucleotide. *Int. J. Biol. Macromol.*, *19*, 9-13.

[72] Forsgren, N., Lamont, R. J. and Persson, K. Two intramolecular isopeptide bonds are identified in the crystal structure of the *Streptococcus gordonii* SspB C-terminal domain. *J. Mol. Biol.*, *397*, 740-751.

[73] Diwan, M. and Park, T. G. (2001). Pegylation enhances protein stability during encapsulation in PLGA microspheres. *J. Control. Release*, *73*, 233-244.

[74] Blomhoff, H. K. and Christensen, T. B. (1983). Effect of dextran and dextran modifications on the thermal and proteolytic stability of conjugated bovine testis beta-galactosidase and human serum albumin. *Biochim. Biophys. Acta*, *743*, 401-407.

[75] Solá, R. J. and Griebenow, K. Glycosylation of therapeutic proteins: an effective strategy to optimize efficacy. *BioDrugs*, *24*, 9-21.

[76] Marfey, P. S., Uziel, M. and Little, J. (1965). Reaction of bovine pancreatic ribonuclease a with 1,5-difluoro-2,4-dinitrobenzene. II. Structure of an intramolecularly bridged derivative. *J. Biol. Chem.*, *240*, 3270-3275.

[77] Lin, S. H., Konishi, Y., Denton, M. E. and Scheraga, H. A. (1984). Influence of an extrinsic cross-link on the folding pathway of ribonuclease A. Conformational and thermodynamic analysis of cross-linked (lysine7-lysine41)-ribonuclease A. *Biochemistry*, *23*, 5504-5512.

[78] Reiner, R., Siebeneick, H.-U., Christensen, I. and Döring, H. (1977). Chemical modification of enzymes II. Conformational stability of cross-linked bovine pancreatic ribonuclease. *J. Mol. Catal.*, *2*, 119-128.

[79] Sheldon, R. A. (2007). Cross-linked enzyme aggregates (CLEAs): stable and recyclable biocatalysts. *Biochem. Soc. Trans.*, *35*, 1583-1587.

[80] Ulbrich, R., Schellenberger, A. and Damerau, W. (1986). Studies on the thermal inactivation of immobilized enzymes. *Biotechnol. Bioeng.*, *28*, 511-522.

[81] Hickey, A. M., Marle, L., McCreedy, T., Watts, P., Greenway, G. M. and Littlechild, J. A. (2007). Immobilization of thermophilic enzymes in miniaturized flow reactors. *Biochem. Soc. Trans.*, *35*, 1621-1623.
[82] Gianfreda, L. and Scarfi, M. R. (1991). Enzyme stabilization: state of the art. *Mol. Cell. Biochem.*, *100*, 97-12.
[83] Vermuë, M. H. and Tramper, J. (1995). Biocatalysis in non-conventional media: Medium engineering aspects. *Pure and Appl. Chem.*, *67*, 345-373.
[84] Illanes, A. (1999). Stability of biocatalysts. *Electron. J. Biotechn.*, *2*, 1-9.
[85] Faria, T. Q., Mingote, A., Siopa, F., Ventura, R., Maycock, C. and Santos, H. (2008). Design of new enzyme stabilizers inspired by glycosides of hyperthermophilic microorganisms. *Carbohydr. Res.*, *343*, 3025-3033.
[86] Urfer, R. and Kirschner, K. (1992). The importance of surface loops for stabilizing an eightfold beta alpha barrel protein. *Protein Sci.*, *1*, 31-45.
[87] Gu, H., Kim, D. and Baker, D. (1997). Contrasting roles for symmetrically disposed beta-turns in the folding of a small protein. *J. Mol. Biol.*, *274*, 588-596.
[88] Leszczynski, J. F. and Rose, G. D. (1986). Loops in globular proteins: a novel category of secondary structure. *Science*, *234*, 849-855.
[89] Fetrow, J. S. (1995). Omega loops: nonregular secondary structures significant in protein function and stability. *FASEB J.*, *9*, 708-717.
[90] Arnold, U., Köditz, J., Markert, Y. and Ulbrich-Hofmann, R. (2005). Local fluctuations*vs.* global unfolding of proteins investigated by limited proteolysis. *Biocatal. Biotransfor.*, *23*, 159-167.
[91] Price, N. C. and Johnson, C. M. (1990). Proteinases as probes of conformation of soluble proteins, in: ed. Beynon, R. J., Bond, J. S., *Proteolytic Enzymes: A practical approach*, p. 163-180, Oxford, IRL Press.
[92] Hubbard, S. J., Eisenmenger, F. and Thornton, J. M. (1994). Modeling studies of the change in conformation required for cleavage of limited proteolytic sites. *Protein Sci.*, *3*, 757-768.
[93] Arnold, U., Rücknagel, K. P., Schierhorn, A. and Ulbrich-Hofmann, R. (1996). Thermal unfolding and proteolytic susceptibility of ribonuclease A. *Eur. J. Biochem.*, *237*, 862-869.
[94] Hubbard, S. J. (1998). The structural aspects of limited proteolysis of native proteins. *Biochim. Biophys. Acta*, *1382*, 191-206.
[95] Park, C. and Marqusee, S. (2004). Probing the high energy states in proteins by proteolysis. *J. Mol. Biol.*, *343*, 1467-1476.

[96] Klee, W. A. (1967). Intermediate stages in the thermally induced transconformation reactions of bovine pancreatic ribonuclease A. *Biochemistry*, *6*, 3736-3742.

[97] Winchester, B. G., Mathias, A. P. and Rabin, B. R. (1970). Study of the thermal denaturation of ribonuclease A by differential thermal analysis and susceptibility to proteolysis. *Biochem. J.*, *117*, 299-307.

[98] Arnold, U. and Ulbrich-Hofmann, R. (1997). Kinetic and thermodynamic thermal stabilities of ribonuclease A and ribonuclease B. *Biochemistry*, *36*, 2166-2172.

[99] Wang, L., Chen, R. X. and Kallenbach, N. R. (1998). Proteolysis as a probe of thermal unfolding of cytochrome c. *Proteins*, *30*, 435-441.

[100] Arnold, U. and Ulbrich-Hofmann, R. (2000). Differences in the denaturation behavior of ribonuclease A induced by temperature and guanidine hydrochloride. *J. Protein Chem.*, *19*, 345-352.

[101] Fontana, A., de Laureto, P. P., Spolaore, B., Frare, E., Picotti, P. and Zambonin, M. (2004). Probing protein structure by limited proteolysis. *Acta Biochim. Pol.*, *51*, 299-321.

[102] Matheson, R. R., Jr. and Scheraga, H. A. (1979). Steps in the pathway of the thermal unfolding of ribonuclease A. A nonspecific photochemical surface-labeling study. *Biochemistry*, *18*, 2437-2445.

[103] Kintses, B., Simon, Z., Gyimesi, M., Tóth, J., Jelinek, B., Niedetzky, C., Kovács, M. and Málnási-Csizmadia, A. (2006). Enzyme kinetics above denaturation temperature: a temperature-jump/stopped-flow apparatus. *Biophys. J.*, *91*, 4605-4610.

[104] Torrent, J., Marchal, S., Ribó, M., Vilanova, M., Georges, C., Dupont, Y. and Lange, R. (2008). Distinct unfolding and refolding pathways of ribonuclease a revealed by heating and cooling temperature jumps. *Biophys. J.*, *94*, 4056-4065.

[105] Ooi, T., Rupley, J. A. and Scheraga, H. A. (1963). Structural Studies of Ribonuclease. VIII. Tryptic Hydrolysis of Ribonuclease a at Elevated Temperatures. *Biochemistry*, *2*, 432-437.

[106] Matthyssens, G. E., Simons, G. and Kanarek, L. (1972). Study of the thermal-denaturation mechanism of hen egg-white lysozyme through proteolytic degradation. *Eur. J. Biochem.*, *26*, 449-454.

[107] Imoto, T., Yamada, H. and Ueda, T. (1986). Unfolding rates of globular proteins determined by kinetics of proteolysis. *J. Mol. Biol.*, *190*, 647-649.

[108] Tams, J. W. and Welinder, K. G. (1996). Unfolding and refolding of *Coprinus cinereus* peroxidase at high pH, in urea, and at high

temperature. Effect of organic and ionic additives on these processes. *Biochemistry*, *35*, 7573-7579.
[109] Arnold, U., Schierhorn, A. and Ulbrich-hofmann, R. (1999). Modification of the unfolding region in bovine pancreatic ribonuclease and its influence on the thermal stability and proteolytic fragmentation. *Eur. J. Biochem.*, *259*, 470-475.
[110] Arnold, U. and Ulbrich-Hofmann, R. (2001). Proteolytic degradation of ribonuclease A in the pretransition region of thermally and urea-induced unfolding. *Eur. J. Biochem.*, *268*, 93-97.
[111] Arnold, U. (2009). Incorporation of non-natural modules into proteins: structural features beyond the genetic code. *Biotechnol. Lett.*, *31*, 1129-1139.
[112] Raines, R. T. (1998). Ribonuclease A. *Chem. Rev.*, *98*, 1045-1066.
[113] Marshall, G. R., Feng, J. A. and Kuster, D. J. (2008). Back to the future: ribonuclease A. *Biopolymers*, *90*, 259-277.
[114] Dubos, R. J. and Thompson, R. H. S. (1938). The decomposition of yeast nucleic acid by a heat-resistant enzyme. *J. Biol. Chem.*, *124*, 501-510.
[115] Kunitz, M. (1940). Crystalline Ribonuclease. *J. Gen. Physiol.*, *24*, 15-32.
[116] Kunitz, M. and McDonald, M. R. (1953). Ribonuclease, in: ed. Snell, E. E., *Biochemical Preparations*, p. 9-19, New York, John Wiley and Sons.
[117] Jones, W. (1920). The action of boiled pancreas extract on yeast nucleic acid. *Am. J. Physiol.*, *52*, 203-207.
[118] Harrington, W. F. and Schellman, J. A. (1956). Evidence for the instability of hydrogen-bonded peptide structures in water, based on studies of ribonuclease and oxidized ribonuclease. *C. R. Trav. Lab. Carlsberg Chim.*, *30*, 21-43.
[119] Hirs, C. H., Moore, S. and Stein, W. H. (1960). The sequence of the amino acid residues in performic acid-oxidized ribonuclease. *J. Biol. Chem.*, *235*, 633-647.
[120] Smyth, D. G., Stein, W. H. and Moore, S. (1963). The sequence of amino acid residues in bovine pancreatic ribonuclease: revisions and confirmations. *J. Biol. Chem.*, *238*, 227-234.
[121] Kartha, G., Bello, J. and Harker, D. (1967). Tertiary structure of ribonuclease. *Nature*, *213*, 862-865.
[122] Saunders, M., Wishnia, A. and Kirkwood, J. G. (1957). The nuclear magnetic resonance spectrum of ribonuclease. *J. Am. Chem. Soc.*, *79*, 3289-3290.

[123] Udgaonkar, J. B. and Baldwin, R. L. (1988). NMR evidence for an early framework intermediate on the folding pathway of ribonuclease A. *Nature*, *335*, 694-699.

[124] Evans, T. C., Jr., Benner, J. and Xu, M. Q. (1998). Semisynthesis of cytotoxic proteins using a modified protein splicing element. *Protein Sci.*, *7*, 2256-2264.

[125] Beintema, J. J., Breukelman, H. J., Carsana, A. and Furia, A. (1997). Evolution of vertebrate ribonucleases: Ribonuclease A superfamily, in: eds. D'Alessio, G., and Riordan, J. F., *Ribonucleases: Structures and functions*, p. 245-269, New York, Academic Press.

[126] Beintema, J. J. and Kleineidam, R. G. (1998). The ribonuclease A superfamily: general discussion. *Cell. Mol. Life Sci.*, *54*, 825-832.

[127] Bennett, M. J., Choe, S. and Eisenberg, D. (1994). Domain swapping: entangling alliances between proteins. *Proc. Natl. Acad. Sci. U. S. A.*, *91*, 3127-3131.

[128] Libonati, M., Gotte, G. and Vottariello, F. (2008). A novel biological actions acquired by ribonuclease through oligomerization. *Curr. Pharm. Biotechnol.*, *9*, 200-209.

[129] Raines, R. T. (1999). Ribonuclease A: from model system to cancer chemotherapeutic, in: eds. Frey, P. A., and Northrop, D. B., *Enzymatic Mechanisms*, p. 235-249, Washington, DC, IOS Press.

[130] Arnold, U. and Ulbrich-Hofmann, R. (2006). Natural and engineered ribonucleases as potential cancer therapeutics. *Biotechnol. Lett.*, *28*, 1615-1622.

[131] Arnold, U. (2008). Aspects of the cytotoxic action of ribonucleases. *Curr. Pharm. Biotechnol.*, *9*, 161-168.

[132] Pace, C. N., Laurents, D. V. and Thomson, J. A. (1990). pH dependence of the urea and guanidine hydrochloride denaturation of ribonuclease A and ribonuclease T1. *Biochemistry*, *29*, 2564-2572.

[133] Klink, T. A., Woycechowsky, K. J., Taylor, K. M. and Raines, R. T. (2000). Contribution of disulfide bonds to the conformational stability and catalytic activity of ribonuclease A. *Eur. J. Biochem.*, *267*, 566-572.

[134] Ramos, C. H. and Baldwin, R. L. (2002). Sulfate anion stabilization of native ribonuclease A both by anion binding and by the Hofmeister effect. *Protein Sci.*, *11*, 1771-1778.

[135] Stelea, S. D., Pancoska, P., Benight, A. S. and Keiderling, T. A. (2001). Thermal unfolding of ribonuclease A in phosphate at neutral pH: deviations from the two-state model. *Protein Sci.*, *10*, 970-978.

[136] Köditz, J., Arnold, U. and Ulbrich-Hofmann, R. (2002). Dissecting the effect of trifluoroethanol on ribonuclease A. Subtle structural changes detected by nonspecific proteases. *Eur. J. Biochem.*, *269*, 3831-3837.

[137] Takeda, K., Sasa, K., Nagao, M. and Batra, P. P. (1988). Secondary structural changes of non-reduced and reduced ribonuclease A in solutions of urea, guanidine hydrochloride and sodium dodecyl sulfate. *Biochim. Biophys. Acta*, *957*, 340-344.

[138] Ahmad, F. (1984). Free energy changes in denaturation of ribonuclease A by mixed denaturants. Effects of combinations of guanidine hydrochloride and one of the denaturants lithium bromide, lithium chloride, and sodium bromide. *J. Biol. Chem.*, *259*, 4183-4186.

[139] Sagar, A. J. and Pandit, M. W. (1983). Denaturation studies on bovine pancreatic ribonuclease. Effect of trichloroacetic acid. *Biochim. Biophys. Acta*, *743*, 303-309.

[140] Ribó, M., Benito, A., Torrent, J., Lange, R. and Vilanova, M. (2006). Pressure as a tool to study protein-unfolding/refolding processes: the case of ribonuclease A. *Biochim. Biophys. Acta*, *1764*, 461-469.

[141] Pace, C. N., Grimsley, G. R., Thomas, S. T. and Makhatadze, G. I. (1999). Heat capacity change for ribonuclease A folding. *Protein Sci.*, *8*, 1500-1504.

[142] Benz, F. W. and Roberts, G. C. (1973). NMR Studies of the unfolding of ribonuclease by guanidine hydrochloride. Evidence for intermediate states. *FEBS Lett.*, *29*, 263-266.

[143] Chen, M. C. and Lord, R. C. (1976). Laser Raman spectroscopic studies of the thermal unfolding of ribonuclease A. *Biochemistry*, *15*, 1889-1897.

[144] Burgess, A. W. and Scheraga, H. A. (1975). A hypothesis for the pathway of the thermally-induced unfolding of bovine pancreatic ribonuclease. *J. Theor. Biol.*, *53*, 403-420.

[145] Plummer, T. H., Jr. and Hirs, C. H. (1963). The isolation of ribonuclease B, a glycoprotein, from bovine pancreatic juice. *J. Biol. Chem.*, *238*, 1396-1401.

[146] Ardelt, W., Mikulski, S. M. and Shogen, K. (1991). Amino acid sequence of an anti-tumor protein from *Rana pipiens* oocytes and early embryos. Homology to pancreatic ribonucleases. *J. Biol. Chem.*, *266*, 245-251.

[147] Puett, D. (1973). Conformational studies on a glycosylated bovine pancreatic ribonuclease. *J. Biol. Chem.*, *248*, 3566-3572.

[148] Joao, H. C. and Dwek, R. A. (1993). Effects of glycosylation on protein structure and dynamics in ribonuclease B and some of its individual glycoforms. *Eur. J. Biochem., 218*, 239-244.

[149] Fu, D., Chen, L. and O'Neill, R. A. (1994). A detailed structural characterization of ribonuclease B oligosaccharides by 1H NMR spectroscopy and mass spectrometry. *Carbohydr. Res., 261*, 173-186.

[150] Woods, R. J., Edge, C. J. and Dwek, R. A. (1994). Protein surface oligosaccharides and protein function. *Nat. Struct. Biol., 1*, 499-501.

[151] Leland, P. A., Staniszewski, K. E., Kim, B. and Raines, R. T. (2000). A synapomorphic disulfide bond is critical for the conformational stability and cytotoxicity of an amphibian ribonuclease. *FEBS Lett., 477*, 203-207.

[152] Arnold, U., Schulenburg, C., Schmidt, D. and Ulbrich-Hofmann, R. (2006). Contribution of structural peculiarities of onconase to its high stability and folding kinetics. *Biochemistry, 45*, 3580-3587.

[153] Anfinsen, C. B., Haber, E., Sela, M. and White, F. H., Jr. (1961). The kinetics of formation of native ribonuclease during oxidation of the reduced polypeptide chain. *Proc. Natl. Acad. Sci. U. S. A., 47*, 1309-1314.

[154] Tsong, T. Y., Baldwin, R. L. and Elson, E. L. (1972). Properties of the refolding and unfolding reactions of ribonuclease A. *Proc. Natl. Acad. Sci. U. S. A., 69*, 1809-1812.

[155] Garel, J. R. and Baldwin, R. L. (1973). Both the fast and slow refolding reactions of ribonuclease A yield native enzyme. *Proc. Natl. Acad. Sci. U. S. A., 70*, 3347-3351.

[156] Schmid, F. X. and Blaschek, H. (1981). A native-like intermediate on the ribonuclease A folding pathway. 2. Comparison of its properties to native ribonuclease A. *Eur. J. Biochem., 114*, 111-117.

[157] Nall, B. T., Garel, J. R. and Baldwin, R. L. (1978). Test of the extended two-state model for the kinetic intermediates observed in the folding transition of ribonuclease A. *J. Mol. Biol., 118*, 317-330.

[158] Schmid, F. X. and Baldwin, R. L. (1978). Acid catalysis of the formation of the slow-folding species of RNase A: evidence that the reaction is proline isomerization. *Proc. Natl. Acad. Sci. U. S. A., 75*, 4764-4768.

[159] Fischer, G. and Bang, H. (1985). The refolding of urea-denatured ribonuclease A is catalyzed by peptidyl-prolyl cis-trans isomerase. *Biochim. Biophys. Acta, 828*, 39-42.

[160] Cook, K. H., Schmid, F. X. and Baldwin, R. L. (1979). Role of proline isomerization in folding of ribonuclease A at low temperatures. *Proc. Natl. Acad. Sci. U. S. A.*, *76*, 6157-6161.

[161] Schmid, F. X. (1981). A native-like intermediate on the ribonuclease A folding pathway. 1. Detection by tyrosine fluorescence changes. *Eur. J. Biochem.*, *114*, 105-109.

[162] Blum, A. D., Smallcombe, S. H. and Baldwin, R. L. (1978). Nuclear magnetic resonance evidence for a structural intermediate at an early stage in the refolding of ribonuclease A. *J. Mol. Biol.*, *118*, 305-316.

[163] Kim, P. S. and Baldwin, R. L. (1980). Structural intermediates trapped during the folding of ribonuclease A by amide proton exchange. *Biochemistry*, *19*, 6124-6129.

[164] Udgaonkar, J. B. and Baldwin, R. L. (1995). Nature of the early folding intermediate of ribonuclease A. *Biochemistry*, *34*, 4088-4096.

[165] Laurents, D. V., Bruix, M., Jamin, M. and Baldwin, R. L. (1998). A pulse-chase-competition experiment to determine if a folding intermediate is on or off-pathway: application to ribonuclease A. *J. Mol. Biol.*, *283*, 669-678.

[166] Kiefhaber, T. and Baldwin, R. L. (1995). Kinetics of hydrogen bond breakage in the process of unfolding of ribonuclease A measured by pulsed hydrogen exchange. *Proc. Natl. Acad. Sci. U. S. A.*, *92*, 2657-2661.

[167] Noronha, M., Lima, J. C., Paci, E., Santos, H. and Maçanita, A. L. (2007). Tracking local conformational changes of ribonuclease A using picosecond time-resolved fluorescence of the six tyrosine residues. *Biophys. J.*, *92*, 4401-4414.

[168] Schmid, F. X., Grafl, R., Wrba, A. and Beintema, J. J. (1986). Role of proline peptide bond isomerization in unfolding and refolding of ribonuclease. *Proc. Natl. Acad. Sci. U. S. A.*, *83*, 872-876.

[169] Juminaga, D., Wedemeyer, W. J. and Scheraga, H. A. (1998). Proline isomerization in bovine pancreatic ribonuclease A. 1. Unfolding conditions. *Biochemistry*, *37*, 11614-11620.

[170] Kiefhaber, T., Labhardt, A. M. and Baldwin, R. L. (1995). Direct NMR evidence for an intermediate preceding the rate-limiting step in the unfolding of ribonuclease A. *Nature*, *375*, 513-515.

[171] Wlodawer, A., Bott, R. and Sjolin, L. (1982). The refined crystal structure of ribonuclease A at 2.0 Å resolution. *J. Biol. Chem.*, *257*, 1325-1332.

[172] Houry, W. A., Rothwarf, D. M. and Scheraga, H. A. (1994). A very fast phase in the refolding of disulfide-intact ribonuclease A: implications for the refolding and unfolding pathways. *Biochemistry*, *33*, 2516-2530.

[173] Houry, W. A. and Scheraga, H. A. (1996). Nature of the unfolded state of ribonuclease A: effect of *cis-trans* X-Pro peptide bond isomerization. *Biochemistry*, *35*, 11719-11733.

[174] Wedemeyer, W. J., Welker, E. and Scheraga, H. A. (2002). Proline cis-trans isomerization and protein folding. *Biochemistry*, *41*, 14637-14644.

[175] Schultz, D. A., Schmid, F. X. and Baldwin, R. L. (1992). Cis proline mutants of ribonuclease A. II. Elimination of the slow-folding forms by mutation. *Protein Sci.*, *1*, 917-924.

[176] Dodge, R. W. and Scheraga, H. A. (1996). Folding and unfolding kinetics of the proline-to-alanine mutants of bovine pancreatic ribonuclease A. *Biochemistry*, *35*, 1548-1559.

[177] Schultz, L. W., Hargraves, S. R., Klink, T. A. and Raines, R. T. (1998). Structure and stability of the P93G variant of ribonuclease A. *Protein Sci.*, *7*, 1620-1625.

[178] Xiong, Y., Juminaga, D., Swapna, G. V., Wedemeyer, W. J., Scheraga, H. A. and Montelione, G. T. (2000). Solution NMR evidence for a cis Tyr-Ala peptide group in the structure of [Pro93Ala] bovine pancreatic ribonuclease A. *Protein Sci.*, *9*, 421-426.

[179] Schultz, D. A., Friedman, A. M., White, M. A. and Fox, R. O. (2005). The crystal structure of the *cis*-proline to glycine variant (P114G) of ribonuclease A. *Protein Sci.*, *14*, 2862-2870.

[180] Muir, T. W., Sondhi, D. and Cole, P. A. (1998). Expressed protein ligation: a general method for protein engineering. *Proc. Natl. Acad. Sci. U. S. A.*, *95*, 6705-6710.

[181] Dawson, P. E., Muir, T. W., Clark-Lewis, I. and Kent, S. B. (1994). Synthesis of proteins by native chemical ligation. *Science*, *266*, 776-779.

[182] Mayo, S. L. and Baldwin, R. L. (1993). Guanidinium chloride induction of partial unfolding in amide proton exchange in RNase A. *Science*, *262*, 873-876.

[183] Neira, J. L., Sevilla, P., Menéndez, M., Bruix, M. and Rico, M. (1999). Hydrogen exchange in ribonuclease A and ribonuclease S: evidence for residual structure in the unfolded state under native conditions. *J. Mol. Biol.*, *285*, 627-643.

[184] Qu, Y. and Bolen, D. W. (2003). Hydrogen exchange kinetics of RNase A and the urea:TMAO paradigm. *Biochemistry*, *42*, 5837-5849.

[185] Kim, K. S., Fuchs, J. A. and Woodward, C. K. (1993). Hydrogen exchange identifies native-state motional domains important in protein folding. *Biochemistry*, *32*, 9600-9608.
[186] Mullins, L. S., Pace, C. N. and Raushel, F. M. (1997). Conformational stability of ribonuclease T1 determined by hydrogen-deuterium exchange. *Protein Sci.*, *6*, 1387-1395.
[187] Matheson, R. R. J. and Scheraga, H. A. (1978). A method for predicting nucleation sites for protein folding based on hydrophobic contacts. *Macromolecules*, *11*, 819-829.
[188] Clarke, J., Hounslow, A. M., Bycroft, M. and Fersht, A. R. (1993). Local breathing and global unfolding in hydrogen exchange of barnase and its relationship to protein folding pathways. *Proc. Natl. Acad. Sci. U. S. A.*, *90*, 9837-9841.
[189] Itzhaki, L. S., Neira, J. L. and Fersht, A. R. (1997). Hydrogen exchange in chymotrypsin inhibitor 2 probed by denaturants and temperature. *J. Mol. Biol.*, *270*, 89-98.
[190] Udgaonkar, J. B. and Baldwin, R. L. (1990). Early folding intermediate of ribonuclease A. *Proc. Natl. Acad. Sci. U. S. A.*, *87*, 8197-8201.
[191] Houry, W. A. and Scheraga, H. A. (1996). Structure of a hydrophobically collapsed intermediate on the conformational folding pathway of ribonuclease A probed by hydrogen-deuterium exchange. *Biochemistry*, *35*, 11734-11746.
[192] Merkley, E. D., Bernard, B. and Daggett, V. (2008). Conformational changes below the Tm: molecular dynamics studies of the thermal pretransition of ribonuclease A. *Biochemistry*, *47*, 880-892.
[193] Loh, S. N., Rohl, C. A., Kiefhaber, T. and Baldwin, R. L. (1996). A general two-process model describes the hydrogen exchange behavior of RNase A in unfolding conditions. *Proc. Natl. Acad. Sci. U. S. A.*, *93*, 1982-1987.
[194] Benz, F. W. and Roberts, G. C. (1975). Nuclear magnetic resonance studies of the unfolding of pancreatic ribonuclease. II. Unfolding by urea and guanidine hydrochloride. *J. Mol. Biol.*, *91*, 367-387.
[195] Rupley, J. A. and Scheraga, H. A. (1963). Structural Studies of Ribonuclease. VII. Chymotryptic Hydrolysis of Ribonuclease A at Elevated Temperatures. *Biochemistry*, *2*, 421-431.
[196] Juneja, J. and Udgaonkar, J. B. (2002). Characterization of the unfolding of ribonuclease a by a pulsed hydrogen exchange study: evidence for competing pathways for unfolding. *Biochemistry*, *41*, 2641-2654.

[197] Grafl, R., Lang, K., Vogl, H. and Schmid, F. X. (1987). The mechanism of folding of pancreatic ribonucleases is independent of the presence of covalently linked carbohydrate. *J. Biol. Chem.*, *262*, 10624-10629.

[198] Schulenburg, C., Martinez-Senac, M. d. M., Löw, C., Golbik, R., Ulbrich-Hofman, R. and Arnold, U. (2007). Identification of three phases in onconase refolding. *FEBS J.*, *274*, 5826-5833.

[199] Schulenburg, C., Löw, C., Weininger, U., Mrestani-Klaus, C., Hofmann, H., Balbach, J., Ulbrich-Hofmann, R. and Arnold, U. (2009). The folding pathway of onconase is directed by a conserved intermediate. *Biochemistry*, *48*, 8449-8457.

[200] Schulenburg, C., Weininger, U., Neumann, P., Meiselbach, H., Stubbs, M. T., Sticht, H., Balbach, J., Ulbrich-Hofmann, R. and Arnold, U. (2010). Impact of the C-terminal disulfide bond on the folding and stability of onconase. *ChemBioChem*, *11*, 978 - 986.

[201] Kolbanovskaya, E., Sathyanarayana, B. K., Wlodawer, A. and Karpeisky, M. (1992). Intramolecular interactions in pancreatic ribonucleases. *Protein Sci.*, *1*, 1050-1060.

[202] Vilà, R., Benito, A., Ribó, M. and Vilanova, M. (2009). Mapping the stability clusters in bovine pancreatic ribonuclease A. *Biopolymers*, *91*, 1038-1047.

[203] Marfey, P. S., Nowak, H., Uziel, M. and Yphantis, D. A. (1965). Reaction of bovine pancreatic ribonuclease a with 1,5-difluoro-2,4-dinitrobenzene. I. Preparation of monomeric intramolecularly bridged derivatives. *J. Biol. Chem.*, *240*, 3264-3269.

[204] Lin, S. H., Konishi, Y., Nall, B. T. and Scheraga, H. A. (1985). Influence of an extrinsic cross-link on the folding pathway of ribonuclease A. Kinetics of folding-unfolding. *Biochemistry*, *24*, 2680-2686.

[205] Reiner, R., Siebeneick, H.-U., Christensen, I. and Lukas, H. (1975/76). Chemical modification of enzymes II. Two-step cross-linking of bovine pancreatic ribonuclease. *J. Mol. Catal.*, *1*, 3-12.

[206] Quirk, D. J., Park, C., Thompson, J. E. and Raines, R. T. (1998). His...Asp catalytic dyad of ribonuclease A: conformational stability of the wild-type, D121N, D121A, and H119A enzymes. *Biochemistry*, *37*, 17958-17964.

[207] Rutkoski, T. J., Kurten, E. L., Mitchell, J. C. and Raines, R. T. (2005). Disruption of shape-complementarity markers to create cytotoxic variants of ribonuclease A. *J. Mol. Biol.*, *354*, 41-54.

[208] Chatani, E., Nonomura, K., Hayashi, R., Balny, C. and Lange, R. (2002). Comparison of heat- and pressure-induced unfolding of ribonuclease a: the critical role of Phe46 which appears to belong to a new hydrophobic chain-folding initiation site. *Biochemistry*, *41*, 4567-4574.

[209] Kadonosono, T., Chatani, E., Hayashi, R., Moriyama, H. and Ueki, T. (2003). Minimization of cavity size ensures protein stability and folding: structures of Phe46-replaced bovine pancreatic RNase A. *Biochemistry*, *42*, 10651-10658.

[210] Markert, Y., Köditz, J., Mansfeld, J., Arnold, U. and Ulbrich-Hofmann, R. (2001). Increased proteolytic resistance of ribonuclease A by protein engineering. *Protein Eng.*, *14*, 791-796.

[211] Markert, Y., Köditz, J., Ulbrich-Hofmann, R. and Arnold, U. (2003). Proline versus charge concept for protein stabilization against proteolytic attack. *Protein Eng.*, *16*, 1041-1046.

[212] Font, J., Benito, A., Lange, R., Ribó, M. and Vilanova, M. (2006). The contribution of the residues from the main hydrophobic core of ribonuclease A to its pressure-folding transition state. *Protein Sci.*, *15*, 1000-1009.

[213] Klink, T. A. and Raines, R. T. (2000). Conformational stability is a determinant of ribonuclease A cytotoxicity. *J. Biol. Chem.*, *275*, 17463-17467.

[214] Pradeep, L., Kurinov, I., Ealick, S. E. and Scheraga, H. A. (2007). Implementation of a k/k(0) method to identify long-range structure in transition states during conformational folding/unfolding of proteins. *Structure*, *15*, 1178-1189.

[215] Thornton, J. M. (1981). Disulphide bridges in globular proteins. *J. Mol. Biol.*, *151*, 261-287.

[216] Rico, M., Santoro, J., Bermejo, F. J., Herranz, J., Nieto, J. L., Gallego, E. and Jiménez, M. A. (1986). Thermodynamic parameters for the helix-coil thermal transition of ribonuclease-S-peptide and derivatives from ^{1}H-NMR data. *Biopolymers*, *25*, 1031-1053.

[217] Fisher, B. M., Ha, J. H. and Raines, R. T. (1998). Coulombic forces in protein-RNA interactions: binding and cleavage by ribonuclease A and variants at Lys7, Arg10, and Lys66. *Biochemistry*, *37*, 12121-12132.

[218] Haigis, M. C., Kurten, E. L., Abel, R. L. and Raines, R. T. (2002). KFERQ sequence in ribonuclease A-mediated cytotoxicity. *J. Biol. Chem.*, *277*, 11576-11581.

[219] Park, C. and Raines, R. T. (2000). Dimer formation by a "monomeric" protein. *Protein Sci.*, *9*, 2026-2033.

[220] Catanzano, F., Graziano, G., Cafaro, V., D'Alessio, G., Di Donato, A. and Barone, G. (1997). From ribonuclease A toward bovine seminal ribonuclease: a step by step thermodynamic analysis. *Biochemistry*, *36*, 14403-14408.

[221] Juminaga, D., Wedemeyer, W. J., Garduno-Juarez, R., McDonald, M. A. and Scheraga, H. A. (1997). Tyrosyl interactions in the folding and unfolding of bovine pancreatic ribonuclease A: a study of tyrosine-to-phenylalanine mutants. *Biochemistry*, *36*, 10131-10145.

[222] Fisher, B. M., Grilley, J. E. and Raines, R. T. (1998). A new remote subsite in ribonuclease A. *J. Biol. Chem.*, *273*, 34134-34138.

[223] delCardayré, S. B. and Raines, R. T. (1995). A residue to residue hydrogen bond mediates the nucleotide specificity of ribonuclease A. *J. Mol. Biol.*, *252*, 328-336.

[224] Fuchs, S. M., Rutkoski, T. J., Kung, V. M., Groeschl, R. T. and Raines, R. T. (2007). Increasing the potency of a cytotoxin with an arginine graft. *Protein Eng. Des. Sel.*, *20*, 505-509.

[225] Catanzano, F., Graziano, G., Capasso, S. and Barone, G. (1997). Thermodynamic analysis of the effect of selective monodeamidation at asparagine 67 in ribonuclease A. *Protein Sci.*, *6*, 1682-1693.

[226] Chatani, E., Tanimizu, N., Ueno, H. and Hayashi, R. (2001). Structural and functional changes in bovine pancreatic ribonuclease a by the replacement of Phe120 with other hydrophobic residues. *J. Biochem.*, *129*, 917-922.

[227] Fujii, T., Ueno, H. and Hayashi, R. (2002). Significance of the four carboxyl terminal amino acid residues of bovine pancreatic ribonuclease A for structural folding. *J. Biochem.*, *131*, 193-200.

Dedicated to Prof. Dr. Renate Ulbrich-Hofmann on the occasion of her 65th birthday.

Edited by Ronald T. Raines.

In: Advances in Proteomics Research ISBN: 978-1-61942-227-8
Editors: Ya Li Huang et al. pp. 159-201

Chapter 5

HETEROLOGOUS PROTEIN FOLDING IN YEAST

Byung-Kwon Choi
GlycoFi, Inc., A Wholly Owned Subsidiary of Merck and Co., Inc., Lebanon, New Hampshire.

ABSTRACT

Yeast is an important platform for the production of therapeutic proteins. It has principally been used for the production of relatively simple proteins that lack *N*-linked glycosylation. However, with recent developments in technologies focused on glycoengineering yeast to produce humanized *N*-glycans, its application to the field of human therapeutics becomes greatly potentiated. A constant challenge in the biotechnology industry is the production of recombinant proteins at high levels. Like other protein expression platforms, productivities in yeast depend on the host strain, its process of cultivation and the type of protein being expressed. In addition, it has been demonstrated that yeast lack some molecular chaperones found in higher eukaryotic cells. Protein folding in the endoplasmic reticulum is a key process that can influence the fate of a protein, directing it either to secretion or ER-associated degradation. Some proteins require specific molecular chaperones for their protein maturation and others require general protein folding chaperones. In this review, yeast folding machinery as well as attempts made to improve protein folding will be discussed.

INTRODUCTION

Yeast is an attractive expression platform for many applications in biologic fields due to several advantages including ease of genetic manipulation, the ability to form disulfide bonds and perform glycosylation, simplicity in cultivation, process development, and relatively low cost of protein production. However, there exist some drawbacks in the field of therapeutic glycoproteins where the presence of fungal type-high mannose *N*-glycan and *O*-glycan structures may affect in vivo efficacy. Many efforts have been made to generate human type *N*-glycans by engineering the glycosylation machinery in yeast. Recent developments of glycoengineered platform allows production of human therapeutic proteins with homogenous and various types of humanized *N*-glycans [1, 2, 3, 4, 5, 6, 7].

Pichia pastoris has been one of mostly used yeast expression systems for protein expression because of high cell density, genetic stability and high secretory capacity besides posttranslational modification. To date, a number of heterologous proteins have been expressed in *P. pastoris* system [8] and other yeasts such as *Saccharomyces cerevisiae*, *Kluyveromyces lactis* and *Hansenula polymorpha* are being used to produce therapeutic proteins in industrial scale [9]. Currently, 21 therapeutic proteins produced from yeast are FDA-approved [10]. In general, the expression of heterologous proteins in yeast is highly protein dependent with productivities ranging from the microgram to gram per liter scale. The highest yields reported from various yeast hosts are as follows; murine collagen (15 g/l) in *P. pastoris*[11], *Aspergillus niger*glucose oxidase (9 g/L) in *S. cerevisiae*[12], human serum albumin(3 g/l) in *K. lactis*[13], and phytase (13.5 g/l) in *H. polymorpha*[14].

It is generally accepted that one of major secretory bottlenecks is the protein folding in the endoplasmic reticulum (ER). Protein folding is a delicate process that is affected by many factors including the properties of the nascent protein, the ER environment including redox potential, the availability of folding enzymes, and molecular chaperones. There have been a number of efforts to enhance protein folding and secretion via genetic modifications (engineering of the ER molecular chaperones and other folding catalysts) and process optimization (temperature, pH, additives, and feeding strategy).

Basically, the primary amino acid sequence of a protein determines the native three-dimensional structure of a protein [15, 16], thus it has a significant impact on overall protein folding. In addition, ER molecular chaperones and folding catalysts are required to facilitate the protein folding and assembly, demonstrating a critical role in protein maturation. The ER folding machinery has been extensively studied to understand the folding of secretory proteins. Many molecular chaperones have been identified in the ER, cytosol, and mitochondria involved in intracellular or secretory protein folding. Therefore, this review will focus on the function of yeast molecular chaperones in the ER and how chaperones improve the folding of heterologous proteins along the secretory pathway, and discusses other approaches.

Co- and Post-Translational Protein Folding

Unlike mammalian cells, translocation of protein into the ER in yeast can occur either cotranslationally or posttranslationally. Yeast have two different types of ribosome-bound Sec61 complexes that are involved in the co-translational pathway. The two types of translocons, the Sec61p complex and the Sshlp complex, differ in their subunit composition. The Sec61p complex consists of Sec61p, Ssh1, and Ssslp, whereas the Sshlp complex contains Sbh1, Sbh2, and Ssslp. Whereas mammalian cells are believed to only have cotranslation as a mechanism for translocation, yeast have the added ability to translocate newly synthesized polypeptides into the ER posttanslationally. This mechanism requires a Sec complex consisting of the Sec61p complex and the Sec62/63 subcomplex (Sec62p, Sec63p, Sec66p, and Sec72p) which is essential. The lumenal ATPase BiP/Kar2p interacts with the Sec63p and provides the energy required for translocation. The co-translational translocation is mediated by a SRP-dependent manner whereas the post-translocation is SRP-independent, but requires a signal peptide. The more hydrophobic the core signal sequence, the more tightly it is bound to SRP. Less hydrophobic sequences do not bind to SRP, and these signal sequences use the posttranslational route [17]. This indicates that the nature of the signal sequence plays a critical role in determining which of the two translocons will be used for protein translocation. The more hydrophobic signal sequence tends to direct protein to the co-translational translocon [18]. Therefore, the choice of a signal sequence for the production of heterologous protein would be an important factor because it determines the type of translocon used in yeast, which may affect the protein folding.

Yeast Folding Machinery

The endoplasmic reticulum (ER) represents a major compartment for the folding of secretory proteins. The ER is rich in folding enzymes, molecular chaperones and co-chaperones that are required for productive protein folding. It has been demonstrated that molecular chaperones play a key role in protein folding and minimizing the degree of misfolded or aggregated proteins. In general, molecular chaperones are structurally diversified by the contribution of various domains having specific roles. Heat shock proteins (HSPs) have been grouped, mainly on the basis of their molecular masses, into specific families that include small HSPs (sHSPs)/alpha-crystallins, HSP10s, HSP40s, HSP60s, HSP70s, HSP90s, HSP100s and HSP110s.

Members of the same family may be located in different cellular compartments. Their expression may vary with time or environmental conditions (developmental, stress, etc.) and substrate specificity (nascent proteins, stress-damaged proteins etc). In mammalian cells, the ER molecular chaperone complex was found in the heavy chain-BiP complex. This chaperone complex includes a number of other ERchaperones and folding enzymes (i.e., BiP, protein disulfideisomerases (P5 and PDI), an ER Hsp40 co-chaperone (ERdj3), GRP94, GRP170, ERp72,cyclophilin B, UDP-glucosyltransferase (UGGT1) and SDF2-L1). Moreover, the multi-chaperone complex also forms in the absence of nascent protein synthesis, indicating that the ER chaperones are present as a pre-formed complex in the ER folding network [19]. However,in yeast, this type of multi-chaperone complex has not been reported.

The key players in the ER molecular chaperones have been identified and functionally characterized in yeast and mammalian cells (Table 1). Yeast lacks some chaperones found in mammalian cells, but contains the major folding machineries; oxidative protein folding via the ERO-PDI pathway, simplified quality control by Cne1p, peptidyl-prolyl isomerases (PPIases), Kar2p and co-chaperones. In addition, an unfolded protein response (UPR) system takes place to deal with the ER stresses caused by misfolded protein, heat shock, and reactive oxygen spices. The ER is also linked to the ER-associated degradation (ERAD) which functions in the disposal of misfolded proteins, thus allowing properly folded proteins to exit the ER.

Oxidative Protein Folding

The multifunctional yeast protein Pdi1p has been extensively characterized. It is essential for cell viability and is the most abundant family member. It constitutes ~0.8% of the total cellular protein in yeast and mammalian cells [20]. The oxidative protein folding by PDI is one of major folding machineries in the endoplasmic reticulum (ER) and catalyzes disulfide bond formation of proteins. Pdi1p also functions to unscramble non-native disulfide bonds for correct disulfide bond formation. Another important function of PDI includes the participation in recognition of some ERAD substrates for degradation of misfolded proteins [21].

Table 1. ER molecular chaperones and co-chaperones for protein folding and assembly

ER molecular chaperones	Yeast (*S. cerevisiae*)	Mammal
Hsp40	Sec63p, Jem1, Scj1, Hlj1, Erj5	ERdj1, ERdj2, ERdj3, ERdj4, ERdj5
Hsp70	Kar2p	BiP
ER molecular chaperones	Yeast (*S. cerevisiae*)	Mammal
Hsp90	-	GRP94
Nuclotide exchange factor (NEF)	Sil1p	BAP
Hsp70/NEF	Lsh1p	GRP170
PPIases	Cpr5p, Fpr2p	Cyclophilin B, FKBP13, FKBP14, FKBP19, FKBP22, FKBP23, FKBP63, FKBP65
PDI family	Pdi1p, Eps1p, Eug1p, Mpd1p, Mpd2	PDI, ERp19, ERp27, ERp29, ERp44, ERp46, ERp57, ERp72, PDIp, P5, ERdj5, PDIR, PDILT, hAG-2, hAG-3, TMX, TMX2, TMX3, TMX4, TMX5
Erv	Erv2p	-
Ero	Ero1p	Ero1α, Ero1β
ER quality control (CNX/CRT cycle)		
CNX	Cne1p	CNX
CRT	-	CRT
ERp57	-	ERp57
UGGT	-	UGGT1

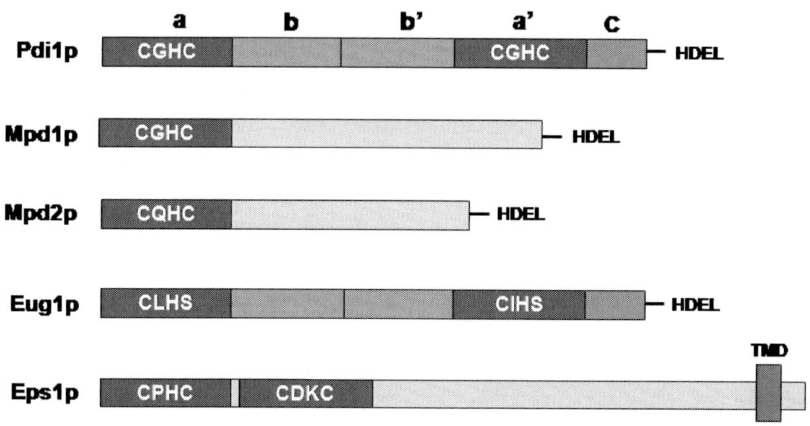

Figure 1. The PDI family in S. cerevisiae. The CXXC motif indicates the thioredoxin active site (a, a').b': substrate binding domain, b: unknown function, Green: acidic region, light blue: unknown function, TMD: transmembrane domain.

In *S. cerevisiae*, there are five PDI homologs including PDI1 and the non-essential members EUG1, MPD1, MPD2, and EPS1 (Figure 1). However, in mammalian cells, 20 PDI homologs (PDI, Erp57, PDIp, ERp72, PDILT, ERp27, PDIr, ERp29, ERdj5, P5, ERp18, ERp44, ERp46, hAG-2, hAG-3, TMX, TMX2, TMX3, and TMX4) have been identified to date and are tissue- and substrate-specific [22]. PDI1p contains four thioredoxin-like domains (a, b, b' and a') where two inactive thioredoxin domains (b and b') are located between two active thioredoxin domains (a and a') followed by an acidic C-terminal domain (c) harboring an ER retention signal (HDEL) [23]. Two active domains contain a catalytically active CGHC motif that is responsible for disulfide bond formation and rearrangement of incorrect disulfide bonds. Unlike other PDI homologs, Eug1p has a CXXS motif at the active sites, but it is unlikely to contribute to oxidative folding as demonstrated by *in vitro* oxidative refolding of proCPY [24].

Besides Pdi1p, the other yeast PDI homologs are not well characterized although some reports suggest that yeast PDI homologs are not functionally interchangeable. These homologs typically carry weak or no isomerase activity. However, based on *in vitro* studies, with the exception of Mpd1p, they all have considerable chaperone activity [25]. Mpd1p is the only homolog capable of complementing the essential functions of Pdi1p in the absence of all PDI homologs, contributing to oxidative protein folding in the ER [26].However, the oxidative activity of Mpd1p is much weaker than Pdi1p.

The PDI family is soluble and carries the ER retention signal (HDEL) at the C-terminus with the exception of Eps1. It has been demonstrated that Eps1p is involved in ER quality control as an ER membrane protein that is linked to the ERAD pathway [27]. Nevertheless, a general role for Eps1p in ERAD pathway has not been established so far.

It has been shown that PDI-mediated oxidative protein folding is most efficient when the reduced Pdi1p is oxidized by the ER oxidoreductin Ero1p, which itself is oxidized by a flavin adenine dinucleotide (FAD), which in turn is oxidized by molecular oxygen (Figure 2).

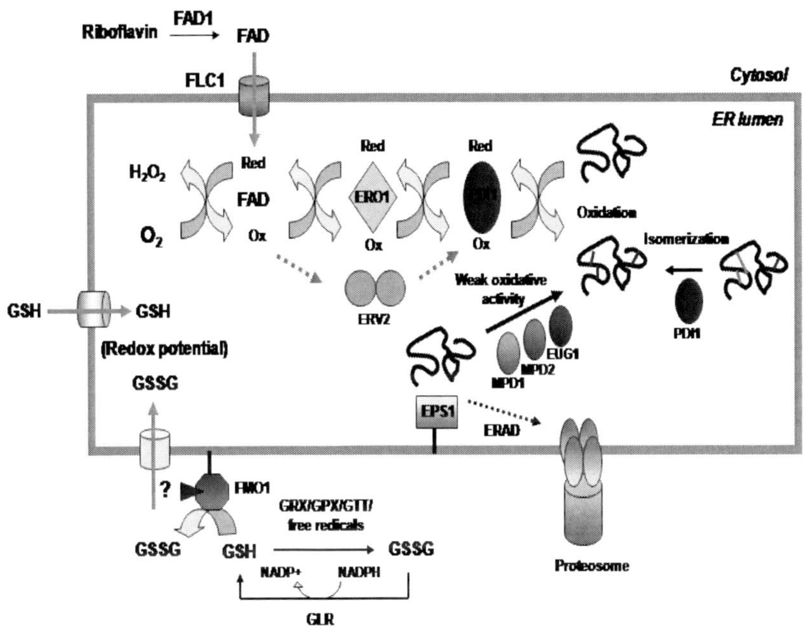

Figure 2. Oxidative protein folding in the ER. GLR: glutathione reductase, GRX: glutaredoxin, GPX: glutathione peroxidase, GTT: glutathione transferase, FLC1: FAD transporter, FMO1: flavin-containing monooxygenase.

Thus, the oxidizing equivalents flow from molecular oxygen to FAD to Ero1p to Pdi1p and on to the substrate[28, 29, 30]. Alternatively, Pdi1p can be re-oxidized independently of Ero1p by the sulfhydryl oxidase Erv2p [31]. Erv2p belongs to the QSOX/ERV family of FAD dependent thiol oxidases that can oxidase substrate thiols to form disulfide bonds with the reduction of oxygen to hydrogen peroxide[32, 33].FAD1 does not act as a direct oxidant on the folding substrate, but instead relies on PDI1 to transfer the oxidizing equivalent. Also, FAD1 is able to directly oxidize the PDI related protein MPD2. However, it does not oxidize all PDI related proteins demonstrating substrate specificity. As a result of the reoxidation of ERO1 via FAD, the electron transfer to molecular oxygen generates a significant proportion of reactive oxygen species (ROS) in the cell, thus providing a source of oxidative stress[29].

The redox potential in the ER lumen plays a crucial role in the production of secretory proteins and protection form oxidative stress. The ER exists normally as an oxidizing environment as compared to the cytosol. The redox potential in eukaryotic cells is principally regulated by the glutathione system at a GSH:GSSG ratio of 30:1-100:1 (~10 mM) in cytosol, and a GSH:GSSG ratio of 1:1-3:1 (~1mM) in the ER [34]. Cytoplasmic GSH is maintained through the action of the ubiquitous enzyme GSH reductase (GLR1), which catalyzes the NADPH-dependent reduction of GSSG to GSH (GSSG+NADPH $+H^+ \rightarrow$ 2 GSH+$NADP^+$) [34].

In contrast to the cytosolic redox buffering system, the regulation of redox potential in the ER has not been well elucidated. However, it has been suggested that reduced GSH and oxidized GSSG are transported from the cytosol to the ER lumen to maintain appropriate redox conditions [35]. Other evidence indicates that only reduced GSH can be transported into the ER. This is supported by the finding that the Ero1p is a major source for delivering oxidizing equivalents to proteins through the Ero1p-Pdi1p pathway and to glutathione in the ER [35]. In addition, it was proposed that oxidized GSSG can be generated by a flavin-containing monooxygenase (Fmo1p) in the ER [36, 37, 38].

The Role of ER HSP70 and HSP40

HSP70 family

HSP70 is a large family of proteins that has been evolutionarily conserved from bacteria (DnaK) to humans. HSP70 proteins were originally classified based upon their size (~70kDa) and their induction through heat-shock. Hsp70 is composed of two major domains, an N-terminal ATPase domain (~40 kDa) and a C-terminal domain containing a substrate-binding domain covered by a removable lid (~25 kDa). *S. cerevisiae* contains at least nine cytosolic forms of HSP70 (encoded by the genes SSA1, SSA2, SSA3, SSA4, SSB1, SSB2, SSE1, SSE2, SSZ1), two HSP70s which are found in the endoplasmic reticulum

(KAR2, LHS1), and three mitochondrial HSP70 proteins (SSC1, SSQ1, ECM10) [39].

Kar2p represents a yeast homolog of the mammalian immunoglobulin heavy chain binding protein (BiP) and is essential for cell survival. Kar2p is involved multiple protein processes including protein translocation across the ER membrane, protein folding in the ER, the unfolded protein response (UPR), the ER-associated degradation (ERAD), and karyogamy[40, 41, 42]. One of key functions of Kar2p is the participation of protein folding and the prevention of misfolded protein aggregation[43]. Kar2p binds in a transient fashion to newly synthesized protein in the ER, where it specifically interacts with patches of hydrophobic amino acids and maintains them in a state competent for subsequent folding and assembly [42]. In particular, BiP has been shown to interact with the CH1 domain of IgG heavy chain, an event critical to the proper assembly of heavy and light chains. Specifically, BiP holds unassembled heavy chains until the light chains assemble. In this way, BiP retains unassembled heavy chains and prevents them from prematurely exiting the ER [42]. Kar2p is also responsible for the translocation of newly synthesized protein into the ER lumen through the translocons [45, 46, 47].

Kar2p is one of the most highly expressed proteins along with PDI under stress conditions. It is regulated by three independent *cis*-acting elements on its promoter; an unfolded protein response element (UPRE), a heat shock element (HSE), and a pyrimidine-rich region that is required for the high level of basal expression [47, 49, 50]. Correctly folded secretory proteins are transported from the ER to the Golgi, but misfolded proteins are retained in the ER and form stable complexes with Kar2p and other molecular chaperones[43]. It has been proposed that Kar2p is a trigger for an unfolded protein response (UPR) mechanism to alleviate ER stress caused by an increased accumulation of misfolded and unfolded proteins in the ER. The UPR mechanism in yeast is well studied. UPR is initiated by dimerization of free Ire1p dissociated from the Ire1p-Kar2p complex, in which Kar2p is sequestered by binding to unfolded proteins [48, 49, 51, 52]. The Ire1p as an RNase activates the HAC1 transcription and the transcription factor Hac1p then up-regulates UPR target genes (ER molecular chaperones and folding catalysts) via binding to the regulatory element UPRE [48, 49, 53, 54]for the transport back across the membrane of aberrant polypeptides destined for degradation by the proteasome[55, 56]. Kar2p is also required during a/a cell mating for the stage of karyogamy that involves fusion of the nuclear membranes, the outer of which is contiguous with the ER membrane [57, 58].

The molecular structure of Kar2p consists of a well conserved N-terminal ATPase domain and a C-terminal substrate binding domain [59]. The intrinsic ATPase activity of all HSP70s is very weak. As such co-chaperones (DnaJ protein/HSP40) are needed to stimulate ATP hydrolysis. Kar2p binds to unfolded proteins in an ATP-regulated cycle via the co-chaperone DnaJ protein [60]. The polypeptide binding affinity of the substrate binding domain (SBD) is allosterically modulated by cycles of ATP binding and hydrolysis at the ATPase domain, which mediates the opening and closure of an α-helical lid over the substrate binding cavity [61].ATP-bound Hsp70 has low substrate affinity, with fast rates of peptide binding and release, whereas ADP-bound Hsp70 has high substrate affinity, with stable peptide association. The low intrinsic Hsp70 ATPase activity is stimulated by co-chaperones such as DnaJ proteins (Scj1p), which contain a conserved 70-aa J domain and increased relative ATP hydrolysis rates, and nucleotide exchange factors (Sil1p) that promote ATP/ADP exchange [62].

LHS1 (CER1/SSI1) encodes a non-essential protein with sequence similarity to the HSP70 family of molecular chaperones. Lhs1p localizes to the ER and shares 24% amino acid identity with the other ER HSP70 protein, Kar2p [63]. These two proteins reciprocally regulate each other; the ATPase activity of Lhs1p is stimulated by Kar2p and Lhs1p enhances the rate of Kar2p ATP turnover by providing specific nucleotide exchange [64]. Lhs1p is also involved in protein translocation and folding. LHS1 expression is induced by UPR, where the UPR element present in the LHS1 promoter is responsible for up-regulation of LHS1 expression. It has been reported that lhs1 null mutation leads to a partial block in ER protein translocation and constitutive activation of UPR [65].

HSP40/DnaJ family

Hsp40/DnaJ is a family of proteins that regulates Hsp70 chaperone activity. Hsp40s stimulate the intrinsically weak ATPase activity of Hsp70 family proteins and facilitate Hsp70 interaction with polypeptide substrates. Hsp70 family members often have multiple Hsp40 partners, and these specific pairings govern Hsp70 chaperone involvement in particular processes [66]. All Hsp40s contain a highly conserved 75-amino acid J domain, which interacts with the ATPase domain of Hsp70 to stimulate ATP hydrolysis[66]. However, there are also other conserved structural domains, and based on the presence or absence of these regions, the Hsp40 family can be divided into three subtypes: type I, type II and type III. In *S. cerevisiae,* 22 DnaJ proteins have been reported: DJ1, XDJ1, APJ1, SIS1, DJP1, ZUO1, SWA2, JJJ1, JJJ2, JJJ3,

CAJ1, CWC23, MDJ1, MDJ2, PAM18, JAC1, JID1, SCJ1, HLJ1, JEM1, SEC63, and ERJ5. They are localized in several compartments including the cytosol, mitochondria, ER, and nucleus. Ten DnaJ proteins are localized in the cytosol to assist cytosol HSP70s (Ssa, Ssb, and Ssz) involved in various cellular functions such as protein folding, translation initiation, peroxisome biogenesis, clathrin uncoating, and possibly endosytosis [67]. Five DnaJ proteins are located in mitochondria for mitochondria biogenesis, protein translocation to mitochondria, protein folding, and iron-sulfur cluster assembly [67]. Two nuclear-associated DnaJ proteins function in mRNA splicing [67]. Five DnaJ proteins have been identified in the ER, in which they are participated in protein translocation of secretory proteins to the ER, protein folding, unfolded protein response (UPR), protein degradation via ER-associated degradation (ERAD), and karyogamy. As mentioned previously, the function of J proteins is to stimulate ATPase activity on HSP70 chaperones[68].Scj1p is a type I DnaJ protein that possesses all three domains: the highly conserved J domain, the glycine-phenylalanine rich region, and a zinc finger-like domain. Scj1 is involved in protein folding with Kar2p [61, 62].Jem1p, Erj5p, and Sec63p are type III DnaJ proteins that only possess the J domain. Scj1, Jem1, and Erj5 are UPR-regulated. Jem1p interacts with Kar2p to promote degradation of misfolded proteins via ERAD and also contributes to karyogamy [69, 70].Sec63p-Kar2p associated with the translocon functions as translocation for newly synthesized proteins into the ER [71]. The function of Erj5 has been proposed that it is not essential but involved in protein folding [72].Hlj1p is a type II DnaJ protein and an integral membrane protein that promotes the ER-associated degradation of integral membrane substrates [73].The ER molecular chaperones and folding catalysts are characterized functionally butthe exact folding process in the ER is still poorly understood. It has not been clearly demonstrated how molecular chaperones and folding catalysts specifically cooperate to assist folding. As shown in the oxidative folding of antibody*in vitro*, BiP plays a critical role in the heavy and light chain assembly, where BiP binds to unfolded antibody and keeps the cysteine residues accessible for PDIp. The cooperation of BiP and PDIp provides for the correct assembly of heavy and light chains [74].

The glucose-regulated protein 94 kDa (GRP94) belongs to the HSP90 family and resides in the ER as a chaperone. Unlike the more general chaperone BiP, the role of GRP94 has been described as a specific chaperone that interacts with only a restricted set of proteins (i.e. a herpes-virus glycoprotein [75], apolipoprotein B [76], collagen[77], thyroglobulin[78], immunoglobulins[79]). It seems that GRP94 binds to advanced folding intermediates and incompletely assembled oligomers during protein maturation. GRP94 is constitutively expressed, butsimilarly to BiP, it is induced by ER stress and increased in the presence of unfolded proteins. Moreover, it was found that GRP94 complexes with other molecular chaperones (BiP, ERp72, and GRP170), and functions in a chaperone complex [78]. The yeast homolog of human GRP94 has not been found in any other yeast.

ER Protein Quality Control System

Under normal conditions, secretory proteins are synthesized and folded in the ER, with only correctly folded proteins being transported to the Golgi apparatus through vesicular transport (COPII vesicles) en route to their final destination. However, misfolded and unfolded proteins are retained in the ER by forming a complex with molecular chaperones with their ultimate degradation in the proteosome via retrotranslocation [80]. The ER quality control (ERQC) mechanism is well characterized in the context of glycoprotein folding as shown in Figure 3. The calnexin/calreticulin (CNX/CRT) cycle is a key element in glycoprotein quality control in the ER. That is, *N*-glycans of newly synthesized glycoproteins are processed by the ER glucosidases I (CWH41) and II (ROT2) and the resulting monoglucosylated proteins enter the calnexin/calreticulin (CNX/CRT) cycle where the correctly folded glycoproteins are transported to the Golgi. However, misfolded glycoproteins are retained in the ER and recognized by a folding sensor, UDP-Glucose:glycoprotein glucosyltransferase (UGT1, UGGT1, GT) and subject to the folding cycle [81]. It has been reported that UGGT recognizes not only hydrophobic patches on misfolded glycoproteins, but also the innermost GlcNAc unit of an N-linked oligosaccharide [82, 83]and adds a glucose molecule to the N-linked glycan.

The enzyme uses UDP-Glc as glycosyl donor and it has been reported that this sugar nucleotide is transported from the cytosol to the ER lumen in mammalian cells [84]. Monoglucosylated non-native glycoproteins re-enter the CNX/CRT cycle where membrane-anchored CNX (CNE1 in yeast) or soluble CRT recognize monoglucosylated glycoprotein [85] and interact with an ER thiol oxidoreductase ERp57 that promotes disulfide bond formation of glycoproteins [86, 87]. In addition, it has been proposed that the CNX/CRT also act as molecular chaperones via protein-protein interaction, preventing aggregation of glycoproteins and non-glycoproteins [88].

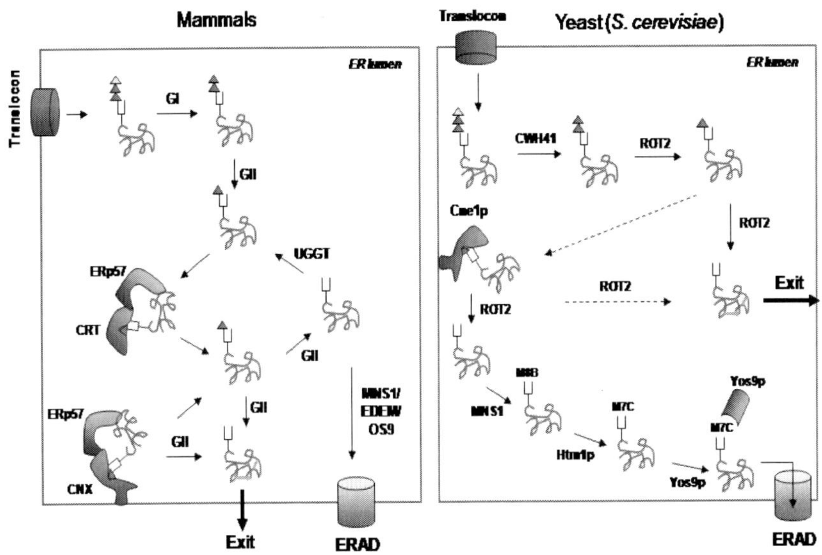

Figure 3. Proposed model for the ER quality control in mammal and S. cerevisiae.GI and CWH41: glucosidase I, GII and ROT2: glucosidase II.

The UGGT activity has been reported in mammalian, insect, protozoan, plant, and fungal (*Mucor rouxii* and *Schizosaccharomyces pombe*) cells. However, UGGT activity has not been detected in *S. cerevisiae*[89]. As such, *S. cerevisiae* lacks the deglucosylation-reglucosylation cycle due to the absence of UGGT [90], calreticulin (CRT) [91], and ERp57. *S. cerevisiae* is known to have only a calnexin-like molecule, Cne1p, which lacks a cytoplasmic tail, and has no calcium-binding capacity. However, the Cnx1p from mammalian cells and *S. pombe* has a cytoplasmic tail and Ca^{2+} binding motif[90]. Cne1p interacts with Glc1Man9GlcNAc2 structure *in vitro*, but it is not essential for the folding of glycoproteins in *S. cerevisiae*[92].In contrast,Cnx1p in *S. pombe* is essential for cell viability, and it is induced in the presence of an accumulation of misfolded glycoproteins [91]. Only Kre5p has high homology to the C-terminal region of UGGT, but it is demonstrated that it does not have UGGT activity. Kre5p is involved in beta-1,6 glucan biosynthesis and is required for the normal vegetative growth of yeast cells [93].Nevertheless, it has been suggested that both calnexin (Cne1p) and monoglucosylated oligosaccharides (Glc1Man9GlcNAc2) generated from Glc3Man9GlcNAc2 by the ER glucosidase I and II are involved in the quality control of glycoprotein folding in *S. cerevisiae* without multiple rounds of folding process via deglucosylation-reglucosylation cycle. Thus, it can be deduced that the folding of glycoprotein should be completed after a single round of Cne1p binding in *S. cerevisiae* [94].It is reasonable that the ER quality control mechanism in *S. cerevisiae* would be quite different from one found in mammalian cells due to lack of UGGT1, ERp57, and CRT (Figure 3).

The CNX/CRT machinery monitors the quality control of glycoprotein folding, and misfolded glycoproteins or non-glycoproteins are retrotranslocated to the cytosol for degradation [80] via the ER associated degradation (ERAD) pathway. It has been demonstrated that ER mannosidase I (MNS1), Htm1p, and Yos9p play key roles in sorting misfolded glycoproteins to the ERAD pathway. The ER Mns1p converts Man9GlcNAc2 to Man8GlcNAc2 (M8B) by trimming a single α-1,2 mannose on the B branch from the N-glycans of misfolded glycoproteins. However, this activity alone is not sufficient to create the ERAD substrate [95, 96]. Subsequently, Htm1p/Mnl1p (EDEM in mammal) interacts with permanently misfolded glycoproteins to generate the ERAD substrate. Htm1p is an α-1,2 specific exomannosidase in the ER that converts Man8GlcNAc2 (M8B) to Man7GlcNAc2 (M7C) by trimming a single α-1,2 Mannose on the C branch of M8B. While Htm1p is not the rate-limiting step in ERAD, deletion of HTM1 reduces the efficiency of the degradation process. It was proposed that the substrate of Htm1p requires a terminal α-1,3 mannose [96]. A recent report indicates that interaction of Pdi1p with the C-terminal domain of Htm1p is essential for the mannosidase activity of Htm1p. This mechanism is believed to occur through Pdi1p catalyzed disulfide bond formation of the N-terminal domain of Htm1p [97]. In addition, it was proposed that stable interaction of Pdi1p with the C-terminal region of Htm1p via disulfide bond formation functions as a reductase for the ERAD substrate [97, 98]. The resulting M7C oligosaccharide is an ERAD substrate signal for ubiquitin-proteosome degradation, where Yos9p (OS-9 in mammal) recognizes the exposed α-1, 6 mannose of M7C [96, 99]. The binding affinity of Yos9p to N-glycans is highest with Man5GlcNAc2 (M5) followed by a group including M8C, M7A, and M6C. However, Glc1Man7GlcNAc2 (G1M7) binds to Yos9p with the lowest affinity, and the binding of M9 or M8B is almost negligible [95, 99]. Yos9p is the ER localized lectin harboring the domain homologous to a mannose 6-phosphate receptor (MRH). Yos9p complex with misfolded glycoprotein is delivered to Hrd3p in the Hrd1complex for proteosomal-mediated degradation [100]. Most ERAD components are up-regulated by UPR to facilitate the degradation of misfolded proteins. ERAD components formmulti-protein complexes on the ER membrane with the ERAD complexes physically interacting with the 26S proteasome in the cytosol. The ERAD system consists of substrate recognition, targeting, retrotranslocation, ubiquitylation and proteasomal degradation. In *S. cerevisiae*, based on localized ERAD substrates, three ERAD systems such as ERAD-lumen (ERAD-L), ERAD-cytosol (ERAD-C), and ERAD-membrane (ERAD-M) are functional to dispose of misfolded proteins. When proteins are misfolded in the ER lumen, they are degraded by the ERAD-L pathway. Similarly, when membrane proteins are misfolded in the membrane spanning domain or the cytosolic domain, they are degraded through the ERAD-M and ERAD-C pathways, respectively [101, 102, 103].It has been described that the ERAD-L pathway comprises Hrd1p (ubiquitin ligase), Hrd3, Der1p, Ubx2p, Usa1p and Ubc/Cue1p (E2 complex). Hrd1p forms a complex with Hrd3p that contains an ER luminal domain with a tetratricopeptide repeat (TPR) motif. Her3p interacts with Yos9p and Kar2p, and recruits misfolded proteins for degradation [104]. Misfolded ERAD-L substrate proteins are retrotranslocated from the ER lumen into the cytosol through Sec61p translocon, where Der1p functions as a component of the translocation channel [105]. Subsequently, misfolded proteins are ubiquitinated and degraded by the proteasome in the cytosol. The ERAD-M pathway is responsible for the degradation of proteins containing misfolded membrane portions that are associated with the ER membrane. The ERAD-M substrates are also transported into the cytosol via the ERAD-M pathway, which contains the Hrd1p/Hrd3p complex but not Der1p and Usa1p [106]. Besides the Hrd1/Her3p complex, additional factors have not been reported in the ERAD-M pathway. The ERAD-C pathway is also required for the degradation of ER membrane proteins with misfolded cytosolic domains, where Doa10p (ubiquitin ligase) is involved, and cytosolic HSP70 and HSP40 chaperones (Ssa1p, Ydj1p, and Hlj1p) were identified with the ERAD-C substrates. Misfolded glycoproteins are directed to the Hrd1p-Hrd3p complex by a Yos9p-mediated route. For the degradation of non glycoproteins via ERAD-L pathway, BiP/Kar2p was identified as a key element in recruiting the ERAD substrates [104]. Molecular chaperones and co-chaperones (Kar2p, Scj1p, Jem1p, Pdi1p, and Eps1p) have also been shown to be associated with the ERAD-L substrates [107].

Peptidyl-Prolyl Isomerases (PPIs)

Peptidyl-prolyl *cis/trans* isomerase (PPIase) enzymes catalyze the *cis-trans* isomerization of peptidyl-prolyl bonds in polypeptides and comprise four structurally unrelated families including a recently identified protein; the cyclophilins (cyclosporin A binding Proteins), FK506-binding proteins (FKBPs), parvulins, and protein phosphatase 2A (PP2A) phosphatase activator (PTPA) [108]. In yeast, PPIases include eight different cyclophilins (Cpr1-Cpr8), four FKBPs (Fpr1-Fpr4), and a single parvulin (Ess1). Four PPIases, Cpr2, Cpr4, Cpr5, and Fpr2, are localized in the secretory pathway with the rest being distributed in the cytosol, mitochondria, and nucleus compartments [109]. Most PPIases that are involved in protein folding contain catalytic domains that have homology to human FKBP12 which are responsible for interacting with unfolded protein [110]. FKBPs have shown that they are highly substrate specific. For example, *in vitro* studies show that human FKBP12 increased isomerization of Phe-Pro by 1,000-fold [111] and Leu-Pro by 12-fold [110], when compared with Glu-Pro. Based on deletion studies to understand the function and role of the PPIs, most of thecyclophilins and FKBPs are not essential and do not affect cell viability [112, 113]. The only exception is Ess1, which is localized in nucleus [114].

It has been reported that Cpr2 and Cpr4 are localized along the secretory pathway, where Cpr4 is localized in vacuole [115]. Cpr5 is a soluble, UPR responsive cyclophilin which harbors an HDEL motif at its C-terminus, presumably to mediate retrograde transport back to the ER [109, 116, 117]. Fpr2, a homolog to human FKBP13, is a 13 kDa membrane-associated protein. Its expression is induced by UPR and heat stress [118]. It was proposed that since most peptide bonds are synthesized in the *trans* isomeric form at the ribosomal stage, the *cis* conformation in peptidyl-prolyl bonds must be acquired during the course of protein folding. There is a relatively large energetic barrier between the *trans* state (lower free energy) and the *cis* state (higher activation energy). As such, the *cis*-to-*trans* conversionis an intrinsically slow reaction that can be a rate-limiting step in protein folding [119, 120].

Unfolded Protein Response (UPR)

The accumulation of misfolded proteins in the ER triggers UPR to alleviate any ER stresses that may disrupt protein folding. The UPR coordinates adaptive responses to these stresses including: the induction of ER resident molecular chaperone and protein foldase expression to increase the protein folding capacity of the ER; induction of phospholipid synthesis; ER expansion; attenuation of general transcription and translation; upregulation of

ER-associated degradation (ERAD) to decrease the unfolded protein load of the ER; and an antioxidant response for detoxification. Upon severe or prolonged ER stress, the UPR induces cell death, or apoptosis, to eliminate unhealthy cells from a population [121].

It has been demonstrated that UPR is initiated via interaction of BiP/Kar2p to unfolded or misfolded proteins which result in Ire1p activation. In an unstressed condition, Ire1p binds to BiP/Kar2p forming an BiP-Ire1p complex. However, upon accumulation of unfolded proteins, BiP/Kar2p release from the BiP-Ire1p complex, leading to Ire1p dimer formation that cascades a signal to the UPR targets through sequential steps. As a ribonuclease (RNase), the active Ire1p and tRNA ligase (Rlg1) process HAC1 mRNA to remove an intron located near the 3' end of the transcript, and enables spliced HAC1 mRNA to be translated into Hac1p, a transcription factor that belongs to the basic leucine zipper (bZIP) family. Hac1p then activates the UPR target genes[122]. Through this Hac1-dependent transcriptional response, UPR increases the folding capacity of the yeast ER and reduces unfolded or misfolded proteins to relieve ER stress.

Under normal growth conditions, IRE1 and HAC1 genes are not essential. However, they are essential for conditions that trigger UPR. Unlike mammalian cells, it has been reported that protein translation is not attenuated under ER stress in yeast cells due to the absence of the PERK pathway, while ER chaperones and the ERAD machinery are induced simultaneously via the UPR due to the absence of ATF6 in yeast [123].

Mammalian cells are able to cope with ER stress in a more sophisticated manner. Mammalian cells possess three functional pathways (IRE1, PERK and ATF6) to alleviate ER stress. These pathways are much more sophisticated than yeast UPR, and are involved in translational and transcriptional control in sequential steps. That is, when unfolded proteins are accumulated in the ER, the existing endogenous ER chaperones participate in the refolding of misfolded proteins without up-regulation of IRE1 and ATF6. However, if misfolded proteins continue to accumulate, the PERK-mediated translational control is shifted to a transcriptional control via the ATF6 pathway. Active ATF6 up-regulates the expression of ER chaperones to refold misfolded proteins. Depending on the presence of unfolded proteins, UPR is terminated or a subsequent UPR pathway, IRE1-XBP1, takes place to target misfolded proteins for degradation. In this case, active XBP1 forms a heterodimer with ATF6 to activate ERAD. Accordingly, the induction of ER chaperones and ERAD cooperate to alleviate ER stresses effectively [123].

In summary, an important functional difference in the UPR system between yeast and mammals is the lack of translational control in yeast. Thus, in the case of overexpression of heterologous protein, yeast continuously synthesizes protein regardless of accumulated misfolded protein, which can be detrimental to the cell. This suggests that the presence of a translational control may provide better control in the folding of aggregation-prone heterologous protein.

Impact of Post-Translation Modifications on Protein Folding

Modification of proteins during transport into the ER can impact protein folding, solubility, and sorting. Post-translational modifications such as *N*-glycosylation and the ability to form disulfide bonds make yeast a good host strain for heterologous proteins. The importance of glycosylation in protein folding, transport, degradation, structure, stability, receptor-recognition, cellular localization, or other biological activities of the glycoproteinshas been demonstrated in a number of cases [124, 125].

In the yeast*S. cerevisiae*, the oligosaccharyltransferase (OST) complex which consists of nine different subunits, co- or post-translationally transfers a lipid-linked precursor dolichol-PP-GlcNAc2Man9Glc3 to an asparagine residue present in a consensus sequon (N-X-S/T, where X is any amino acid except P) on nascent peptides, depending on two different types of translocons on the ER membrane. Among nine subunits, Ost1p, Ost2p, Stt3p, Wbp1p, and Swplp areessential for the viability of the cell. Other subunits, Ost3p, Ost5p, and Ost6p are not essential, but are required for maximal activity of OST [126]. As discussed earlier, yeast contains two functional translocons (Sec61p and Ssh1), and the OST complexes interact with these translocons to enable *N*-glycosylation of newly synthesized proteins. It has been proposed that the OST complex is associated with Sec61 translocon (Sec61p, Sbh1p, and Sss1p) via the Ost3p-Sbh1p interaction, and the Ssh1 translocon (Ssh1p, Sbh2p, and Sss1p) is associated with the OST complex via the Ost6p-Sbh2p interaction [127]. Two different types of translocons determine co- or post-translational translocation of proteins, leading to co- or post-translational glycosylation, respectively. In general, it has been shown that the *N*-glycan occupancy of the glycoproteins produced from yeast is not the same as that of mammalian cells [128]. As a consequence, the portion of unoccupied N-linked sites on proteins may result in potential conformational changes, causing misfolding, decreased solubility, and aggregation[129]. As demonstrated in the mutational analysis of human tripeptidyl-peptidase I (TPP I), human TPP I was misfolded when it was not fully *N*-glycosylated in human embryonic kidney 293 cells [129], suggesting that *N*-glycosylation plays a critical role in protein folding.

In addition to high-mannose type N-glycosylation, yeast*O*-mannosylation is initiated in the ER, where the protein *O*-mannosyltransferase (PMT) gene family transfers Dol-P-mannose to serine or threonine residues of secretory proteins[130]. Yeast *O*-mannosylation has been extensively studied in *S. cerevisiae.* Seven PMT family members (Pmt1p-Pmt7p) have been identified [131]and are divided into three subfamilies: the PMT1, PMT2, and PMT4 subfamily. In *S. cerevisiae* and *C. albicans*, the PMT1 and PMT2 subfamilies are redundant (two or more members of each subfamily) whereas only a single member of the PMT4 subfamily is present [131, 132]. Members of the PMT1 subfamily (Pmt1p andPmt5p) form heterodimeric complexes with members of thePMT2 subfamily (Pmt2p, Pmt3p). The heterodimers, Pmt1p-Pmt2p and Pmt5p-Pmt3p complexes,are formed, and the Pmt1p-Pmt2p complex is responsible for the majority of mannosyl transfer activity. Unlikethe PMT1/PMT2 subfamily members, Pmt4p acts as a homomericcomplex [133]. In *S. cerevisiae*, the PMT family members transfer a single mannose to S/T residues of secretory proteins in the ER and further extension of the *O*-linked mannose residues occurs in the Golgi apparatus by three α1,2-mannosyltrasferases of the KTR family (Kre2p, Ktr1p, and Ktr3p), which catalyze the stepwise addition of α1,2-linked mannose in the medial Golgi compartment. Moreover, phosphomannose is added to *O*-linked glycans by a mannosylphosphate trnasferase (Mnn6p) [134].Further addition of α1,3-linked mannose residues by α1,3-mannosyltrasferases (Mnn1p, Mnt2p, and Mnt3p) takes place in the medial and *trans*-Golgi [135].

In contrast to N-glycosylation, the consensus motif for *O*-mannosylation has not been identified in yeast and higher eukaryotes [136, 137]. However, it has been proposed that *O*-mannosylation is affected by an extended β-turn in the protein secondary structure in higher eukaryotes [138, 139, 140]. In general Thr is more frequently modified than Ser and this is influenced by the neighboring amino acids[141]. In *S. cerevisiae*, it was demonstrated that the substrate specificity for the Pmt1p-Pmt2p complex and Pmt4p is different and therefore they can catalyze *O*-mannosylation on either different regions of a protein or on different target proteins[131, 142]. For instance, the Pmt1p-Pmt2p complex exclusively *O*-mannosylates a subset of proteins such as Aga2p, Bar1p, Kre9p, and Pir2p, whereas the Pmt4p preferentially *O*-mannosylates a group of proteins including Axl2p, Fus1p, Gas1p, and Kex2p. However, other proteins (the WSC family members, Mid2p, and Sccw5p) are

O-mannosylated by two PMT subfamily (Pmt1p-Pmt2p complex and Pmt4p) [142, 143].

It has been proposed that *O*-mannosylation plays a critical role in the control of heterologous protein folding in the ER [144].As shown in the variability of N-glycan occupancy of heterologous protein in yeast, it has been reported that heterologous protein, which is not *O*-glycosylated in higher eukaryotes, can be *O*-mannosylated in yeast [145, 146]. The *O*-mannosylation of heterologous proteins was shown to negatively impact productive protein folding. In an attempt to minimize yeast specific *O*-mannosylation, the addition of a chemical inhibitor of PMT partially suppressed PMT enzymatic activity and increased the secretion of assembled antibody. This study suggests that there is a correlation between abnormal *O*-mannosylation and decreased antibody folding and assembly [144]. In other cases, the inactivation of the *H. polymorpha* PMT1 gene has shown a decrease in aggregation and improvement in human urokinase-typeplasminogen activator secretion, suggesting an enhancement in protein folding by inhibiting *O*-mannosylation [147].Moreover, *O*-linked mannosylation was found in human plasma antithrombin III (pATIII) produced in *P. pastoris*. Unlike native plasma ATIII, *O*-mannosylation reduced the inhibitory activity of recombinant ATIII, indicating suboptimal protein folding due to *O*-glycosylation[148]. In addition to *N*-glycan occupancy, the control of *O*-mannose occupancy may also play a role in the folding of heterologous proteins in yeast. Where *O*-glycosylation has been shown to negatively impact protein folding or activity, its control may prove valuable.

Improvements of Protein Folding

Molecular Chaperone Engineering

In yeast, potential secretion bottlenecks have been identified along the secretory pathway. There have been significant efforts to improve heterologous protein production by engineering transcription of gene of interest, translation, translocation, folding (molecular chaperones), secretory vesicles, sorting, and proteolysis. Protein folding in the ER is recognized as a key rate-limiting step and is highly protein specific. A general control for protein folding is a difficult task because of the complexity of protein folding control mechanisms and the disparate nature of secreted proteins. To date, there is no universal approach to improve protein folding. Several efforts have been made to improve protein folding in the ER using overexpression or deletion of ER molecular chaperones, chemical chaperones, modulation of UPR and ERAD, fusion partners, modification of *O*-mannosylation, and the optimization of process conditions [149].

The unfolded protein response (UPR) is well studied and it is necessary to cope with various stresses for the survival of cells. In the ER, the increase in unfolded and misfolded proteins trigger the UPR to up-regulate the ER molecular chaperones to facilitate protein folding and promote the ERAD pathway to eliminate permanently misfolded proteins. It has been demonstrated that the constitutive up-regulation of the UPR by overexpression of Hac1p can promote folding of heterologous proteins [150].Interestingly, the constitutive expression of *S. cerevisiae* Hac1p in *P. pastoris* has shown to be effective in the up-regulation of UPR and improved Fab secretion[151]. In contrast, inactivation of HAC1 resulted in the reduced secretion of recombinant α-amylase[150].This confirms that up-regulation of UPR contributes to protein folding by increasing the ER folding capacity via overexpression of molecular chaperones and activation of the ERAD system.

The CNX/CRT cycle is known as the ER quality control of mainly glycoproteins, and due to the lack of GT1 in *S. cerevisiae*, it was proposed that the glycoprotein quality control is relatively simpler than one in other eukaryotes harboring UGT1. The overexpression of *H. polymorpha* Cne1p improved secretion of non-glycoproteins as well as glycoproteins, indicating the direct contribution of Cne1p to the protein folding via an increased Cne1p function. In the case of human serum albumin, which is not glycosylated, it is likely that Cne1p functions as a molecular chaperone [152]. In contrast to overexpression of Cne1p, disruption of the CNE1 gene improved secretion of a1-antitrypsin [153]and an unstable lysozyme[154], which suggests that some proteins are not dependent of Cne1p for protein folding.

As a multifunctional protein, Kar2p/BiP plays an important role in protein folding by interacting with the hydrophobic regions of unfolded protein. It is well known that this interaction stabilizes protein and prevent aggregation until it is properly folded. The overexpression of Kar2p/BiP increases availability of BiP required for unfolded proteins, whereas excess BiP may attenuate necessary UPR. As shown in many studies, overexpression of BiP enhanced the secretion of bovine prochymosin [155]and hirudin [156], but had no effect on that of plant thaumatin [157]and actually reduced the expression of β-glucosidase [158]and manganese peroxidase [159].Unlike PDI, overexpression of BiP does not lead to a consistently positive outcome presumably due to the complexity of the biological function of BiP. This could be also explained in part that BiP interaction may depend on the folding kinetics of individual protein, where a slow-folding protein has more interaction with BiP than a fast-folding protein. BiP requires a DnaJ protein and a nucleotide exchange factor to be functional. In some cases, the co-chaperones (Jem1p, Scj1p, Sil1p, Lhs1p) were overexpressed to activate Kar2p function via stimulating ATPase cycle, resulting in overall enhancement of protein folding and secretion with human serum albumin, GM-CSF, and human transferring [160].The co-expression of *S. cerevisiae* Kar2p and Pdi1p synergistically improved G-CSF secretion by 6.5-fold [161].

As shown in Kar2p/BiP studies, an increasing body of evidence suggests that the impact of PDI on the folding of heterologous proteins plays a significant role in protein secretion. Thus, the PDI overexpression has been successfully used for recombinant protein secretion as a good tool. Since PDI is essential, many overexpression studies including yeast Pdi1p and other PDIs and homologs derived other species have been performed to improve protein folding in the presence of endogenous Pdi1p in yeast. Overexpression of yeast or human PDIs resulted in substantial enhancement of secretion of human platelet-derived growth factor, acid phosphatase [162], bovine follicle-stimulating hormone (bFSH) [163]and human serum albumin (HSA) [164], but did not provide benefit in improving secretion of human interleukin-1β [162] and mammalian G-protein-coupled receptors [165].On the other hand, constitutive overexpression of *S. cerevisiae* Pdi1p was reported to improve Fab folding and assembly in *P. pastoris* [166].In another report, the secretion of the *Necator americanus*secretory protein Na-ASP1 showed a strong correlation with increased PDI1 copy number, where *P. pastoris* Pdi1p was overexpressed under the control of the AOX1 promoter. That is, when the gene dosage of Na-ASP1 was increased, more intracellular aggregation was observed. However, as the expression of Pdi1p increased with higher copy number, the secretion of Na-ASP1 increased proportionally. This suggests that the overexpression of a protein of interest saturates the available Pdi1p and the ER folding machinery, which becomes a rate-limiting step in protein secretion [167]. This type of a folding bottleneck was also observed with bovine pancreatic trypsin inhibitor (BPTI) when it was expressed at high levels in *S. cerevisiae*[168].In some cases, co-overexpression of Pdi1p with Kar2p impacted the secretion of recombinant proteins in a synergistic manner. As demonstrated in single-chain antibody fragment (scFv) expression, overexpression of rat Pdip or yeast Kar2p elevated scFv secretion 2.3 and 2.4-fold, respectively, whereas combination of Pdip and Kar2p resulted in 8-fold increase in secretion [169, 170]. The results are in good agreement with *in vitro* studies that showed cooperative function of BiP and PDI [74]. Increasing levels of Pdi1p improved β-glucosidase secretion that is not a disulfide bonded protein, indicating that chaperone activity of Pdi1p possibly contributed to its folding [158]. The chaperone activity of Pdi1p may be protein specific because it did not affect secretion of human interleukin 1 β, a protein that contains no disulfide bonds[171]. The ER oxidase, Ero1p, is known to oxidize Pdi1p and its overexpression is detrimental to the cells due to hyperoxidation of the ER [172]. However, overexpression of Ero1p is beneficial when HSA, a disulfide bond rich protein, is overexpressed. HSA secretion was accelerated and cell growth improved in *K. lactis*[171]. In another example, yeast Ero1p was identified as a key folding enhancer from a yeast cDNA overexpression study, where secretion of a single-chain T-cell receptor (scTCR) was greatly enhanced [173].

Codon Optimization and Protein Folding

It is well established that codon usage influences the rate of protein translation, where the rare codon patches control the protein translation. Some reports indicate that the rare codon cluster plays a functional role in promoting protein folding by introducing translational pausing between functional domains on a nascent polypeptide [174, 175, 176, 177]. It has been known that the rate of protein translation varies depending on the distribution of high frequent codons and rare codons. Thus, codon optimization has been an effective tool for protein expression. The location of rare codon cluster in mRNA is intriguing and it was demonstrated experimentally that rare codon cluster plays a critical role in protein folding as shown in *S. cerevisiae* TRP3 gene. The yeast TRP3 contains ten rare codon clusters between functional domains and with the removal of the translational pause, TRP3 activity was reduced by 1.5 fold. This suggests that translational pause is an important factor for productive folding [178]. In addition, the impact of rare codon clusters on protein folding was observed for a fatty acid binding protein, where replacement of three rare codons with more frequent codons resulted in misfolding [179]. As shown in several cases [180, 181, 182, 183, 184], the location of a rare codon cluster is functionally important in protein folding, thus this should be considered in expression of heterologous proteins when codon optimization is required.

Chemical Chaperones

Chemical chaperones, low-molecular weight compounds, are known to improve protein folding in the ER [185]. The function of chemical chaperones are not fully understood but it has been proposed that chemical chaperones contribute to stabilization of unfolded protein, prevention of intracellular accumulation and aggregation, and modulation of endogenous chaperone activity [185]. Chemical chaperones include 4-phenylbutyrate (PBA) and tauroursodeoxycholic acid (TUDCA), polyols (glycerol, sucrose, sorbitol), DMSO, trimethylamines such as trimethylamine N-oxide (TMAO) and amino acid and derivatives (proline, glycine betaine, trehalose), 6-aminohexanoic acid (6-AH), and hapten. Among the chemical chaperones, 4-PBA and TUDCA are FDA-approved for human treatment to rescue mutant proteins caused by genetic mutation [186]. Glycerol has been reported to facilitate protein folding of the common mutant in cysticfibrosis transmembrane conductance regulator (CFTR) [187]. In yeast, a group of chemical chaperones have been successfully used to improve protein folding in which the activity of several mutants in human cystathionine beta-synthase were enhanced by adding individual glycerol, DMSO, trimethylamine-N-oxide, dimethylsulfoxide, proline or sorbitol to yeast media. Moreover, the combined chemical chaperones have been shown to be more effective than any of the individual chemical chaperones. In this study, it was demonstrated that chemical chaperones are directly involved in protein folding process in the ER [188]. It was found that trehalose suppresses the aggregation of denatured proteins as well as stabilizing proteins during heat shock. Therefore, the resulting unfolded proteins can be refolded by molecular chaperones into properly folded proteins [189]. Another example shows that 10% glycerol in media increased human P-glycoprotein dramatically in yeast [190].Some chemical chaperones are nonspecific, which have a promiscuous effect on various types of proteins, whereas other chemical chaperones have a narrow substrate specificity. As a specific chemical chaperone, the use of the cognate hapten ligand, *p*-nitrophenylphosphocholine(NPPC), led to a marked secretion of anti-phenylphosphocholine antibodies up to 27-fold in transfected PCG1-1 cells. This indicates that the antibody-specific antigen can be possibly used to enhance the folding and assembly of heavy and light chains by co-expressing antigens [191].Chemical chaperones have been successfully used to promote the folding of heterologous proteins, and have potentials in combined application with molecular chaperones.

Other Environmental Factors

Bioprocess conditions (temperature, pH, media composition, and feeding strategy) have a profound impact on the overall heterologous production in yeast by minimizing proteolysis and aggregation, stabilizing protein, and controlling growth rate. However, it is not clear that those process conditions are associated with protein folding in the ER.

It has been demonstrated that temperature has a significant impact on heterologous protein folding and secretion. For instance, the secretion of herring antifreeze protein was substantially increased by lowering the induction temperature from 30°C to 23°C [192], suggesting that the protein folding is favored at the temperature in which the original host species grows rather than the growth temperature of the host yeast. In another case, the culture temperature shift from 37°C to 30°C in *H. polymorpha* reduced aggregation of the human urokinase-type plasminogen activator (uPA) and increased protein secretion by 10-fold, indicating that the control of temperature can be utilized to remove one of the secretion bottlenecks along the secretory pathway [147]. A comprehensive proteomic analysis of the temperature effect on protein secretion in *P. pastoris* indicates that multiple cellular changes contribute synergistically to enhanced protein secretion. It can also be speculated that the lower temperature may decrease protein aggregation by stabilizing heterologous protein [193]. The application of using a lower temperature for folding improvement of heterologous proteins does not seem to be a general strategy, but it could be considered based on the property of protein of interest.

CONCLUSION

Yeast has been an important expression system for the production of heterologous proteins for many years. However, the folding and assembly of heterologous proteins in yeast has been a challenge due to non-native, suboptimal conditions and folding machinery in the ER. Protein folding and maturation is a complicated and controlled process, thus overexpression of a foreign protein can lead to misfolding and aggregation that are resulted from overloading of folding machinery in the ER. The optimization of protein expression is required for productive protein folding. In addition, since protein folding is generally protein specific, the rational engineering of customized folding machinery and ER environment would be indispensable for the enhancement of heterologous protein-specific folding. In addition, yeast ER quality control of glycoproteins via the CNE1 pathway may not be optimal for foreign glycoprotein folding compared with the mammalian CNX/CRT system. The engineering of yeast quality control may provide enhanced quality control that is more optimized for folding of recombinant proteins. With the

ER folding machinery, the UPR is a key element to cope with the ER stresses, and augments the ER folding capacity. However, the yeast UPR pathway lacks a translation control that is required to control the ER overloading when misfolded protein is accumulated. The integration of translation control that lacks in yeast UPR pathway could result in a better controlled folding of recombinant proteins with the transcriptional control of UPR targets that up-regulate the ER chaperones and folding catalysts including induction of ERAD components.

ACKNOWLEDGMENTS

I would like to thank Terrance A. Stadheim for his critical review of this manuscript.

REFERENCES

[1] Chiba, Y., Suzuki, M., Yoshida, S., Yoshida, A., Ikenaga, H., Takeuchi, M., Jigami, Y. and Ichishima, E. (1998). Production of human compatible high mannose-type (Man5GlcNAc2) sugar chains in *Saccharomyces cerevisiae*. *J. Biol. Chem., 273,* 26298-26304.

[2] Choi, B. K., Bobrowicz, P., Davidson, R. C., Hamilton, S. H , Kung, D. H, Li, H., Miele, R. G, Nett, J. H., Wildt, S. and Gerngross, T. U. (2003). Use of combinatorial genetic libraries to humanize N-linked glycosylation in the yeast. *Pichia pastoris*. *Proc. Natl. Acad. Sci. USA, 100*, 502-5027.

[3] Hamilton, S. R., Bobrowicz, P., Bobrowicz, B., Davidson, R. C, Li, H., Mitchell, T., Nett, J. H., Sebastian Rausch, Terrance A. Stadheim, Wischnewski, H., Wildt, S. andGerngross, T. U. (2003). Yeast Production of Complex Human Glycoproteins in Yeast. *Science*, *301,* 244-246.

[4] Bobrowicz, P., Davidson, R. C., Li, H., Potgieter, T. I., Nett, J. H., Hamilton, S. R., Stadheim, T. A., R, Miele, R. G., Bobrowicz, B., Mitchell, T., Rausch, S., Renfer, E. and Wildt, S. (2004). Engineering of an artificial glycosylation pathway blocked in core oligosaccharide assembly in the yeast*Pichia pastoris*: production of complex humanized glycoproteins with terminal galactose. *Glycobiology, 14,* 757-766.

[5] Hamilton, S. R., Davidson, R. C., Sethuraman, N., Nett, J. H., Jiang, Y., Sandra Rios, Bobrowicz, P., Stadheim, T. A., Li, H., Choi, B. K., Hopkins, D., Wischnewski, H., Roser, J., Mitchell, T., Strawbridge, R. R., Hoopes, J., Wildt, S. andGerngross, T. U. (2006). Humanization of Yeast to Produce Complex Terminally Sialylated Glycoproteins. *Science, 313,* 1441-1443.

[6] Kuroda, K., Kobayashi, K., Tsumura, H., Komeda, T., Chiba, Y. and Jigami, Y. (2006). Production of Man5GlcNAc2- type sugar chain by the methylotrophic yeast*Ogataeaminuta*. *FEMS Yeast Res., 6,* 1052-1062.

[7] Li, H., Sethuraman, N., Stadheim, T. A., Zha, D., Prinz, B., Ballew, N., Bobrowicz, P., Choi, B. K, Cook, W. J., Cukan, M., Houston-Cummings, N. R., Davidson, R., Gong, B., Hamilton, S. R., Hoopes, J. P., Jiang, Y., Kim, N., Mansfield, R., Nett, J. H., Rios, S., Strawbridge, R., Wildt. S.and Gerngross, T. U. (2006). Optimization of humanized IgGs in glycoengineering *Pichia pastoris*. *Nature Biotech., 24*, 210-215.

[8] Lin Cereghino J. L. andCregg J. M. (2000). Heterologous protein expression in the methylotrophic yeast*Pichia pastoris*. *FEMS Microbiol. Rev., 24,* 45-66.

[9] Schmidt, F. R. (2004). Recombinant expression systems in the pharmaceutical industry. *Appl. Microbiol. Biotechnol.,65,* 363-372.

[10] Rader, R. A. (2007). *Biopharmaceutical products in the US and European markets*. 6th Edition. Rockville,M.D.: BioPlan Associates Inc.

[11] Werten, M. W., Bosch, T. J. van den, Wind, R.D., Mooibroek, H. and Wolf, F. A. de (1999). High-yield secretion of recombinant gelatins by *Pichia pastoris*. *Yeast, 15,* 1087-1096.

[12] Park, E. H., Shin, Y. M., Lim, Y. Y., Kwon, T. H., Kim, D. H. and Yang, M. S. (2000). Expression of glucose oxidase by using recombinant yeast. *J. Biotechnol., 81,* 35-44.

[13] Fleer, R., Yeh, P., Amellal, N., Maury, I., Fournier, A., Bacchetta, F., Baduel, P., Jung, G., L'HôteH. and Becquart, J. (1991b). Stable multicopy vectors for high level secretion of recombinant human serum albumin by *Kluyveromyces lactis*. *Bio/technology, 9,* 968-975.

[14] Mayer, A. F., Hellmuth, K., Schlieker, H., Lopez-Ulibarri, R., Oertel, S., Dahlems, U., Strasser, A. W. M. and van Loon, A. P. (1999). An expression system matures: a highly efficient and cost-effective process for phytase production by recombinant strains of *Hansenula polymorpha*. *Biotechnol. Bioeng., 63,* 373-381.

[15] Anfinsen, C. B. (1972). The formation and stabilization of protein structure. *Biochem. J., 128,* 737-749.

[16] Anfinsen, C. B. (1973). Principles that govern the folding of protein chains. *Science,181,* 223-230.

[17] Ng, D. T. W., Brown, J. D., and Walter, P. (1996). Signal Sequences Specify the Targeting Routeto the Endoplasmic Reticulum Membrane. *J. Cell Biol. 134,* 269-278.

[18] Rapoport, T. A., Jungnickel, B. and Kutay, U. (1996). Protein transport across the eukaryotic endoplasmic reticulum and bacterial inner membranes. *Annu. Rev. Biochem.,65,* 271-303.

[19] Meunier, L., Usherwood, Y. K., Chung, K. T., andHendershot, L. M. (2002). A Subset of Chaperones and Folding Enzymes FormMultiprotein Complexes in Endoplasmic Reticulum toBind Nascent Proteins. *Mol. Biol. Cell, 13,* 4456-4469.

[20] Ferrari, D. and Söling, H. D. (1999). The protein disulphide-isomerase family: unravelling a string of folds. *Biochem. J., 339,* 1-10.

[21] Gillece, P., Luz, J. M., Lennarz, W. J., de la Cruz, F. J. and Romisch, K. (1999). Export of a cysteine-free misfolded secretory protein from the endoplasmic reticulum for degradation requires interaction with protein disulfide isomerase. *J. Cell Biol., 147,* 1443-1456.

[22] Hatahet. F. and Ruddock, L. W. (2009). Protein Disulfide Isomerase: A Critical Evaluationof its Function in Disulfide Bond Formation. *Antioxid. Redox Signal., 11,* 2807-2850.

[23] Tian, G., Xiang, S., Noiva, R., Lennarz, W. J., and Schindelin, H. (2006). The Crystal Structure of Yeast Protein Disulfide Isomerase Suggests Cooperativity between Its Active Sites. *Cell, 124,* 61-73.

[24] Tachibana, C. and Stevens, T. H. (1992). The yeast EUG1 gene encodes an endoplasmic reticulum protein that is functionally related to protein disulfide isomerase. *Mol. Cell. Biol., 12,* 4601-4611.

[25] Kimura, T., Hosoda, Y., Kitamura, Y., Nakamura, H.,Horibe, T. and Kikuchi, M. (2004). Functional differences between human and yeast proteindisulfide isomerase family proteins. *Biochem. Biophys. Res. Commun., 320,* 359-365.

[26] Nørgaard, P., Westphal, V., Tachibana, C., Alsøe, L., Holst, B. and Winther, J. R.(2001). Functional Differences in Yeast Protein Disulfide Isomerases. *J. Cell Biol., 152,* 553-562.

[27] Wang, Q. and Chang, A. (2003). Substrate recognition in ER-associated degradation mediated by Eps1, a member of the protein disulfide isomerase family. *EMBO J., 22,* 3792-3802.

[28] Frand, A. R. and Kaiser, C. A. (1999). Ero1p oxidizes protein disulfide isomerase in a pathway for disulfide bond formation in the endoplasmic reticulum. *Mol. Cell., 4,* 469-477.

[29] Tu, B. P., Ho-Schleyer, S. C., Travers, K. J. and Weissman, J. S. (2000). Biochemical basis of oxidative protein folding in the endoplasmic reticulum. *Science, 290,* 1571-1574.

[30] Sevier, C. S. and Kaiser, C. A. (2002). Formation and transfer of disulphide bonds in living cells. *Nature Rev.Mol. Cell Biol., 3,* 836-847.

[31] Sevier, C. S., Cuozzo, J. W., Vala, A., Aslund, F. and Kaiser, C. A. (2001). A flavoprotein oxidase defines a new endoplasmic reticulum pathway for biosynthetic disulphide bond formation. *Nature Cell Biol., 3,* 874-882.

[32] Lisowsky, T. (1992). Dual function of a new nuclear gene for oxidative phosphorylation and vegetative growth in yeast. *Mol. Gen. Genet., 232,* 58-64.

[33] Thorpe, C., Hoober, K. L., Raje, S., Glynn, N. M., Burnside, J., Turi, G. K. and Coppock, D. L. (2002). Sulfhydryl oxidases: emerging catalysts of protein disulfide bond formation in eukaryotes. *Arch. Biochem. Biophys., 405,* 1-12.

[34] Hwang, C., Sinskey, A. J. and Lodish, H. F. (1992). Oxidized redox state of glutathione in the endoplasmic reticulum. *Science, 257,*1496-1502.

[35] Cuozzo, J. W. and Kaiser, C. A. (1999). Competition between glutathione and protein thiols for disulphide-bond formation. *Nat. Cell Biol., 1,* 130-135.

[36] Suh, J. K., Poulsen, L. L., Ziegler, D. M. and Robertus, J. D. (1996). Molecular Cloning and Kinetic Characterization of a Flavin-Containing Monooxygenase from *Saccharomyces cerevisiae. Arch. Biochem. Biophys., 336,*268-274.

[37] Suh, J. K., Poulsen, L. L., Ziegler, D. M. and Robertus, J. D. (1999). Yeast flavin-containing monooxygenase generates oxidizing equivalents that control protein folding in the endoplasmic reticulum. *Proc. Natl. Acad. Sci. USA, 96,*2687-2691.

[38] Suh, J. K. and Robertus, J. D. (2000). Yeast flavin-containing monooxygenase is induced by the unfolded protein response. *Proc. Natl. Acad. Sci. USA, 97,* 121-126.

[39] Werner-Washburne, M, Stone, D. E. and Craig, E. A. (1987).Complex interactions among members of an essential subfamily of hsp70 genes in *Saccharomyces cerevisiae. Mol. Cell Biol.7,* 2568-77.

[40] Vogel, J. P., Misra, L. M., and Rose, M. D. (1990). Loss of BiP/GRP78 function blocks translocation of secretory proteins in yeast. *J. Cell Biol., 110,* 1885-1895.

[41] Te Heesen, S. and Aebi, M. (1994). The genetic interaction of kar2 and wbp1 mutations. Distinct functions of binding protein BiP and N-linked glycosylation in the processing pathway of secreted proteins in *Saccharomyces cerevisiae. Eur. J. Biochem., 222,* 631-637.

[42] Simons, J. F., Ferro-Novick, S., Rose, M. D. and Helenius, A. (1995). BiP/Kar2p serves as a molecular chaperone during carboxypeptidase Y folding in yeast. *J. Cell Biol., 130,* 41-49.

[43] Gething, M. J. and Sambrook, J. F. (1992). Protein folding in the cell. *Nature, 355,* 33-45.

[44] Hendershot, L., Bole, D., Köhler, G. and Kearney, J. F. (1987). Assembly and Secretion of Heavy Chains that Do Not Associate Posttranslationally with Immunoglobulin Heavy Chain-binding Protein. *J. Cell Biol, 104,* 761-767.

[45] Young, B. P., Craven, R. A., Reid, P. J., Willer, M. and Stirling, C. J. (2001). Sec63p and Kar2p are required for the translocation of SRP-dependent precursors into the yeast endoplasmic reticulum in vivo. *EMBO J., 20,* 262-271.

[46] Corsi, A. K., Schekman, R. (1997). The lumenal domain of Sec63p stimulates the ATPase activity of BiP and mediates BiP recruitment to the translocation in *Saccharomyces cerevisiae. J. CellBiol., 137,* 1483-1493.

[47] McClellan, A. J., Endres, J. B., Vogel, J. P., Palazzi, D., Rose, M. D. and Brodsky, J. L. (1998). Specific molecular chaperone interactions and an ATP-dependent conformational change are required during post-translational protein translocation into the yeastER. *Mol. Biol. Cell, 9,* 3533-3545.

[48] Mori, K., Sant, A., Kohno, K., Normington, K, Gething, M. J. and Sambrook, J. F. (1992). A 22-bp cis-acting element is necessary and sufficient for the induction of the yeastKAR2 (BiP) gene by unfolded proteins. *EMBO J., 11,* 2583-2593.

[49] Kohno, K., Normington, K., Sambrook, J., Gething, M. J. and Mori, K. (1993). The promoter region of the yeastKAR2/BiP.gene contains a regulatory domain that responds to the presence of unfolded proteins in the endoplasmic reticulum. *Mol. Cell Biol., 13,* 877-890.

[50] Mori, K., Ogawa, N., Kawahara, T., Yanagi, H. and Yura, T. (1998). Palindrome with spacer of one nucleotide is characteristic of the cis-

acting unfolded protein response element in *Saccharomycescerevisiae. J. Biol. Chem., 730,* 9912-9920.

[51] Okamura, K., Kimata, Higashio, Y. H., Tsuru, A. and Kohno, K.. (2000). Dissociation of Kar2p/BiP from an ER sensory molecule, Ire1p, triggers the unfolded protein response in yeast. *Biochem. Biophys. Res. Commun., 279,* 445-450.

[52] Kimata, Y., Oikawa, D., Shimizu, Y., Ishiwata-Kimata, Y. and Kohno, K. (2004). A role for BiP as an adjustor for the endoplasmic reticulum stress-sensing protein Ire1. *J. Cell Biol., 167,* 445-456.

[53] Cox, J. S. and Walter, P. (1996). A novel mechanism for regulatingactivity of a transcription factor that controls the unfolded protein response. *Cell, 87,*391-404.

[54] Mori, K., Kawahara, T., Yoshida, H., Yanagi, H. and Yura, T. (1996). Signalling from endoplasmic reticulum to nucleus: Transcription factor with a basic-leucine zipper motif is required for the unfolded protein-response pathway. *Genes Cells, 1,*803-817.

[55] Plemper, R. K., Bohmler, S., Bordallo, J., Sommer, T. and Wolf, D. H. (1997). Mutant analysis links the translocon and BiP to retrograde protein transport for ER degradation. *Nature, 388,* 891-895.

[56] Brodsky, J. L., Werner, E. D., Dubas, M. E., Goeckeler, J. L., Kruse, K. B. and McCracken, A. A. (1999). The requirement for molecular chaperones during endoplasmic reticulum-associated protein degradation demonstrates that protein export and import are mechanistically distinct. *J. Biol. Chem., 274,* 3453-3460.

[57] Rose, M. D., Misra, L. M. and Vogel, J. P. (1989). KAR2, a karyogamy gene, is the yeast homologue of mammalian BiP/GRP78. *Cell, 57,* 1211-1221.

[58] Ng, D. T. W. and Walter, P. (1996). ER membrane protein complex required for nuclear fusion. *J. Cell Biol., 132,* 499-509.

[59] McKay, D. B. (1993). Structure and mechanism of 70-kDa heatshock-related proteins. *Adv. Prot. Chem., 44,* 67-80.

[60] Schlenstedt, G., Harris, S., Risse, B., Lill, R. and Silver, P. A. (1995). A yeast DnaJ homologue, Scj1p, can function in the endoplasmic reticulum with BiP/Kar2p via a conserved domain that specifies interactions with Hsp70s. *J. Cell Biol., 129,* 979-988.

[61] Zhu, X., Zhao, X., Burkholder, W. F., Gragerov, Ogata, C. M., Gottesman, M. E. and Hendrickson, W. A. (1996). Structural Analysis of Substrate Binding by the Molecular Chaperone DnaK. *Science, 272,* 1606-1614.

[62] Silberstein, S., Schlenstedt, G., Silver, P. A. and Gilmore, R. (1998). A role for the DnaJ homologue Scj1p in protein folding in the yeast endoplasmic reticulum. *J. Cell Biol., 143,* 921-933.

[63] Baxter, B. K., James, P., Evans., T. and Craig, E. A. (1996). *SSI1* Encodes a Novel Hsp70 of the *Saccharomyces cerevisiae* Endoplasmic Reticulum. *Mol. Cell. Biol., 16,* 6444-6456.

[64] Craven, R. A., Egerton, M. and Stirling, C. J. (1996).A novel Hsp70 of the yeast ER lumen is required for the efficient translocation of a number of protein precursors. *EMBO J.,15*, 2640-2650.

[65] Bukau, B. and Horwich, A. L. (1998).The Hsp70 and Hsp60 chaperone machines. *Cell*, *92*, 351-66.

[66] Qiu X. B., Shao, Y. M., Miao, S. and Wang, L. (2006.) The diversity of the DnaJ/Hsp40 family, the crucial partners for Hsp70 chaperones. *Cell Mol. Life Sci.,* 63, 2560-2570.

[67] Walsh, P., Bursac, D., Law, Y. C., Cyr, D. and Lithgow, T. (2004). The J-protein family: modulating protein assembly, disassembly and translocation. *EMBO J.,* 5, 567-571.

[68] Greene, M. K., Maskos, K. and Landry, S. J. (1998). Role of the J-domain in the cooperation of Hsp40 with Hsp70. *Proc. Natl. Acad. Sci. USA, 95,*6108-6113.

[69] Nishikawa, S. and Endo, T. (1997). The yeast Jem1p is a DnaJ-like protein of the endoplasmic reticulum membrane required for nuclear fusion. *J. Biol. Chem., 272,*12889-12892.

[70] Nishikawa, S., Terazawa, Y., Nakayama, T., Hirata, A., Makio, T. and Endo, T. (2003). Nep98p is a component of the yeast spindle pole body and essential for nuclear division and fusion. *J. Biol. Chem., 278,*9938-9943.

[71] Corsi, A. K. and Schekman, R. (1997). The lumenal domain of Sec63p stimulates the ATPase activity of BiP and mediates BiP recruitment to the translocon in*Saccharomyces cerevisiae*. J. *Cell Biol., 137,*1483-1493.

[72] Famá, M. C., Raden, D., Zacchi, N., Lemos, D. R., Robinson, A. S. and Silberstein, S. (2007). The *Saccharomyces cerevisiae* YFR041C/ERJ5 gene encoding a type I membrane protein with a J domain is required to preserve the foldingcapacity of the endoplasmic reticulum. *Biochim Biophys Acta, 1773,* 232-242.

[73] Beilharz, T., Egan, B., Silver, P. A., Hofmann, K. and Lithgow, T. (2003). Bipartite signals mediate subcellular targeting of tail-anchored membrane proteins in *Saccharomyces cerevisiae. J. Biol. Chem., 278,* 8219-8223.

[74] Mayer, M., Kies, U., Kammermeier, R. and Buchner, J. (2000). BiP and PDI cooperate in the oxidative folding of antibodies in vitro. *J. Biol. Chem. 275,* 29421-29425.

[75] Ramakrishnan, M., Tugizov, S., Pereira, L. and Lee, A. S. (1995). Conformation-defective herpes simplex virus 1 glycoprotein B activates the promoter of the grp94 gene that codes for the 94-kD stress protein in the endoplasmic reticulum. *DNA Cell Biol., 14,* 373-384.

[76] Linnik, K. M. and Herscovitz, H. (1998). Multiple molecular chaperones interact with apolipoprotein B during its maturation. The network of endoplasmic reticulum-resident chaperones (ERp72, GRP94, calreticulin, and BiP) interacts with apolipoprotein b regardless of its lipidation state. *J. Biol. Chem., 273,* 21368-21373.

[77] Ferreira, L. R., Norris, K., Smith, T., Hebert, C. and Sauk, J. J. (1994). Association of Hsp47, Grp78, and Grp94 with procollagen supports the successive or coupled action of molecular chaperones. *J. Cell Biochem., 56,* 518-526.

[78] Kuznetsov, G., Chen, L. B. and Nigam, S. K. (1997). Multiple Molecular Chaperones Complex with Misfolded Large Oligomeric Glycoproteins in the Endoplasmic Reticulum. *J. Biol. Chem., 272,* 3057-3063.

[79] Melnick, J., Dul, J. L. and Argon, Y. (1994). Sequential interaction of the chaperones BiP and GRP94 with immunoglobulin chains in the endoplasmic reticulum. *Nature, 370,* 373-375.

[80] Tsai, B., Ye, Y. and Rapoport, T. A. (2002). Retro-translocation of proteins from the endoplasmic reticulum into cytosol. *Nat. Rev. Mol. Cell Biol., 3,* 246-255.

[81] Taylor, S. C., Thibault, P., Tessier, D. C., Bergeron, J. J. M. and Thomas, D. Y. (2003). Glycopeptide specificity of the secretory protein folding sensor UDP-glucose glycoprotein:glucosyltransferase. *EMBO Rep., 4,* 405-411.

[82] Sousa, M. and Parodi, A. J. (1995). The molecular basis for the recognition of misfolded glycoproteins by the UDP-Glc:glycoprotein glucosyltransferase. *EMBO J. 14,* 4196-4203.

[83] Caramelo, J. J., Castro, O. A., Alonso, L. A., de Prat-Gay, G. and Parodi, A. J. (2003). UDP-Glc:glycoprotein glucosyltransferase recognizes structured and solvent accessible hydrophobic patches in molten globule-like folding intermediates. *Proc. Natl. Acad. Sci. USA,100,* 86-91.

[84] Perez, M. and Hirschberg, C. B. (1986). Topography of glycosylation reactions in the rough endoplasmic reticulum membrane. *J. Biol. Chem., 261,* 6822-6830.

[85] Hebert, D. N., Foellmer, B. and Helenius, A. (1995). Glucose trimming and reglucosylation determine glycoprotein association with calnexin in the endoplasmic reticulum. *Cell, 81,* 425-433.

[86] Oliver, J. D., Roderick, H. L., Llewellyn, D. H. and High, S. (1999). ERp57 functions as a subunit of specific complexes formed with the ER lectins calreticulin and calnexin. *Mol. Biol. Cell., 10,* 2573-2582.

[87] Frickel, E. M., Frei, P., Bouvier, M., Stafford, W. F., Helenius, A., Glockshuber, R. and Ellgaard, L. (2004). ERp57 is a multifunctional thioldisulfide oxidoreductase. *J. Biol. Chem., 279,* 18277-18287.

[88] Ware, F. E., Vassilakos, A., Peterson, P. A., Jackson, M. R., Lehrman, M. A. and Williams, D. B. (1995). The molecular chaperone calnexin binds Glc1Man9GlcNAc2 oligosaccharide as an initial step in recognizing unfolded glycoproteins.*J. Biol. Chem., 270,* 4697-4704.

[89] Parodi, A. J. (1999). Reglucosylation of glycoproteins and quality control of glycoprotein folding in the endoplasmic reticulum of yeast cells. *Biochimica et Biophysica Acta, 1426,* 287-295.

[90] Fernändez, F., Trombetta, S. E., Hellman, U. and Parodi, A. J. (1994). Purification to homogeneity of UDP-glucose: glycoprotein glucosyltransferase from *Schizosaccharomyces pombe* and apparent absence of the enzyme from *Saccharomyces cerevisiae. J. Biol. Chem., 269,* 30701-30706.

[91] Parlati, F., Dignard, D., Bergeron, J. J. M. and Thomas, D. Y. (1995). The calnexin homologue cnx1+ in *Schizosaccharomyces pombe*, is an essential gene which can be complemented by its soluble ER domain.*EMBO J., 14,* 3064-3072.

[92] Xu, X., Kanbara, K., Azakami, H. and Kato, A. (2004).Expression and Characterization of Saccharomyces cerevisiae Cne1p, a Calnexin Homologue. *J. Biochem.* 135, 615-618.

[93] Meaden, P., Hill, H., Wagner, J., Slipetz, D., Sommer, S. S. and Bussey, H. (1990). The Yeast KRE5 Gene Encodes a Probable Endoplasmic Reticulum Protein Required for (1 >6)-13-D-Glucan Synthesis and Normal Cell Growth. *Mol. Cell. Biol., 10,* 3013-3019.

[94] Solda, T., Galli, C., Kaufman, R. J. and Molinari, M. (2007). Substrate-specific requirements for UGT1-dependent release from calnexin. *Mol. Cell, 27,* 238-249.

[95] Quan, E. M., Kamiya, Y., Kamiya, D., Denic, V., Weibezahn, J., Kato, K. and Weissman, J. S. (2008). Defining the glycan destruction signal for endoplasmic reticulum-associated degradation. *Mol. Cell, 32,* 870-877.

[96] Clerc, S., Hirsch, C., Oggier, D. M., Deprez, P., Jakob, C., Sommer, T. and Aebi, M. (2009). Htm1 protein generates the N-glycan signal for glycoprotein degradation in the endoplasmic reticulum. *J. Cell Biol., 184,* 159-172.

[97] Sakoh-Nakatogawa,M., Nishikawa, S. and Endo, T. (2009). Roles of Protein-disulfide Isomerase-mediated Disulfide Bond Formation of Yeast Mnl1p in Endoplasmic Reticulum-associated Degradation. *J. Biol. Chem., 284,* 11815-11825.

[98] Gillece, P., Luz, J. M., Lennarz, W., de la Cruz, F. J. and Römisch. K. (1999). Export of a cysteine-free misfolded secretory protein from the endoplasmic reticulum for degradation requires interaction with protein disulfide isomerase. *J. Cell Biol., 147,* 1443-1456.

[99] Jakob, C. A., Burda, P., Roth, J. and Aebi, M. (1998). Degradation of misfolded endoplasmic reticulum glycoproteins in *Saccharomyces cerevisiae* is determined by a specific oligosaccharide structure. *J. Cell Biol., 142*, 1223-1233.

[100] Gauss , R., E. Jarosch, T. Sommer, and Hirsch. C. (2006a). A complex of Yos9p and the HRD ligase integrates endoplasmic reticulum quality control into the degradation machinery. *Nat. Cell Biol.,* 8, 849 - 854.

[101] Bonifacino, J. S., Suzuki, C. K. and Klausner, R. D. (1990). A peptide sequence confers retention and rapid degradation in the endoplasmic reticulum. *Science, 247,* 79 - 82.

[102] Taxis, C., Hitt, R., Park, S. H., Deak, P. M., Kostova, Z. and Wolf, D. H. (2003). Use of modular substrates demonstrates mechanistic diversity and reveals differences in chaperone requirement of ERAD. *J. Biol. Chem., 278,* 35903 - 35913.

[103] Vashist, S. and Ng, D. T. (2004). Misfolded proteins are sorted by a sequentialcheckpoint mechanism of ER quality control. *J. Cell Biol.,* 165, 41 - 52.

[104] Hoseki, J., Ushioda, R. and Nagata, K. (2010). Mechanism and components of endoplasmic reticulum associated Degradation. *J. Biochem., 147,* 19-25.

[105] Scott, D. C. and Schekman, R. (2008). Role of Sec61p in the ER-associated degradation of short-lived transmembrane proteins. *J. Cell Biol., 181,* 1095-1105.

[106] Carvalho, P., Goder, V. and Rapoport, T. A. (2006). Distinct ubiquitin-ligase complexes define convergent pathways for the degradation of ER proteins. *Cell, 126,* 361-373.

[107] Nakatsukasa, K. and Brodsky, J. L. (2008). The Recognition and Retrotranslocation of Misfolded Proteins from the Endoplasmic Reticulum. *Traffic, 9,* 861-870.

[108] Magnusdottir, A., Stenmark, P., Flodin, S., Nyman, T., Hammarström, M., Ehn, M., Bakali, H. M. A., Berglund, H. and Nordlund, P. (2006). The Crystal Structure of a Human PP2A Phosphatase Activator Reveals a Novel Fold and Highly Conserved Cleft Implicated in Protein-Protein Interactions. *J. Biol. Chem., 281,* 22434-22438.

[109] Pemberton, T. J. and Kay, J. E. (2005). Identification and comparative analysis of the peptidyl-prolyl *cis/trans* isomerase repertoires of *H. sapiens, D. melanogaster,C. elegans, S. cerevisiae and Sz. pombe. Comp. Funct. Genom., 6,* 277-300.

[110] Jakoba, R. P., Zoldáka, G., Aumüllerb, T. and Schmid, F. X. (2009). Chaperone domains convert prolyl isomerases into generic catalysts of protein folding. *Proc. Natl. Acad. Sci. USA, 106,* 20282-20287.

[111] Harrison, R. K. and Stein, R. L. (1990). Substrate specificities of the peptidyl prolyl cis-trans isomerase activities of cyclophilin and FK-506 binding protein: evidence for the existence of a family of distinct enzymes. *Biochemistry,29,* 3813-3816.

[112] Dolinski, K., Muir, S., Cardenas, M., Heitman, J. (1997a). All cyclophilins and FK506 binding proteins are, individually and collectively, dispensable for viability in *Saccharomycescerevisiae. Proc. Natl. Acad. Sci. USA,94,* 13093-13098.

[113] Hemenway, C. and Heitman J. (1993). Proline isomerases in microorganisms and small eukaryotes. *Ann. N.Y. Acad. Sci. 696,* 38-46.

[114] Hanes, S. D., Shank, P. R. and Bostian, K. A. (1989). Sequence and mutational analysis of ESS1, a gene essential for growth in *Saccharomyces cerevisiae. Yeast,5,* 55-72.

[115] Huh, W. K., Falvo, J. V., Gerke, L. C., Carroll, A. S., Howson, R. W., Weissman, J. S. and O'shea, E. K. (2003). Global analysis of protein localization in budding yeast. *Nature, 425,* 686-869.

[116] Frigerio, G. and Pelham, H. R. (1993). A *Saccharomyces cerevisiae* cyclophilin resident in the endoplasmic reticulum. *J. Mol. Biol.,233,*183-188.

[117] Kumar, A., Agarwal, S., Heyman, J. A., Matson, S., Heidtman, M., Piccirillo, S., Umansky, L., Drawid, A., Jansen, R., Liu, Y., Cheung, K.

H., Miller, P., Gerstein, M., Roeder, G. S. and Snyder, M. (2002). Subcellular localization of the yeast proteome. *Genes Dev., 16,* 707-719.

[118] Partaledis, J. and Berlin, V. (1993). The *FKB2* gene of *Saccharomyces cerevisiae*, encoding the immunosuppressant- binding protein FKBP-13, is regulated in response to accumulation of unfolded proteins in the endoplasmic reticulum. *Proc. Natl. Acad. Sci. USA, 90,* 5450-5454.

[119] Schmid, F. X., Mayr, L. M., Mucke, M. and Schonbrunner, E. R. (1993). Prolyl isomerases: role in protein folding. *Adv. Protein Chem.,44,* 25-66.

[120] Lu, K. P., Finn, G., Lee, T. H. and Nicholson, L. K. (2007). Prolyl *cis-trans* isomerization as a molecular Timer. *Nature chem. Biol., 3,* 619-629.

[121] Schröder, M. (2006). The Unfolded Protein Response. *Mol. Biotch., 34,* 279-290.

[122] Korennykh, A. V., Egea1, P. F., Korostelev, A. A., Finer-Moore, J., Zhang, C., Shokat, K. M., Stroud, R. M. and Walter, P.(2009). The unfolded protein response signals through high-order assembly of Ire1. *Nature, 457,* 687-693.

[123] Mori , K. (2009). Signalling Pathways in the Unfolded Protein Response: Development from Yeast to Mammals. *J. Biochem., 146,* 743-750.

[124] Helenius, A. and Aebi, M. (2001). Intracellular functions of N-linked glycans. *Science, 291,* 2364-2369.

[125] Mitra, N., Sinha, S., Ramya, T. N. C. and Surolia, A. (2006) N-linked oligosaccharides as outfitters for glycoprotein folding form and function. *Trends Biochem. Sci., 31,* 156-163.

[126] Knauer, R. and Lehle, L. (1999b). The oligosaccharyltransferase complex from yeast. *Biochim. Biophys. Acta, 1426,* 259-273.

[127] Yan, A. and Lennarz, W. J. (2005). Two oligosaccharyl transferase complexes exist in yeast and associate with two different translocons. *Glycobiology, 15,* 1407-1415.

[128] Choi, B. K., Actor, J. K., Rios, S. d'Anjou, M., Terrance A. Stadheim, T. A., Warburton, S., Giaccone, E., Cukan, M., Li, H., Kull, A., Sharkey, N., Gollnick, P., Kocięba, M., Artym, J., Zimecki, M., Kruzel, M. L. and Wildt, S. (2008). Recombinant human lactoferrin expressed in glycoengineered Pichia pastoris: effect of terminal N-acetylneuraminic acid on in vitro secondary humoral immune response. *Glycoconj. J., 25,* 581-593.

[129] Wujek, P., Kida, E., Walus, M., Wisniewski, K. E., and Golabek, A. A. (2004). N-glycosylation is crucial for folding, trafficking, and stability of human tripeptidyl-peptidase I. *J. Biol. Chem. 279,* 12827-12839.

[130] Strahl-Bolsinger, S., Immervoll, T., Deutzmann, R. and Tanner, W. (1993). PMT1, the gene for a key enzyme of protein O-glycosylation in *Saccharomyces cerevisiae. Proc. Natl, Acad. Sci. USA, 90,* 8164-8168.

[131] Gentzsch, M. and Tanner, W. (1996). The *PMT* gene family: protein Oglycosylation in *Saccharomyces cerevisiae* is vital. *EMBO J., 15,* 5752- 5759.

[132] Prill, S. K., Klinkert, B., Timpel, C., Gale, C. A., Schroppel, K., and Ernst, J. F. (2005). PMT family of *Candida albicans*: Five protein mannosyltransferase isoforms affect growth, morphogenesis and antifungal resistance. *Mol. Microbiol. 55,* 546-560.

[133] Girrbach, V. and Strahl, S. (2003). Members of the evolutionarily conserved PMT family of protein *O*-mannosyltransferases form distinct protein complexes among themselves. *J Biol Chem. 278,* 12554-12562.

[134] Jigami, Y. and Odani, T. (1999). Mannosylphosphate transfer to yeast mannan. *Biochim Biophys Acta, 1426,* 335-345.

[135] Graham, T. R., Seeger, M., Payne, G. S., MacKay, V. L. and Emr, S. D. (1994). Clathrin dependent localization of alpha 1,3 mannosyltransferase to the Golgi complex of *Saccharomyces cerevisiae. J. Cell Biol.,127,* 667-678.

[136] Elliott, S., Bartley, T., Delorme, E., Derby, P., Hunt, R., Lorenzini, T., Parker, V., Rohde, M. F. and Stoney, K. (1994). Structural requirements for addition of *O*-linked carbohydrate to recombinant erythropoietin. *Biochemistry, 33,* 11237-1145.

[137] Kirnarsky, L., Nomoto, M., Ikematsu, Y., Hassan, H., Bennett, E. P., Cerny, R. L., Clausen, H., Hollingsworth, M. A. and Sherman, S. (1998). Structural analysis of peptide substrates for mucin-type *O*-glycosylation. *Biochemistry, 37,* 12811-12817.

[138] Hansen, J. E., Lund, O., Engelbrecht, J., Bohr, H. and Nielsen, J. O. (1995). Prediction of *O*-glycosylation of mammalian proteins: specificity patterns of UDP-GalNAc:polypeptide N-acetylgalactosaminyl transferase. *Biochem. J., 308,* 801-813.

[139] Gentzsch, M. and Tanner, W. (1997). Protein-O-glycosylation in yeast: protein-specific mannosyltransferases. *Glycobiology, 7,* 481-486.

[140] Thanka Christlet, T. H. and Veluraja, K. (2001). Database analysis of *O*-glycosylation sites in proteins. *Biophys. J., 80,* 952-960.

[141] Strahl-Bolsinger, S. and Tanner, W. (1991). Protein *O*-glycosylation in *Saccharomyces cerevisiae*. Purification and characterization of the dolichyl-phosphate-dmannose-protein *O*-d-mannosyltransferase. *Eur. J. Biochem. 196,* 185-190.

[142] Ecker, M., Mrsa, V., Hagen, I., Deutzmann, R., Strahl, S. and Tanner, W. (2003). *O*-Mannosylation precedes and potentially controls the *N*-glycosylation of a yeast cell wall glycoprotein. *EMBO Rep., 4,* 628-632.

[143] Lommel, M. and Sabine Strahl, S. (2009). Protein *O*-mannosylation: Conserved from bacteria to humans. *Glycobiology, 19,* 816-828.

[144] Kuroda, K., Kobayashi, K., Kitagawa, Y., Nakagawa, T., Tsumura, H., Komeda, T., Shinmi, D., Mori, E., Motoki, K., Fuju, K., Sakai, T., Nonaka, K., Suzuki, T., Ichikawa, K., Chiba, Y. and Jigami, Y. (2008). Efficient Antibody Production upon Suppression of O Mannosylation in the Yeast *Ogataea minuta. Appl. Environ. Microbiol., 74,* 446-453.

[145] Harty, C., Strahl, S. and Römisch, K. (2001). O-mannosylation protects mutant alpha-factor precursor from endoplasmic reticulum-associated degradation. *Mol. Biol. Cell, 12,* 1093-1101.

[146] Nakatsukasa, K., Okada, S., Umebayashi, K., Fukuda, R., Nishikawa, S. and Endo, T. (2004). Roles of O-mannosylation of aberrant proteins in reduction of the load for endoplasmic reticulum chaperones in yeast. *J. Biol. Chem. 279,* 49762-49772.

[147] Agaphonov, M. O., Sokolov, S. S., Romanova, N. V., Sohn, J. H., Kim, S. Y., Kalebina, T. S., Choi, E. S. and Ter-Avanesyan, M. D. (2005). Mutation of the protein-*O*-mannosyltransferase enhances secretion of the human urokinase-type plasminogen activator in *Hansenula polymorpha, Yeast, 22,* 1037-1047.

[148] Mochizuki, S., Hamato, N., Hirose, M., Miyano, K., Ohtani, W., Kameyama, S., Kuwae, S., Tokuyama, T. and Ohi, H. (2001). Expression and Characterization of Recombinant Human Antithrombin III in *Pichia pastoris.Protein. Expr. Purif., 23,*55-65.

[149] Idiris A., Tohda H., Kumagai, H. and Takegawa, K. (2010). Engineering of protein secretion in yeast: strategies and impact on protein production. *Appl. Microbiol. Biotechnol., 86,* 403-417.

[150] Valkonen, M., Penttilä, M. and Saloheimo, M. (2003). Effects of inactivation and constitutive expression of the unfolded- protein response pathway on protein production in the yeast*Saccharomyces cerevisiae. Appl. Environ. Microbiol.,69,*2065-2072.

[151] Gasser, B., Maurer, M., Gach, J., Kunert, R., Mattanovich, D. (2006). Engineering of *Pichia pastoris* for improved production of antibody fragments. *Biotechnol. Bioeng.,94,*353-361.

[152] Klabunde, J., Kleebank, S., Piontek, M., Hollenberg, C. P., Hellwig, S. and Degelmann, A. (2007). Increase of calnexin gene dosage boosts the secretion of heterologous proteins by *Hansenula polymorpha. FEMS Yeast Res. 7,* 1168-1180.

[153] Parlati, F., Dominguez, M., Bergeron, J. J. and Thomas, D. Y. (1995). *Saccharomyces cerevisiae* CNE1 encodes an endoplasmic reticulum (ER) membrane protein with sequence similarity to calnexin and calreticulin and functions as a constituent of the ER quality control apparatus. *J. Biol. Chem., 270,* 244-253.

[154] Arima, H., Kinoshita, T., Ibrahim, H., Azakami, H. and Kato, A. (1998). Enhanced secretion of hydrophobic peptide fused lysozyme by the introduction of N-glycosylation signal and the disruption of the calnexin gene in *Saccharomyces cerevisiae. FEBS Lett., 440,* 89-92.

[155] Harmsen, M. M., Bruyne, M. I., Raue, H. A. and Maat, J. (1996). Overexpression of binding protein and disruption of the PMR1 gene synergistically stimulate secretion of bovine prochymosin but not plant thaumatin in yeast. *Appl. Microbiol. Biotechnol., 46,* 365-370.

[156] Kim, M. D., Han, K. C., Kang, H. A., Rhee, S. K. and Seo, J. H. (2003). Coexpression of BiP increased antithrombotic hirudin production in recombinant *Saccharomyces cerevisiae. J. Biotechnol., 101,* 81-87.

[157] Harmsen, M. M., Bruyne, M. I., Raue, H. A. and Maat, J. (1996). Overexpression of binding protein and disruption of thePMR1 gene synergistically stimulate secretion of bovine prochymosin but not plant thaumatin in yeast. *Appl. Microbiol. Biotechnol., 46,* 365-370.

[158] Smith, J. D., Tang, B. C. and Robinson, A. S. (2004). Protein disulfide isomerase, but not binding protein, overexpression enhances secretion of a non-disulfide-bonded protein in yeast. *Biotechnol. Bioeng., 85,* 340-350.

[159] Conesa, A., Jeenes, D., Archer, D. B., van den Hondel, C. A. and Peter J. Punt, P.J. (2002). Calnexin Overexpression Increases Manganese Peroxidase Production in *Aspergillus niger. Appl. Environ. Microbiol., 68,* 846-851.

[160] Payne, T., Finnis, C., Evans, L. R., Mead, D. J., Avery, S. V., Archer, D. B., Sleep, D. (2008). Modulation of chaperone gene expression in mutagenized *Saccharomyces cerevisiae* strains developed for recombinant human albumin production results in increased production

of multiple heterologous proteins. *Appl. Environ. Microbiol. 74,* 7759-7766.

[161] Zhang, W., Zhao, H. L., Xue, C., Xiong, X. H., Yao, X. Q., Li, X. Y.,Chen, H. P. and Liu, Z. M. (2006). Enhanced Secretion of Heterologous Proteins in *Pichia pastoris* FollowingOverexpression of *Saccharomyces cerevisiae* Chaperone Proteins. *Biotechnol. Prog. 22,* 1090-1095.

[162] Robinson, A. S., Hines, V. and Wittrup, K. D. (1994). Protein disulfide overexpression enhances secretion of foreign proteins in *Saccharomyces cerevisiae. Bio/Technology, 12,* 381-384.

[163] Huo, X., Liu, Y., Wang, X., Ouyang, P., Niu, Z., Shi, Y., Qiu, B. (2007). Co-expression of human protein disulfide isomerase (hPDI) enhances secretion of bovine follicle-stimulating hormone (bFSH) in *Pichia pastoris. Protein Expr. Purif., 54,* 234-239.

[164] Bao, W. G. and Fukuhara, H. (2001). Secretion of human proteins from yeast: stimulation by duplication of polyubiquitin and protein disulfide isomerase genes in *Kluyveromyces lactis. Gene 272,* 103-110.

[165] Butz, J. A., Niebauer, R. T. and Robinson, A. S. (2003) Co-expression of molecular chaperones does not improve the heterologous expression of mammalian G-protein coupled receptor expression in yeast. *Biotechnol. Bioeng. 84,* 292-304.

[166] Gasser, B., Maurer, M., Gach, J., Kunert, R., Mattanovich, D. (2006). Engineering of *Pichia pastoris* for Improved Production of Antibody Fragments. *Biotechnol. Bioeng., 94,* 353-361.

[167] Inan, M., Aryasomayajula, D., Sinha, J. and Meagher, M. M. (2006). Enhancement of Protein Secretion in *Pichia pastoris* by Overexpression of Protein Disulfide Isomerase. *Biotechnol. Bioeng., 93,* 771-778.

[168] Parekh, R., Forrester, K., Wittrup, D. (1995). Multicopy overexpression of bovine pancreatic trypsin inhibitor saturates the protein folding and secretory capacity of *Saccharomyces cerevisiae. Protein Expr. Purif., 6,* 537 545.

[169] Shusta, E. V., Raines, R. T., Plückthun, A. and Wittrup, K. D. (1998). Increasing the secretory capacity of *Saccharomyces cerevisiae* for production of single-chain antibody fragments. *Nat. Biotechnol., 16,* 773-777.

[170] Xua, P., Radena, D., Doyle IIIb, F. J. and Robinson, A. S. (2005). Analysis of unfolded protein response during single-chain antibody expression in *Saccharomyces cerevisiae* reveals different roles for BiP and PDI in folding. *Metab. Eng., 7,* 269-279.

[171] Lodi, T., Neglia, B. and Donnini, C. (2005). Secretion of human serum albumin by *Kluyveromyces lactis* overexpressing KlPDI1 and KlERO1. *Appl. Environ. Microbiol. 71,* 4359-4363.

[172] Sevier, C. S., Qu, H., Heldman, N., Gross, E., Fass, D. and Kaiser, C. A. (2007). Modulation of Cellular Disulfide-Bond Formation and the ER Redox Environment by Feedback Regulation of Ero1. *Cell, 129,* 333-344.

[173] Wentz, A. E. and Shusta, E. V. (2007). A Novel High-Throughput Screen Reveals Yeast Genes That Increase Secretion of Heterologous Proteins. *Appl. Environ. Microbiol., 73,* 1189-1198.

[174] Komar, A. A. and Jaenicke, R. (1995). Kinetics of translation of g B crystallin and its circularly permutated variant in an in vitro cell-free system: possible relations to codon distribution and protein folding. *FEBS Lett. 376,* 195-198.

[175] Purvis, I. J., Andrew J. E. Bettany, A. J. E., Santiago, T. C., Coggins, J. R., Duncan, K. Eason, R. and Brown, A. J. P. (1987). The efficiency of folding of some proteins is increased by controlled rates of translation in vivo. A hypothesis. *J. Mol. Biol. 193,* 413-417.

[176] Krasheninnikov, I. A., Komar, A. A. and Adzhubeĭ, I. A. (1989). Frequency of using codons in mRNA and coding of the domain structure of proteins. *Dokl. Akad. Nauk. SSSR, 305,* 1006-1012.

[177] Thanaraj, T. A. and Argos, P. (1996). Ribosome-mediated translational pause and protein domain organization. *Protein. Sci., 5,* 1594-1612.

[178] Crombie, T., Swaffield, J. C. and Brown, A. J. (1992). Protein Folding within the Cell Is Influenced by Controlled Rates of Polypeptide Elongation, *J. Mol. Biol., 228,* 7-12.

[179] Cortazzo, P., Cervenansky, C., Marin, M., Reiss, C., Ehrlich, R. and Deana, A. (2002). Silent mutations affect in vivo protein folding in *Escherichiacoli. Biochem. Biophys. Res. Commun. 293,*537-541.

[180] Thanaraj, T. A. and Argos, P. (1996). Protein secondary structural types are differentially coded on messenger RNA. *Protein Sci., 5,*1973-1983.

[181] Komar, A. A., Lesnik, T. and Reiss, C. (1999). Synonymous codon substitutions affect ribosome traffic and protein folding during in vitro translation. *FEBS Lett. 462,*387-391.

[182] Makhoul, C. H. and Trifonov, E. N. (2002). Distribution of rare triplets alongmRNA and their relation to protein folding. *J. Biomol. Struct. Dyn., 20,*413-420.

[183] Zhou, Z., Schnake, P., Xiao, L. and Lal, A. A. (2004). Enhanced expression of a recombinant malaria candidate vaccine in Escherichia coli by codon optimization. *Protein Expr. Purif., 34,*87-94.

[184] Widmann, M., Clairo, M., Dippon, J. and Pleiss, J. (2008). Analysis of the distribution of functionally relevant rare codons. *BMC Genomics*, 9, 207-214.

[185] Perlmutter, D. H. (2002). Chemical chaperones: a pharmacological strategy for disorders of protein folding and trafficking. *Pediatr. Res. 52,* 832-836.

[186] Gaetani, S. (2009). A sideway glance: a new role for endoplasmic reticulum chemical chaperones as leptin sensitizers. *Genes Nutr., 4,* 157-159.

[187] Sato, S., Ward, C. L., Krouse, M. E., Wine, J. J. and Kopito, R. R. (1996). Glycerol reverses the misfolding phenotype of the most common cystic fibrosis mutation. *J. Biol. Chem., 271,* 635-638.

[188] Singh, L. R., Chena, X., Kožich, V. and Kruger, W. D. (2007). Chemical chaperone rescue of mutant human cystathionine β-synthase. *Mol. Genet. Metab., 91,* 335-342.

[189] Singer, M. A. and Lindquist, S. (1998). Multiple Effects of Trehalose on Protein Folding In Vitro and In Vivo. *Molecular Cell, 1,* 639-648.

[190] Figler, R. A., Omote, H., Nakamoto, R. K. and Al Shawi, M. K. (2000). Use of Chemical Chaperones in the Yeast *Saccharomyces cerevisiae* to Enhance Heterologous Membrane ProteinExpression: High-Yield Expression and Purification of Human P-Glycoprotein. *Arch. Biochem. Biophys., 376,* 34-46.

[191] Wiens, G. D., O'Hare, T., Rittenberg, M. B. (2001). Recovering antibody secretion using a hapten ligand as a chemical chaperone. *J. Biol. Chem. 276,* 40933-40939.

[192] Li, Z., Xiong, F., Lin, Q., d'Anjou, M., Daugulis, A. J., Yang, D. S., Hew, C. L. (2001). Low temperature increases the yield of biologically active herring antifreeze protein in *Pichia pastoris.Protein Expr. Purif., 21,*438-445.

[193] Dragosits, M., Stadlmann, J., Albiol, J., Baumann, K., Maurer, M., Gasser, B., Sauer, M., Altmann, F., Ferrer, P. and Mattanovich, D. (2008). The Effect of Temperature on the Proteome of Recombinant *Pichia pastoris. J. Proteome Res.,8,* 1380-1392.

In: Advances in Proteomics Research
Editors: Ya Li Huang et al. pp. 203-221 ISBN: 978-1-61942-227-8

Chapter 6

PROTEIN KINASE INHIBITORS IN THE TREATMENT OF MALIGNANT LIVER AND KIDNEY TUMORS

Panagiotis Samaras and Frank Stenner*
Department of Oncology, UniversityHospitalZurich,
Raemistrasse 100, 8091 Zurich, Switzerland.

ABSTRACT

Treatment options for cancer have increased in the last years due to the ongoing research and development of new therapeutics. A focus shift from formerly undirected cytostatic agents to more targeted therapies, mainly antibodies and protein kinase inhibitors has taken place. New agents directed against receptors which control proliferation, migration and angiogenesis of tumor cells have been developed. Mainly specific antibodies directed against the extracellular ligand binding domain of various receptor tyrosine kinases, and protein kinase inhibitors targeting the intracellular protein kinase domain of receptors or cytoplasmic signalling proteins have been increasingly developed in the past years. In this chapter we will address the current treatment options with protein kinase inhibitors exemplarily for hepatocellular carcinoma and renal cell

* Corresponding author: Phone: +41 (0) 44 255 2214 Fax: +41 (0)44 255 45 48 frank.stenner@usz.ch

cancer. We will further give an insight into the actual research perspectives and the conception of incorporating new drugs into clinical trials as single agent treatment or combined with "classical" chemotherapy. The first part elucidates the molecular pathways of carcinogenesis and depicts the mode of action of these new agents in the treatment of hepatocellular carcinoma, the second part illustrates the pathogenesis of renal cell cancer and the resulting therapeutic options by targeting these pathways.

INTRODUCTION

Much progress was achieved in the last decade regarding cancer treatment. The completion of the Human Genome Project (1990 – 2003) and the analysis of the kinome, the protein kinase complement of the human genome, in 2002, were the basis for understanding the mechanisms of cell signalling pathways and their impact on cancer development. These achievements finally paved the way to the development of small molecules and specific antibodies [1]. Protein kinases are enzymes that control key functions of the cell. As today, over 500 kinases have been identified in the human genome, coding 1.7% of all proteins, but controlling the activity of approximately 30% of all proteins by transferring phosphate groups.

Protein kinases play a critical role in cell proliferation, migration and tumor angiogenesis and represent promising targets for specific therapies, mainly with antibodies and small molecules. The first breakthrough was the development and approval of imatinib (Gleevec©, Novartis) for the treatment of chronic myelogenous leukemia (CML) in 2001. A seminal mechanism in the development of CML is a cytogenetic mutation, the translocation of the short arm of chromosome 9 to chromosome 22 (t(9;22)(q34;q11)). The affected gene of the so called "Philadelphia-chromosome" encodes bcr-abl, an abnormal fusion protein with a continuously activated abl tyrosine kinase. Imatinib is a phenylaminopyrimidine which functions by binding to the ATP binding site of the tyrosine kinase and blocking its activity completely. Imatinib proved highly efficient in clinical trials compared with conventional chemotherapy and is currently considered standard of care in Philadelphia-positive CML [2].

Tyrosine kinase inhibitors targeting the intracellular protein kinase domain of receptors or cytoplasmic downstream signalling proteins with kinase activity have been increasingly developed in the past years. Researchers were trying to design specific inhibitors against a single kinase that may deploy a pivotal effect in a given disease, with the goal to reduce toxicity. The key caveat of single-kinase inhibition may be a rapid development of resistance thus reducing efficacy of the drug. Agents targeting several pathways at once were developed and tested in the last years. These so-called multi-kinase inhibitors proved to be efficient in different tumors without a significant increase of toxicity.

As today, numerous agents received approval for the treatment of different neoplasms. Here we will focus on hepatocellular and renal cell carcinoma to highlight the impact of protein kinase inhibition for the treatment of these malignancies.

Pathogenesis of Hepatocellular Carcinoma and Current Treatment Options Offered by Tyrosine Kinase Inhibitors

Hepatocellular carcinoma (HCC) is the sixth most common cancer worldwide and its incidence is increasing. It is the third most common cause of cancer mortality and a growing cause of cancer related death [3]. Complete resection of the tumor and liver transplantation are the only treatment modalities with curative intent. Most patients have unresectable disease, either at presentation or in the further course. Patients with advanced or metastatic HCC who are not candidates for curative resection have a poor prognosis with a 5-year survival rate of 7% [4].

The incidence of HCC varies among geographic regions, being most frequent in Eastern Asia and Africa, where more than 80% of all cases occur. In general, men are contracting HCC more often than women. This may be due to a higher incidence of hepatitis infections and higher alcohol consumption in men, but animal models and clinical studies suggest that androgen levels may also have an influence on carcinogenesis[5-7].

Underlying cirrhosis due to chronic liver damage is the most important risk factor for HCC. The main reasons for the development of cirrhosis are chronic hepatitis B and C, heavy alcohol consumption or iron overload [8].

Different models of hepatocarcinogenesis have been discussed in the past years. However, HCC development is a complex process with numerous alterations involved. It is assumed that a chronic inflammatory state may cause different genetic changes in the hepatocytes. These changes induce phenotypical alterations of the hepatocytes and may produce monoclonal populations of dysplastic cells in the further course. HCC finally develops after a pre-neoplastic period of 10-20 years due to accumulation of irreversible DNA-damage [9].

Loss of liver mass and reduction of liver function during cirrhosis may further activate growth-stimulating pathways and produce a proinflammatory state, thus promoting HCC formation [10].

In accordance with the role of inflammation for carcinogenesis, intake of non-steroidal anti-inflammatory drugs (NSAID) was found to reduce the incidence of various tumors in the general population. Cyclooxigenase-2 (COX-2) is overexpressed in HCC and application of COX-2 inhibitors blocks tumor growth*in vitro* and *in vivo* due to reduction of proliferation and induction of apoptosis[11-13]. The selective COX-2 inhibitor celecoxib is tested in ongoing clinical studies in combination with biologicals or conventional chemotherapy as a consequence of these findings (Table 2).

In some cases, HCC may occur in patients with chronic viral hepatitis without underlying cirrhosis due to oncogenic properties of viral proteins. The HBV X protein (HBx) is considered to promote HCC development by increasing insulin-like growth factor II (IGF-II) expression [14]. In addition, this effect may be enhanced by concomitant mutations of PTEN, a tumor suppressor gene product inducing apoptosis by inhibiting the Akt signalling pathway [15].

Beside PTEN, numerous oncogenic pathways are involved in up to 60% of cases, including phosphatidylinositol 3-kinase/Akt, c-myc, β-catenin, MET and hedgehog [16-20].

Furthermore, different molecular alterations of cell cycle and apoptosis pathways have been identified [6]. HCC formation results from a combination of inactivated suppressor genes and activated oncogenes. As today, more than 20 genes have been identified to be linked with HCC formation. The p53 tumor suppressor gene, which is considered “the guardian of the genome”, is altered in up to 50% of cases [21]. Common changes associated with the p53 pathway are overexpression of the MDM2 and Gankyrin [22, 23]. The p16/ retinoblastoma/ cyclin D1 pathway is impaired frequently, resulting in reduced cell cycle control[24].

A therapeutically interesting finding is overexpression of insulin-like growth factor I and II (IGF-I and IGF-II) and insulin-like growth factor I receptor (IGF-IR) [25]. IGF-IR-mediated signaling promotes tumor growth through cell cycle progression and reduction of apoptosis. On the other hand, the M6P/ insulin-like growth factor II receptor (IGF-2R) pathway, which degradates IGF-II, is compromised [26]. NVP-AEW541, a novel IGF-IR tyrosine kinase inhibitor, has been tested in hepatocellular carcinoma cell lines. NVP-AEW541 reduced tumor growth in a time- and dose-dependent manner by induction of apoptosis. It reduced the expression of the antiapoptotic proteins bcl-2 and survivin and caused cell cycle arrest at the G1/S phase[27].

Based on the existing *in vitro* data, NVP-AEW541 may be a promising agent for further clinical testing in combination with cytotoxic agents or small molecules.

The limited efficacy seen in trials with conventional chemotherapy so far may be at least in part attributable to the well known resistance of HCC against various cytostatics (Table 1). Hepatocellular carcinoma cells overexpress the multidrug resistance gene 1 (MDR1) product P-glycoprotein (MDR P-gp) and MDR-associated protein 1 (MRP-1), making this tumor chemotherapy resistant by enhancing drug efflux, as demonstrated in numerous studies [28-31]. Reversion of resistance was attempted in the past decade by transfection of hepatocellular carcinoma cells with antisense RNA or anti-MDR1 ribozymes[32-34]. Different inhibitors of MDR also were tested, i.e. calcium channel blockers, immunosuppressants like cyclosporine and calmodulin antagonists. However, efforts to enhance chemotherapy efficacy were unsuccessful or remained experimental so far.

HCC is a highly vascularized tumor with enhanced microvessel density. Vascular endothelial growth factor (VEGF), a key protein for endothelial cell growth and angiogenesis, is overexpressed in human hepatocellular carcinoma cells [35]. As a consequence, reducing the vascularization of the tumor by targeting VEGF appears to be a promising treatment approach. In a non-randomized, single-arm phase II study, systemic chemotherapy with gemcitabine and oxaliplatin – a regimen with activity in pancreaticobiliary tumors – was combined with bevacizumab (Avastin©, Roche), a humanized monoclonal antibody targeting VEGF. The objective response rate was 20%, and 27% of the patients achieved stable disease. The median overall survival was 9.6 months and the median progression free survival was 5.3 months. This trial showed promising efficacy in the treatment of HCC by utilizing an antiangiogenic agent compared to historical results with chemotherapy alone or best supportive care (Table 1).

HCC also is associated with interferences in the Raf-1 - MAPK/ERK kinase (MEK) - extracellular signal regulated kinase (ERK) pathway (Raf/ MEK/ ERK pathway). Overexpression and enhanced activity of MAPK was detected in HCC tumors, resulting in growth and migration of the tumor.

A novel specific MEK1/2 inhibitor, AZD6244, was found to inhibit growth of HCC effectively *in vitro* and *in vivo*by inactivating ERK1/2 and inducing apoptosis[36]. AZD6244 is a promising new kinase inhibitor and is currently tested in phase II studies (Table 2).

Table 1. Selected phase II and III trials of systemic treatment in hepatocellular carcinoma

Author	Therapy	Patients (n)	DCR (%)	OS (months)	p
Kouroumalis et al. [57]	Octreotide Placebo	28 30	32 0	13 4	0.002
Becker et al. [58] (HECTOR trial)	Octreotide Placebo	60 59	0 0	4.7 5.3	n.s.
Yeo et al. [59]	PIAF Doxorubicin	94 94	21 11	8.7 6.8	0.83
Llovet et al. [38] (SHARP trial)	Sorafenib Placebo	299 303	43 32	10.7 7.9	0.0006
Barbare et al. [60]	Tamoxifen Placebo	210 210	n.a. n.a.	4.8 4.0	0.17
Hsu et al. [61]	BEV/Capecitabine	45	60	10.7	n.a.
Thomas et al. [62]	BEV/Erlotinib	29	50	19	n.a.
Zhu et al. [63]	BEV/GEMOX	33	47	9.6	n.a.
Sun et al. [64]	BEV/CAPOX	30	77	10.6	n.a.
Philip et al. [45]	Erlotinib	38	59	13	n.a.
Thomas et al. [44]	Erlotinib	40	43	10.8	n.a.
Abou-Alfa et al. [42]	Sorafenib/Dox. Doxorubicin	47 49	81 57	13.7 6.5	0.013

DCR, disease control rate; BEV, bevacizumab; PIAF, cisplatin, interferon, doxorubicin, 5-fluorouracil; GEMOX, gemcitabine and oxaliplatin; CAPOX, capecitabine and oxaliplatin; n.a., not available; n.s., not significant; Dox, Doxorubicin.

The best studied substance so far is sorafenib (Nexavar©, Bayer). Sorafenib is an oral multi-kinase inhibitor which hampers tumor cell proliferation by blocking the Raf/ MEK/ ERK pathway as well as tumor angiogenesis by blocking VEGFR-2, VEGFR-3 and platelet derived growth factor receptor beta (PDGFR-β).

The multi-kinase inhibition of sorafenib leads to induction of apoptosis in HCC tumors*in vitro* and *in vivo* in preclinical studies [37] (Figure 1).

The results of a large international placebo-controlled randomized trial (SHARP-trial) were published recently. Patients with advanced HCC, good performance status and Child-Pugh status A were treated with sorafenib 400 mg BID (n = 299) and compared to patients who received placebo (n = 303).

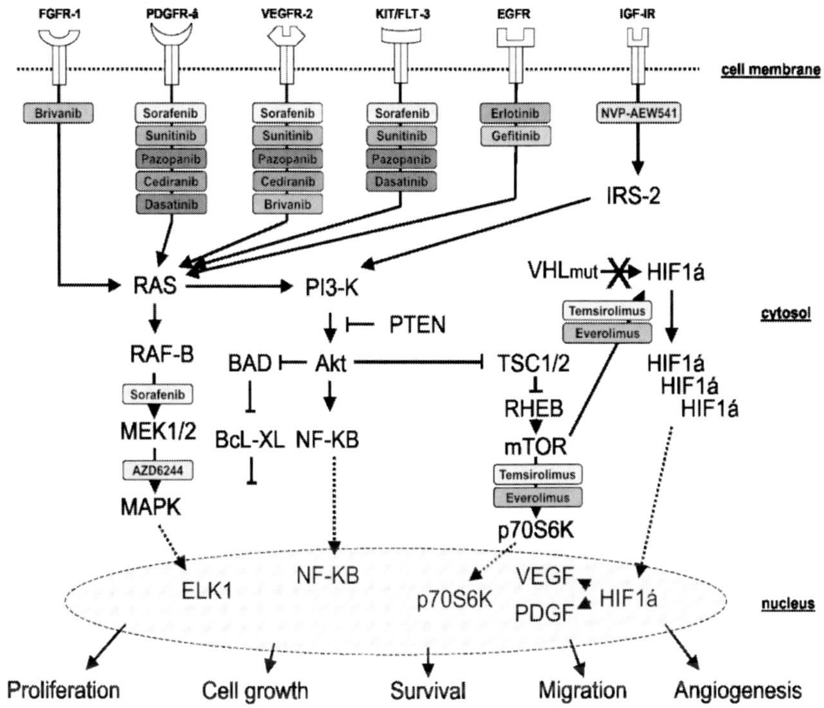

Figure 1. Simplified illustration of seminal pathways in human carcinogenesis. Depicted are the Ras-, Akt-, mTOR- and VHL pathway. Activation of these pathways – either via extracellular growth factor receptor stimulation or mutations of their intracellular tyrosine kinase domain or downstream signalling proteins – leads to increased proliferation, migration, survival and angiogenesis of the cell. Protein kinase inhibitors may reduce these effects by targeting receptor tyrosine kinases or cytoplasmic protein kinases.

Treatment with sorafenib significantly prolonged overall survival (10.7 versus 7.9 months) and time to progression (5.5 versus 2.8 months). The treatment was well tolerated, the most frequent grade 3/4 toxicities were diarrhea, hand-foot skin reaction (HFSR) and fatigue[38]. Two randomized controlled studies, in different populations (patients coming from Europe and Asia) demonstrated a significant benefit from targeted therapy in HCC after many years of disillusion, making sorafenib the new standard of care in patients with unresectable HCC.

Other new tyrosin kinase inhibitors with antiangiogenic properties recently developed may be good candidates for studies with HCC patients (Table 2). Pazopanib is an oral multikinase inhibitor targeting VEGFR1-3, PDGFR and stem cell factor receptor (c-KIT). It is currently under investigation in the treatment of renal cell cancer and other solid tumors, and early clinical trials with HCC patients have been initiated [39]. Cediranib (Recentin©, Astra Zeneca) is a potent inhibitor of VEGR1-3 and is currently tested in large phase III studies in the treatment of non-small cell lung cancer and colorectal carcinoma combined with chemotherapy. A non-randomized phase II study is ongoing testing its efficacy in hepatocellular carcinoma patients as single agent therapy.

Table 2. Ongoing clinical studies with new drugs for the treatment of patients with advanced unresectable HCC registered in "clinical trials.gov"

Study center / sponsor	Drugs	Phase	randomized
M.D. Anderson / Genentech	Erlotinib and bevacizumab	II	no
GlaxoSmithKline	Pazopanib	I	no
UCSF / NCI	Celecoxib and erlotinib	I/II	no
H.LeeMoffittCancerCenter / Pfizer	Sunitinib	II	no
Massachusetts GeneralHospital / NCI	Cediranib	II	no
California Cancer Consortium	Dasatinib	II	no
H.LeeMoffittCancerCenter	AZD6244	II	no
Pfizer	Arm A: sunitinib Arm B: sorafenib	III	yes
Bristol-Myers Squibb	Brivanib	II	no
Italian trial in med. oncology	Sorafenib and 5-fluorouracil	II	no
NationalTaiwanUniversity	Sorafenib and tegafur/uracil	II	no
ECOG / NCI	Gefitinib	II	no
M.D. Anderson / NCI	Erlotinib	II	no
ChicagoCancerCenter / NCI	Celecoxib and epirubicin	II	no
MahidolUniv.Bangkok / Bayer	Sorafenib and gemcitabine	II	no
HOG / Sanofi-Aventis / OSI	Erlotinib and docetaxel	II	no

UCSF, University of California, San Francisco; NCI, National Cancer Institute; ECOG, Eastern Cooperative Oncology Group; HOG, Hoosier Oncology Group; OSI, OSI Pharmaceuticals.

Brivanib is a dual tyrosine kinase inhibitor of VEGFR2 and fibroblast growth factor receptor 1 (FGFR1). In vivo studies with athymic mice bearing L2987 human tumor xenografts proved the ability of brivanib to inhibit tumor growth due to its antiangiogenic properties [40]. A clinical phase II trial utilizing brivanib for the treatment of patients with advanced HCC is ongoing. Dasatinib (Sprycel©, Bristol Myers Squibb) is a multi-kinase inhibitor of bcr-abl, numerous tyrosine kinases of the proto-oncogenic SRC family, and also of cKIT and PDGFR-β. It is approved for use in patients with chronic myelogenous leukemia after failure of imatinib treatment. It is being evaluated for the use in advanced HCC in one ongoing clinical trial (Table 2).

Sunitinib (Sutent©, Pfizer) is a multi-kinase inhibitor targeting PDGFR-β, VEGFR1-3, c-KIT, fms-like tyrosin kinase-receptor 3 (flt3) and the RET tyrosin kinase. Currently, sunitinib is being tested in different trials for the treatment of advanced HCC. A randomized international multi-center phase III trial is testing sunitinib in patients with HCC compared to sorafenib. Sunitinib may prove equally effective, since both drugs have a similar spectrum of activity and both are effective in the treatment of advanced renal cell cancer. Multi-kinase inhibitors are effective in the treatment of HCC as monotherapy, and combination therapy is tested in various clinical studies. Preclinical data suggest that combination with other agents may improve the results achieved in the SHARP trial. Doxorubicin demonstrated synergistic effects with sorafenib in preclinical models, while antimetabolites like gemcitabine, fluorouracil and capecitabine seemed to reduce the efficacy of sorafenib. The latter finding may be explained by the different mechanisms of action: sorafenib induces apoptosis and leads to a cell cycle arrest in the G1/G0-transition, while antimetabolites are effective in the S-phase of the cell cycle [41]. The results of a randomized phase II study testing sorafenib in combination with doxorubicin compared to doxorubicin alone were presented in 2007 (ECCO, European Cancer Conference, Barcelona). Patients were enrolled to receive doxorubicin 60 mg/m² every 3 weeks alone (n=49) or combined with sorafenib 400 mg BID (n=47). The median progression free survival was 6.9 months in the combination arm compared with 2.8 months in the doxorubicin arm. The median overall survival was 13.7 months and 6.5 months, respectively (Table 1) [42]. However, the explanatory power of this study is limited since the investigational arm was not compared with sorafenib, but with doxorubicin alone. Patients treated with doxorubicin alone did worse compared to the patients receiving placebo in the SHARP trial (median OS 6.5 months and 7.9 months, respectively), taking the shortcoming of cross comparison between different studies into account. However, combination therapy of sorafenib with doxorubicin needs to be compared with the present standard of care sorafenib before use in clinical praxis can be recommended.

Epidermal growth factor receptor (EGFR) and its ligands epidermal growth factor (EGF), IGF-I and TGF-β are overexpressed in hepatocellular carcinoma[43]. Therefore, EGFR may be a good candidate protein for targeted therapy. Two non-randomized phase II studies evaluated the antitumoral activity of erlotinib (Tarceva©, Roche), a selective inhibitor of the EGFR/ HER-1 tyrosine kinase, in advanced HCC. Erlotinib inhibits tumor cell growth and induces cell cycle arrest in the G1 phase. Treatment with erlotinib modestly prolonged PFS and OS compared to historical controls with acceptable toxicity[44, 45] (Table 1). Blockage of EGFR/ HER-1 is a promising treatment option, and numerous ongoing phase II trials are testing erlotinib either alone or in combination with other agents (bevacizumab, docetaxel, celecoxib). However, larger randomized trials should be conducted as interpretation and explanatory power of single-arm phase II trials is limited.

Efficacy also was observed with gefitinib (Iressa©, Astra Zeneca), a similar selective EGFR tyrosine kinase inhibitor, in preclinical models [46]. Two non-randomized trials are ongoing investigating efficacy of gefitinib monotherapy in HCC patients.

Table 2 gives an overview of ongoing clinical studies currently testing protein kinase inhibitors in the treatment of hepatocellular carcinoma patients. The sites of action of approved and still evaluated tyrosin kinase inhibitors are depicted in Figure 1. Taking into account that HCC formation is a multi-step process with numerous genes involved, one can speculate that targeting multiple pathways may be more effective than selective blockage of only one catalyzing enzyme. This assumption is supported by the documented efficacy of sorafenib, a multi-kinase inhibitor with a broad spectrum activity against numerous signalling proteins. The improvement of treatment efficacy by defining ideal combination partners without compromising the toxicity profile at the same time remains a challenge for clinical researchers.

Pathogenesis of Renal Cell Carcinoma and Current Treatment Options Offered by Tyrosine Kinase Inhibitors

Renal cell carcinoma (RCC) is the most common form of kidney cancer in adults. 36.000 patients are newly affected by RCC in the US and about 12.000 patients will die of this disease in one year [47]. 5 year survival has been traditionally poor with some rare exceptions. The latter have been attributed to incipient immunological responses, a situation when the immune system regains control of the tumor, sometimes ultimately destroying the malignant clone. Based on these observations, clinical research in RCC focused on modulation of the immune system in the past two decades. Interleukin-2 and interferon (IFN) have been widely applied in clinical practice in an effort to overcome an immunological absence [48]. Even allogeneic stem cell transplantation has been used to exchange a failing immune system with a functional one [49]. Though seemingly rational approaches, the median survival with chemo- and/or immunotherapy hardly exceeded 10 months [50]. Thus, novel treatments were overdue.

Basic research delineated two major intracellular pathways as the key players in RCC pathogenesis. On the one hand side the hypoxia response pathway controlled by the von-Hippel-Lindau (VHL) tumor suppressor gene and on the other side the mammalian target of rapamycin (mTOR) pathway. Activation of either pathway results in transcriptional events promoting proliferation of cells and malignant transformation.

Mainly responsible for RCC development are the transcription factors HIF1α and HIF2α, and their target genes, which are involved in anaerobic energy metabolism, angiogenesis, cell survival and cell invasion.

The expression of HIF proteins is regulated by an ubiquitin ligase complex involving VHL protein. VHL targets HIF, thus enabling ubiquitination and degradation of the protein under normoxic conditions. This degradation is hampered and HIF stabilized and overexpressed in case of hypoxia due to inhibition of VHL binding. Downstream pathways responsible for angiogenesis are activated subsequently (Figure 1). High protein levels of these transcription factors are found in many human tumors and underscore their importance in carcinogenesis.

The VHL gene is mutated or lost in the majority of clear cell RCC leading to a permanent stabilization of HIF proteins. This results in a permanent "on" switch for several pathways, namely those of vascular endothelial growth factor (VEGF), platelet derived growth factor (PDGF) and transforming growth factorα (TGF-α). Consequently, different protein kinase inhibitors targeting these pathways were evaluated increasingly in the last years.

Sorafenib was the first drug to be approved by the FDA for RCC in second line treatment. A large randomized placebo controlled international multicenter trial has shown a significantly better progression free survival for patients treated with 400 mg sorafenib BID (24 weeks with sorafenib versus 12 weeks without, $P<0.001$) [51].

It has to be noted that the response rate was only 2% and overall survival (19.3 months TKI arm versus 15.9 months placebo arm) was not statistically significant, the latter possibly due to cross over events from the placebo into the sorafenib arm.

In a head to head comparison with interferon-α in first line treatment, sorafenib showed equal efficacy (PFS 5.7 and 5.6 months) (ASCO 2007 Annual Meeting, Chicago). A few phase II trials have been published showing increasing efficacy of combination therapies (sorafenib plus interferon), but the additive toxicities thwart a combined use outside clinical trials so far.

Sunitinib has also shown superior results over IFN treatment in a randomized phase III trial in RCC and was subsequently approved for first line treatment of this disease [52]. Response rates were 31% versus 6% in the IFN control arm and PFS was 11 months versus 5 month ($P<0.001$). Side effects were similar to sorafenib treatment, but grades 3 and 4 were seen in less than 10%. Thus, sunitinib 50 mg daily, given in a 4 weeks on / 2 weeks off schedule is the current standard treatment for metastasized renal cell carcinoma.

Direct VEGF inhibition with bevacicumab in combination with IFN has shown similar results in a recent study and could represents an alternative treatment for patients with RCC in the intermediate risk group [53].

The mTOR pathway is the other important pathogenetic factor in RCC. The mammalian target of rapamycin (mTOR) is a serine/ threonine protein kinase that regulates cell growth and proliferation. Activation of mTOR leads to HIF1α expression and stabilization, resulting in angiogenic downstream events. Rapamycin was found to inhibit mTOR through directly binding the mTOR complex 1, subsequently reducing HIF1α transcription[54].

Temsirolimus (CCI-779, Torisel©, Wyeth pharmaceuticals) and everolimus (RAD-001, Certican©, Novartis) are derivatives of rapamycin inhibiting mTOR selectively. The former has shown beneficial value for "poor-risk" patients in a phase III trial compared to standard IFN treatment. Interestingly, no synergism between the two approaches was seen, the combination therapy arm (temsirolimus plus interferon) of the study showed inferiority with regard to overall survival compared to mTOR inhibition with temsirolimus alone [55].

A recently published double-blind, randomized study compared everolimus with placebo in patients with clear cell RCC who progressed after treatment with sorafenib, sunitinib, or both. Patients who received 10 mg everolimus daily had a significantly prolonged PFS compared with placebo (4.0 and 1.9 months, $P < 0.001$) [56].

Four large randomized trials with TKIs and targeted therapy have shaped a new standard of care for renal cell carcinomas[51, 52, 55, 56]. Nevertheless, many questions remain unanswered.

Can higher efficacy be achieved with dose escalation or different application schedules?

What is the optimal sequence of these novel therapies in the course of the disease?

What is the optimal usage of TKI in non-clear cell RCCs (papillary and chromophobe carcinomas)?

Another important aspect is how to handle the side effects of these drugs. Several trials addressing these problems have been initiated and their results will give us a better understanding of these fascinating new drugs.

REFERENCES

[1] Manning, G; Whyte, DB; Martinez, R; Hunter, T; Sudarsanam, S. The protein kinase complement of the human genome. *Science*, 2002 Dec 6, 298(5600), 1912-34.

[2] O'Brien, SG; Guilhot, F; Larson, RA; Gathmann, I; Baccarani, M; Cervantes, F; et al. Imatinib compared with interferon and low-dose cytarabine for newly diagnosed chronic-phase chronic myeloid leukemia. *The New England journal of medicine,* 2003 Mar 13, 348(11), 994-1004.

[3] Parkin, DM; Bray, F; Ferlay, J; Pisani, P. Global cancer statistics, 2002. CA: a cancer *journal for clinicians,* 2005 Mar-Apr., 55(2), 74-108.

[4] Bosch, FX; Ribes, J; Diaz, M; Cleries, R. Primary liver cancer: worldwide incidence and trends. *Gastroenterology*, 2004 Nov., 127(5 Suppl 1), S5-S16.

[5] Rudolph, KL; Chang, S; Millard, M; Schreiber-Agus, N; DePinho, RA. Inhibition of experimental liver cirrhosis in mice by telomerase gene delivery. *Science*, 2000 Feb 18, 287(5456), 1253-8.

[6] El-Serag, HB; Rudolph, KL. Hepatocellular carcinoma: epidemiology and molecular carcinogenesis. *Gastroenterology*, 2007 Jun., 132(7), 2557-76.

[7] Yu, MW; Chen, CJ. Elevated serum testosterone levels and risk of hepatocellular carcinoma. *Cancer Res.*, 1993 Feb 15, 53(4), 790-4.

[8] Chen, CJ; Yu, MW; Liaw, YF. Epidemiological characteristics and risk factors of hepatocellular carcinoma. *J Gastroenterol Hepatol,* 1997 Oct., 12(9-10), S294-308.

[9] Thorgeirsson, SS; Grisham, JW. Molecular pathogenesis of human hepatocellular carcinoma. *Nat Genet*, 2002 Aug., 31(4), 339-46.

[10] Giannelli, G; Bergamini, C; Fransvea, E; Sgarra, C; Antonaci, S. Laminin-5 with transforming growth factor-beta1 induces epithelial to mesenchymal transition in hepatocellular carcinoma. *Gastroenterology*, 2005 Nov., 129(5), 1375-83.

[11] Koga, H; Sakisaka, S; Ohishi, M; Kawaguchi, T; Taniguchi, E; Sasatomi, K; et al. Expression of cyclooxygenase-2 in human hepatocellular carcinoma: relevance to tumor dedifferentiation. *Hepatology*, 1999 Mar., 29(3), 688-96.

[12] Bae, SH; Jung, ES; Park, YM; Kim, BS; Kim, BK; Kim, DG; et al. Expression of cyclooxygenase-2 (COX-2) in hepatocellular carcinoma and growth inhibition of hepatoma cell lines by a COX-2 inhibitor, NS-398. *Clin. Cancer Res.,* 2001, May, 7(5), 1410-8.

[13] Leng, J; Han, C; Demetris, AJ; Michalopoulos, GK; Wu, T. Cyclooxygenase-2 promotes hepatocellular carcinoma cell growth through Akt activation: evidence for Akt inhibition in celecoxib-induced apoptosis. *Hepatology,* 2003 Sep., 38(3), 756-68.

[14] Lee, YI; Lee, S; Lee, Y; Bong, YS; Hyun, SW; Yoo, YD; et al. The human hepatitis B virus transactivator X gene product regulates Sp1 mediated transcription of an insulin-like growth factor II promoter 4. *Oncogene*, 1998 May 7, 16(18), 2367-80.

[15] Kang-Park, S; Lee, YI; Lee, YI. PTEN modulates insulin-like growth factor II (IGF-II)-mediated signaling; the protein phosphatase activity of PTEN downregulates IGF-II expression in hepatoma cells. *FEBS Lett.*, 2003 Jun 19, 545(2-3), 203-8.

[16] De La Coste, A; Romagnolo, B; Billuart, P; Renard, CA; Buendia, MA; Soubrane, O., et al. Somatic mutations of the beta-catenin gene are frequent in mouse and human hepatocellular carcinomas. *Proc Natl Acad Sci U S A.* 1998 Jul 21, 95(15), 8847-51.

[17] Sicklick, JK; Li, YX, Jayaraman, A; Kannangai, R; Qi, Y; Vivekanandan, P; et al. Dysregulation of the Hedgehog pathway in human hepatocarcinogenesis. *Carcinogenesis,* 2006 Apr., 27(4), 748-57.

[18] Kaposi-Novak, P; Lee, JS; Gomez-Quiroz, L; Coulouarn, C; Factor, VM; Thorgeirsson, SS. Met-regulated expression signature defines a subset of human hepatocellular carcinomas with poor prognosis and aggressive phenotype. *J. Clin. Invest,* 2006, Jun., 116(6), 1582-95.

[19] Chen, RH; Su, YH; Chuang, RL; Chang, TY. Suppression of transforming growth factor-beta-induced apoptosis through a phosphatidylinositol 3-kinase/Akt-dependent pathway. *Oncogene*, 1998 Oct 15, 17(15), 1959-68.

[20] Wang, Y; Wu, MC; Sham, JS; Zhang, W; Wu, WQ; Guan, XY. Prognostic significance of c-myc and AIB1 amplification in hepatocellular carcinoma. A broad survey using high-throughput tissue microarray. *Cancer*, 2002 Dec 1., 95(11), 2346-52.

[21] Tannapfel, A; Busse, C; Weinans, L; Benicke, M; Katalinic, A; Geissler, F; et al. INK4a-ARF alterations and p53 mutations in hepatocellular carcinomas. *Oncogene*, 2001 Oct 25, 20(48), 7104-9.

[22] Endo, K; Ueda, T; Ohta, T; Terada, T. Protein expression of MDM2 and its clinicopathological relationships in human hepatocellular carcinoma. *Liver*, 2000, Jun., 20(3), 209-15.

[23] Umemura, A; Itoh, Y; Itoh, K; Yamaguchi, K; Nakajima, T; Higashitsuji, H; et al. Association of gankyrin protein expression with early clinical stages and insulin-like growth factor-binding protein 5 expression in human hepatocellular carcinoma. *Hepatology*, 2008, Feb., 47(2), 493-502.

[24] Azechi, H; Nishida, N; Fukuda, Y; Nishimura, T; Minata, M; Katsuma, H; et al. Disruption of the p16/cyclin D1/retinoblastoma protein pathway in the majority of human hepatocellular carcinomas. *Oncology*, 2001, 60(4), 346-54.

[25] Scharf, JG; Braulke, T. The role of the IGF axis in hepatocarcinogenesis. *Horm Metab Res.*, 2003 Nov-Dec., 35(11-12), 685-93.

[26] Yamada, T; De Souza, AT; Finkelstein, S; Jirtle, RL. Loss of the gene encoding mannose 6-phosphate/insulin-like growth factor II receptor is an early event in liver carcinogenesis. *Proc. Natl. Acad. Sci. USA*. 1997 Sep 16, 94(19), 10351-5.

[27] Hopfner, M; Huether, A; Sutter, AP; Baradari, V; Schuppan, D; Scherubl, H. Blockade of IGF-1 receptor tyrosine kinase has

antineoplastic effects in hepatocellular carcinoma cells. *Biochem. Pharmacol.*, 2006 May 14, 71(10), 1435-48.

[28] Chenivesse, X; Franco, D; Brechot, C. MDR1 (multidrug resistance) gene expression in human primary liver cancer and cirrhosis. *J. Hepatol.*, 1993 Jun., 18(2), 168-72.

[29] Soini, Y; Virkajarvi, N; Raunio, H; Paakko, P. Expression of P-glycoprotein in hepatocellular carcinoma: a potential marker of prognosis. *J. Clin. Pathol.,* 1996 Jun., 49(6), 470-3.

[30] Chen, CJ; Chin, JE; Ueda, K; Clark, DP; Pastan, I; Gottesman, MM; et al. Internal duplication and homology with bacterial transport proteins in the mdr1 (P-glycoprotein) gene from multidrug-resistant human cells. *Cell*, 1986 Nov 7, 47(3), 381-9.

[31] Chin, JE; Soffir, R; Noonan, KE; Choi, K; Roninson, IB. Structure and expression of the human MDR (P-glycoprotein) gene family. *Molecular and cellular biology*., 1989 Sep., 9(9), 3808-20.

[32] Chan, JY; Chu, AC; Fung, KP. Inhibition of P-glycoprotein expression and reversal of drug resistance of human hepatoma HepG2 cells by multidrug resistance gene (mdr1) antisense RNA. *Life Sci.*, 2000 Sep 15, 67(17), 2117-24.

[33] Wang, H; Chen, XP; Qiu, FZ. Overcoming multi-drug resistance by anti-MDR1 ribozyme. *World J. Gastroenterol,* 2003 Jul., 9(7), 1444-9.

[34] Li, B; Ye, T; Zhao, L; Li, DH; Gou, XH; Zhao, LY; et al. Effects of multidrug resistance, antisense RNA on the chemosensitivity of hepatocellular carcinoma cells. *Hepatobiliary Pancreat Dis. Int.* 2006 Nov., 5(4), 552-9.

[35] Suzuki, K; Hayashi, N; Miyamoto, Y; Yamamoto, M; Ohkawa, K; Ito, Y; et al. Expression of vascular permeability factor/vascular endothelial growth factor in human hepatocellular carcinoma. *Cancer Res.*, 1996 Jul 1, 56(13), 3004-9.

[36] Huynh, H; Soo, KC; Chow, PK; Tran, E. Targeted inhibition of the extracellular signal-regulated kinase kinase pathway with AZD6244 (ARRY-142886) in the treatment of hepatocellular carcinoma. *Mol. Cancer Ther.*, 2007 Jan., 6(1), 138-46.

[37] Liu, L; Cao, Y; Chen, C; Zhang, X; McNabola, A; Wilkie, D; et al. Sorafenib blocks the RAF/MEK/ERK pathway, inhibits tumor angiogenesis, and induces tumor cell apoptosis in hepatocellular carcinoma model PLC/PRF/5. *Cancer Res.*, 2006 Dec 15, 66(24), 11851-8.

[38] Llovet, JM; Ricci, S; Mazzaferro, V; Hilgard, P; Gane, E; Blanc, JF; et al. Sorafenib in advanced hepatocellular carcinoma. *The New England journal of medicine,* 2008 Jul 24, 359(4), 378-90.

[39] Harris, PA; Boloor, A; Cheung, M; Kumar, R; Crosby, RM; Davis-Ward, RG; et al. Discovery of 5-[[4-[(2,3-Dimethyl-2H-indazol-6-yl)methylamino]-2-pyrimidinyl]amino]-2-m ethyl-benzenesulfonamide (Pazopanib), a Novel and Potent Vascular Endothelial Growth Factor Receptor Inhibitor. *J Med Chem.*, 2008 Jul. 12.

[40] Ayers, M; Fargnoli, J; Lewin, A; Wu, Q; Platero, JS. Discovery and validation of biomarkers that respond to treatment with brivanib alaninate, a small-molecule VEGFR-2/FGFR-1 antagonist. *Cancer research,* 2007 Jul 15, 67(14), 6899-906.

[41] Huether, A; Hopfner, M; Baradari, V; Schuppan, D; Scherubl, H. Sorafenib alone or as combination therapy for growth control of cholangiocarcinoma. *Biochem Pharmacol*, 2007 May 1, 73(9), 1308-17.

[42] Abou-Alfa GK, JP; Knox, J; Davidenko, I; Lacava, J; Leung, T; Mori, A; Le Berre, M; Voliotis, D; Saltz, L. Final results from a phase II (PhII), randomized, double-blind study of sorafenib plus doxorubicin (S+D) versus placebo plus doxorubicin (P+D) in patients (pts) with advanced hepatocellular carcinoma (AHCC). *Gastrointestinal Cancers Symposium.* Orlando, Florida 2008.

[43] Ito, Y; Takeda, T; Higashiyama, S; Sakon, M; Wakasa, KI; Tsujimoto, M; et al. Expression of heparin binding epidermal growth factor-like growth factor in hepatocellular carcinoma: an immunohistochemical study. *Oncol .Rep.*, 2001 Jul-Aug., 8(4), 903-7.

[44] Thomas, MB; Chadha, R; Glover, K; Wang, X; Morris, J; Brown, T; et al. Phase 2 study of erlotinib in patients with unresectable hepatocellular carcinoma. *Cancer*, 2007 Sep 1, 110(5), 1059-67.

[45] Philip, PA; Mahoney, MR; Allmer, C; Thomas, J; Pitot, HC; Kim, G; et al. Phase II study of Erlotinib (OSI-774) in patients with advanced hepatocellular cancer. *J Clin Oncol,* 2005 Sep 20, 23(27), 6657-63.

[46] Ueda, S; Basaki, Y; Yoshie, M; Ogawa, K; Sakisaka, S; Kuwano, M; et al. PTEN/Akt signaling through epidermal growth factor receptor is prerequisite for angiogenesis by hepatocellular carcinoma cells that is susceptible to inhibition by gefitinib. *Cancer Res.*, 2006 May 15, 66(10), 5346-53.

[47] Jemal, A; Siegel, R; Ward, E; Hao, Y; Xu, J, Murray, T; et al. *Cancer statistics*, 2008, CA: *A cancer journal for clinicians,* 2008 Mar-Apr., 58(2), 71-96.

[48] Pantuck, AJ; Zisman, A; Belldegrun, AS. The changing natural history of renal cell carcinoma. *The Journal of urology,* 2001 Nov., 166(5), 1611-23.

[49] Childs, R; Chernoff, A; Contentin, N; Bahceci, E; Schrump, D; Leitman, S; et al. Regression of metastatic renal-cell carcinoma after nonmyeloablative allogeneic peripheral-blood stem-cell transplantation. *The New England journal of medicine,* 2000 Sep 14, 343(11), 750-8.

[50] Motzer, RJ; Mazumdar, M; Bacik, J; Berg, W; Amsterdam, A; Ferrara, J. Survival and prognostic stratification of 670 patients with advanced renal cell carcinoma. *J. Clin. Oncol,* 1999 Aug., 17(8), 2530-40.

[51] Escudier, B; Eisen, T; Stadler, WM; Szczylik, C; Oudard, S; Siebels, M; et al. Sorafenib in advanced clear-cell renal-cell carcinoma. *The New England journal of medicine,* 2007 Jan 11, 356(2), 125-34.

[52] Motzer, RJ; Hutson, TE; Tomczak, P; Michaelson, MD; Bukowski, RM; Rixe, O; et al. Sunitinib versus interferon alfa in metastatic renal-cell carcinoma. *The New England journal of medicine,* 2007 Jan 11, 356(2), 115-24.

[53] Escudier, B; Pluzanska, A; Koralewski, P; Ravaud, A; Bracarda, S; Szczylik, C; et al. Bevacizumab plus interferon alfa-2a for treatment of metastatic renal cell carcinoma: a randomised, double-blind phase III trial. *Lancet*, 2007 Dec 22, 370(9605), 2103-11.

[54] Hudson, CC; Liu, M; Chiang, GG; Otterness, DM; Loomis, DC; Kaper, F; et al. Regulation of hypoxia-inducible factor 1alpha expression and function by the mammalian target of rapamycin. *Molecular and cellular biology,* 2002 Oct., 22(20), 7004-14.

[55] Hudes, G; Carducci, M; Tomczak, P; Dutcher, J; Figlin, R; Kapoor, A; et al. Temsirolimus, interferon alfa, or both for advanced renal-cell carcinoma. *The New England journal of medicine,* 2007 May 31, 356(22), 2271-81.

[56] Motzer, RJ; Escudier, B; Oudard, S; Hutson, TE; Porta, C; Bracarda, S; et al. Efficacy of everolimus in advanced renal cell carcinoma: a double-blind, randomised, placebo-controlled phase III trial. *Lancet*, 2008 Aug 9, 372(9637), 449-56.

[57] Kouroumalis, E; Skordilis, P; Thermos, K; Vasilaki, A; Moschandrea, J; Manousos, ON. Treatment of hepatocellular carcinoma with octreotide: a randomised controlled study. *Gut*. 1998 Mar., 42(3), 442-7.

[58] Becker, G; Allgaier, HP; Olschewski, M; al. e. Long-acting octreotide versus placebo for treatment of advanced HCC: a randomized controlled double-blind study. *Hepatology*, 2007 Jan., 45(1), 9-15.

[59] Yeo, W; Mok, TS; Zee, B; Leung, TW; Lai, PB; Lau, WY; et al. A randomized phase III study of doxorubicin versus cisplatin/interferon alpha-2b/doxorubicin/fluorouracil (PIAF) combination chemotherapy for unresectable hepatocellular carcinoma. *J. Natl. Cancer Inst.,* 2005 Oct 19, 97(20), 1532-8.

[60] Barbare, JC; Bouche, O; Bonnetain, F; Raoul, JL; Rougier, P; Abergel, A; et al. Randomized controlled trial of tamoxifen in advanced hepatocellular carcinoma. *J. Clin. Oncol,* 2005 Jul 1, 23(19), 4338-46.

[61] Hsu, C; Yang; T; Toh, T. Modified-dose capecitabine + bevacizumab for the treatment of advanced/metastatic hepatocellular carcinoma (HCC): A phase II, single-arm study. Journal of Clinical Oncology, 2007 *ASCO Annual Meeting Proceedings Part I.* Vol 25, No. 18S (June 20 Supplement), 2007, 15190. 2007.

[62] Thomas, MB; Chadha, R; Iwasaki, M. The combination of bevacizumab (B) and erlotinib (E) shows significant biological activity in patients with advanced hepatocellular carcinoma (HCC). *Journal of Clinical Oncology*, 2007 ASCO Annual Meeting Proceedings Part I. Vol 25, No. 18S (June 20 Supplement), 2007, 4567, 2007.

[63] Zhu, AX; Blaszkowsky, LS; Ryan, DP; Clark, JW; Muzikansky, A; Horgan, K; et al. Phase II study of gemcitabine and oxaliplatin in combination with bevacizumab in patients with advanced hepatocellular carcinoma. *J. Clin. Oncol.,* 2006 Apr 20, 24(12), 1898-903.

[64] Sun, W; Haller, DG; Mykulowycz, K. Combination of capecitabine, oxaliplatin with bevacizumab in treatment of advanced hepatocellular carcinoma (HCC): A phase II study. *Journal of Clinical Oncology,* 2007 ASCO Annual Meeting Proceedings Part I. Vol 25, No. 18S (June 20 Supplement), 2007, 4574. 2007.

In: Advances in Proteomics Research ISBN: 978-1-61942-227-8
Editors: Ya Li Huang et al. pp. 223-252

Chapter 7

PARADIGM OF PROTEIN FOLDING IN NEURODEGENERATIVE DISEASES

Pratibha Mehta Luthra *

University of Delhi, Delhi, India.

ABSTRACT

The most abundant molecules in nature other than water are proteins, which are involved to stimulate or control virtually every chemical process. Majority of proteins must be converted into tightly folded compact structures in order to function and their ability to fold to a unique structure generate enormous selectivity and diversity in their functions. Conformational changes in proteins result in misfolding, aggregation, and intra- or extraneuronal accumulation of amyloid fibrils in many neurodegenerative disorders. Proteins appear to fold by diverse pathways, the rates of folding are largely determined by the topology of the native structure. In general, secondary structure is inherently unstable and its stability is enhanced by tertiary interactions. The most conspicuous feature of many neurodegenerative disorders, including Alzheimer's, Parkinson's, and Huntington's disease, is the occurrence of protein aggregates in ordered fibrillar structures known as amyloid found inside and outside of brain cells. The appearance of aggregates in diseased brains implies an underlying incapacity in the cellular machinery

* Division of Medicinal Chemistry, Dr. B.R. Ambedkar Centre for Biomedical Research, University of Delhi, Delhi 110007, India, Phone: 91-11-27666272, Fax : 91-11-27666248, Email: pmluthra@acbr.du.ac.in, pmlsci@yahoo.com

of molecular chaperones that normally functions to prevent the accumulation of misfolded proteins. Molecular chaperones provide a first line of defense against misfolded, aggregation-prone proteins, and are among the most potent suppressors of neurodegeneration known for animal models of human disease. A detailed understanding of the molecular basis of protection by chaperones against neurodegeneration might lead to the development of therapies for neurodegenerative disorders that are associated with protein misfolding and aggregation.

In this review, the advances on the protein folding in neurodegenrative disorder and unfolding the role of molecular chaperones in neuroprotection has been discussed.

1. Introduction

Neuro-degenerative disorders such as Alzheimer's disease (AD), Parkinson's disease (PD), Huntington's disease (HD), amyotrophic lateral sclerosis (ALS) are characterized by neuronal damage caused due to toxic, aggregation-prone proteins. The aggregates usually consist of fibers containing mis-folded protein with β-sheet conformation. A major effect of mutations in the genes is the abnormal processingand accumulation of mis-folded protein in neuronal inclusions andplaques. Aggregates and protein misfolding due to mutations are the major cause of neurodegenerative diseases. Increased accumulation of abnormal proteins and their toxic effects play vital role in development of Parkinson's disease (PD) occurs due to degeneration of dopaminergic neurons in substantia nigra of the brain. Clusters of alpha-synuclein protein have been found throughout the brain of PD patients, which are involved in the formation of Lewy bodies. Misfolded proteins and aggregates cause molecular stress and interfere with cellular function. The energetics of protein association could not be simply interpreted by that of the exothermic reactions, aggregation – would be always highly susceptible to pressure and low temperatures. Molecular chaperones provide a first line of defense against misfolded, aggregation-prone proteins, and are among the most potent suppressors ofneurodegeneration, because of their ability to modulate the earliest aberrantprotein interactions that trigger pathogenic cascades. To decrease amyloid burden and neurotoxicity in neurodegenerative disorders, advanced knowledge of cellular mechanisms fordisposal of abnormal proteins and effects of toxic proteinaccumulation on neuronal survival may allow the development ofrational, effective treatment to fight these disorders.

2. BRAIN LESIONS IN NEURODEGENERATIVE DISEASE

The most common apparent feature of neurodegerative disorders such as Alzheimer's disease (AD), Huntington's disease (HD), Parkinson's disease (PD), amyotrophic lateral sclerosis (ALS), and transmissible spongiform encephalopathies (TSEs or prion diseases) is the occurrence of lesions in brains. The inclusion bodies frequently contain the disease protein in a fibrillar aggregated form called amyloid [Eanes and Glenner 1968; Sunde and Blake 1998; Makin and Serpell 2005] and also may contain other material. Intra- and extrecellular accumulation of misfolded, aggregated, and ubiquitinated proteins form lesions [Ross and Michelle 2005] that are associated with neurodegeneration (Figure 1).The lesions observed in AD are intracellular neurofibrillary tangles that contain the protein tau and extracellular plaques that contain β-amyloid (βA) peptides [Selkoe 2001].

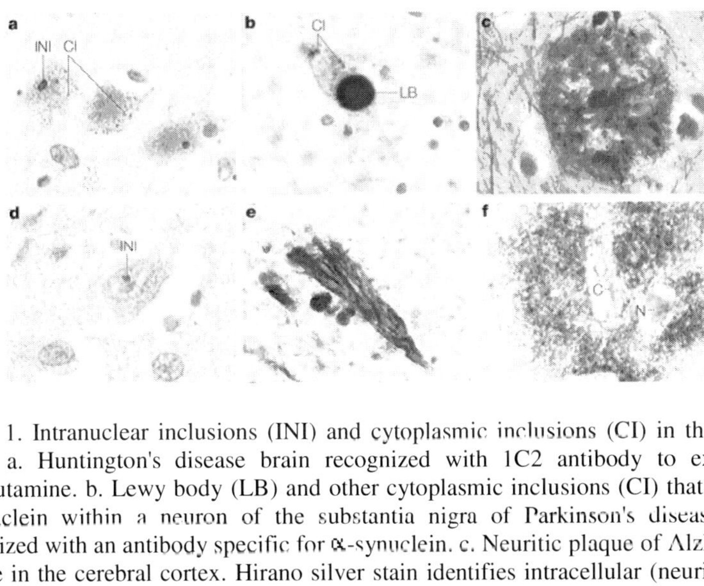

Figure 1. Intranuclear inclusions (INI) and cytoplasmic inclusions (CI) in the motor cortex a. Huntington's disease brain recognized with 1C2 antibody to expanded polyglutamine. b. Lewy body (LB) and other cytoplasmic inclusions (CI) that contain α-synuclein within a neuron of the substantia nigra of Parkinson's disease brain recognized with an antibody specific for α-synuclein. c. Neuritic plaque of Alzheimer's disease in the cerebral cortex. Hirano silver stain identifies intracellular (neuritic) and extracellular protein aggregates. d. Intranuclear inclusion in the frontal cortex of Huntington's disease brain recognized with anti-ubiquitin antibody. e. Neurofibrillary tangles of Alzheimer's disease in the hippocampus immunostained with antibody specific for phosphorylated tau. f. Diffuse plaque of Alzheimer's disease in the cerebral cortex. Amyloid β(Aβ)-specific antibody recognizes extracellular deposits of Aβ (surrounding a neuron (N) and a capillary (C)). Figure provided by O. Pletnikova and J. C. Troncoso, John Hopkins University, Baltimore, USA. Reproduced from: Ross andMichelle [2005].doi:10.1038/nrm1742.

In PD, the lesions are called Lewy bodies, are found in cytoplasm, and are composed primarily of α-synuclein [Goedert 2001]. In HD, the lesions are observed as intranuclear and cytoplasmic inclusion bodies that contain the protein huntigtin [Lorenzetti et al. 2000] All these protein lesions have tendency to form an ordered fibrillar structure called amyloid [Rochet and Lansbury 2000].

Amyloid formation is thought to arise from partial unfolding and exposure to hydrophobic surfaces that are normally buried in the core of a folded protein, thus increasing attractive forces among protein molecules. Mutations that increase the production of amyloid cause rare, early on-set of forms of AD and PD. In HD, the length of polyglutamine correlates directly with kinetics of amyloid formation and indirectly with age of onset and severity of the disease. The other common feature of AD, PD and HD is the presence of molecular chaperones and components of the ubiquitin-proteasome degradation system in the brain lesions characteristics of each disease [Clark and Muchowski 2000; Huang et al. 2001].

3. Pre-Fibrillar Intermediates (Protofibrils) and Neurotoxicity

In neurodeg\enerative diseases, theaccumulation of intracellular or extracellular protein leads to formation of aggregates in tissue. The aggregates may consist of fibrillar structures containing β-sheet-rich misfolded protein, termed amyloids, are characterized by their ability to bind aromatic dyes. Most neurotoxic protein aggregates cause cell death by impairment of various cellular functions and eventually lead to degeneration of brain regions. The quantity of such aggregates can be almost un-dectectable in some cases, whilst in systemic diseases kilograms of protein can be found in such deposits [Goedert 1997]. A monomer might misfold into various distinct conformations each of which could then give rise to a distinct higher-order assembly (spherical, annular or amorphous aggregates or a fibril). Because protein aggregation may be a generic property of polypeptide chains that does not depend on specific amino acid sequence and the toxic effects of pre-fibrillar organisation results from common structural features rather that from specific sequences of side chains it is likely that the formation of toxic oligomeric structures formed by different proteins show structural similarities and these have indeed been observed (for example, Aβ, synuclein and a fragment of huntingtin form annular oligomers). Studies of polyglutamine[Kazantsev et al.

1999; Preisinger et al. 1999; McCampbell et al. 2000; Chen et al. 2001; Nucifora et al. 2001; McNaught et al. 2004] demonstrated the relationship between aggregation and toxicity. The toxicity depends on interactions with, and possibly recruitment of, other cellular constituents during the aggregation process (Figure 2). Therefore, perhaps no single species is toxic *per se*, but instead the active process of aggregation, and interactions with other proteins in the cell, causes toxicity [Dobson 2003; Lashuel et al. 2002; Quist et al. 2005].

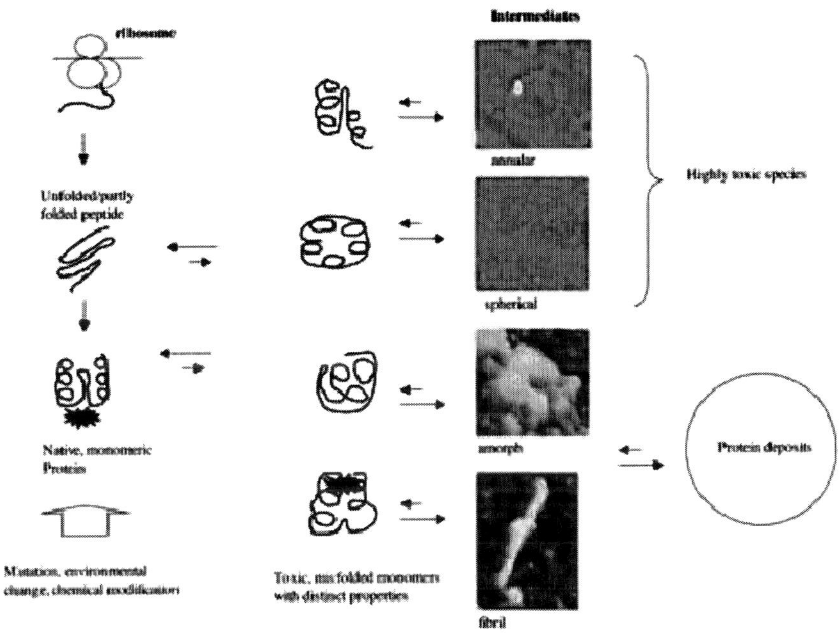

Figure 2.Formation of intra- or extracellularly accumulation of the protein deposits. Various factors cause formation of misfolded monomers leading to neurotoxic misfolded aggregates. www.ncbi.nlm.nih.gov/bookshelf/br.fcgi?book=e...

Defect in complex I inhibition causes aggregation of α-synuclein leading to the demise of dopamineneurons, and may be the central cause of sporadic PD. Several environmental toxins (e.g., herbicides, insecticides such as rotenone) are selectively neurotoxic to dopaminergic neurons and inhibit complex I of the electron transfer chain within mitochondria. These toxins also lead to the formation of LBs. ROS/RNS play a critical role during PD leading to modulate PD toxicity (Figure 3). Increased oxidative damage and altered mitochondrial activity (probably because of decreased complex IV activity) has been reported in AD [Anderson 2004].

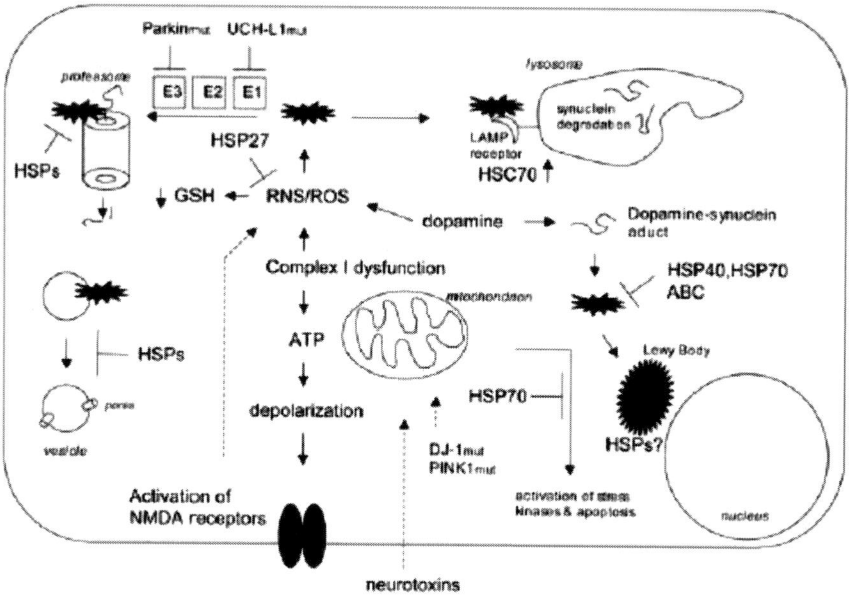

Figure 3. Neurotoxicity in PD. Impairment of complex I of the electron transfer chain within mitochondria may contribute to the demise of dopamine neurons through direct proteasome impairment by α-synuclein assemblies or indirectly via mutations in parkin and UCH-L1. http://www.ncbi.nlm.nih.gov/bookshelf/br.fcgi.

"Senile plaques" and "tangles" in stained sections from the postmortem brain were composed of fibrils formed by the aggregation of short peptides, which were mostly 40 and 42 aa long [Glenner and Wong 1984; Sisodia et al. 1990]. These peptides had a perfectly normal amino acid sequence (common to both peptides) and represented a part of a much larger common transmembrane "amyloid precursor protein" (APP) of unknown function. These peptides are greatly over-produced in AD, the two overproduced peptides, Aβ1-40 and Aβ1-42, when liberated from their parent APP, refold ("misfold") and aggregate spontaneously to a neurotoxic, β-sheet-containing fibrillar form [Blanchard et al. 2004].

In the HD brain, oxidative damage has been detected together with a decreased mitochondrial complex II and IV activity [Browne et al. 1999] and in HD mouse models free radical damage has been observed [Tabrizi et al. 2000]. Each amyloid disease involves the aggregation of a specific protein although a range of other components, including other proteins and carbohydrates, is also incorporated into the deposits when they form *in vivo*. The characteristics of the soluble forms of the 20 or so proteins involved in the well-defined amyloidoses are varied—they range from intact globular proteins to largely unstructured peptide molecules—but the aggregated forms have many common characteristics [Ravikumar et al. 2004]. Extracellular aggregates might lead to apoptosis by interacting with specific cellular receptors, thereby inducing cellular stress and activation of NF-κB [Yan et *al.* 2000]. Intracellular aggregates might damage cells by modulating the cell viability leading to the fibrillar aggregates. Components of the proteasome, chaperone proteins, cytoskeletal proteins and transcription factors have been found in huntingtin and α-synuclein aggregates[Cummings et al. 1998]. Membrane disruption and depolarization mediated by ion-channel formation, resulting in alteration of ion homeostasis and disregulation of cellular signal transduction, leading to cell death due to Aβ and PrP neurotoxicity [Lin et al. 1997]. Finally, protein aggregates might induce oxidative stress by producing free radical species, resulting in protein and lipid oxidation, elevation of intracellular calcium and mitochondrial disfunction [Behl et al. 1994; Hsu et al. 2000].

4. Mechanism of Protein Folding

The most fundamental biochemical processes in protein folding arises from the challenge of understanding the wrapping of the protein sequences. Even small proteins folding on a sub-second timescale may pass through structural intermediates en route to the native state [Brockwell and Radford 2007; Bartlett and Radford 2009], that either represent on-pathway 'stepping stones' toward the native state or kinetically stable, misfolded conformations that may require substantial reorganization before the native state can be reached. The formation of meta-stable, non-native interactions during folding is interpreted as a consequence of the ruggedness of folding energy [Onuchic and Wolynes 2004; Jahn and Radford 2005], irrespective of whether proteins are thought to fold through multiple downhill routes or through preferred pathways defined by the sequential assembly of elementary folding units, so-called 'foldons' [Englander etal. 2007; Lindberg and Oliveberg 2007] The protein-folding has been divided into two parts i) prediction of the three-dimensional structure from the amino acid sequence and ii) understanding the relation between protein sequences and mechanisms of folding.

Two distinct mechanisms have classically been used to describe the folding of small single-domain proteins, DC (diffusion-condensation) and NC (nucleation-condensation) model. DC model [Karplus and Weaver 1976; 1994] assumes that a protein molecule is divided into parts such that the information contained in the amino acid sequence of each part is sufficient to fold autonomously. Folding proceeds as a series of coalescence events that might either follow a unique order (sequential folding pathways) or explore different routes (parallel folding pathways), whose dominant components might be affected by solvent conditions or primary structure compositions for different homologous proteins. DC model is based on the existence of fluctuating quasi-particles, the "micro-domains", which may be portions of incipient secondary structure. DC model reduces the dynamics of the folding process to the diffusion events of discrete pre-formed micro-domains of nascent secondary structure elements. Chymotrypsin inhibitor 2 (CI2), a small, single domain protein without additional chemical complexity from disulfide bridges, metals, or other cofactor showed a distorted version of the native state and the protein seemed to fold as a single cooperative unit, thus challenging the concept of pre-existing micro-domains postulated by the DC (diffusion-condensation) model (**Fig. 4**).The NC (nucleation-condensation) model postulates the existence of a folding nucleus, about which the transition state is constructed [Abkevich et al. 1994]. A significant portion of the structure must collapse (or condense) to an approximately correct conformation for the discontinuous network of interactions in the nucleus to come together. Formation of the nucleus (nucleation) is coupled with a more extended formation of structure (condensation) [Fersht 1995].

Interestingly, despite the weakness of the folding nucleus implied by the NC model, ingenious experiments based on topological mutations of CI2, including circular permutation (Itzhaki et. al 1995) and splitting of the protein [Neira et al.1996], suggest that the position of the nucleus is quite conserved in proteins following the pure NC model.

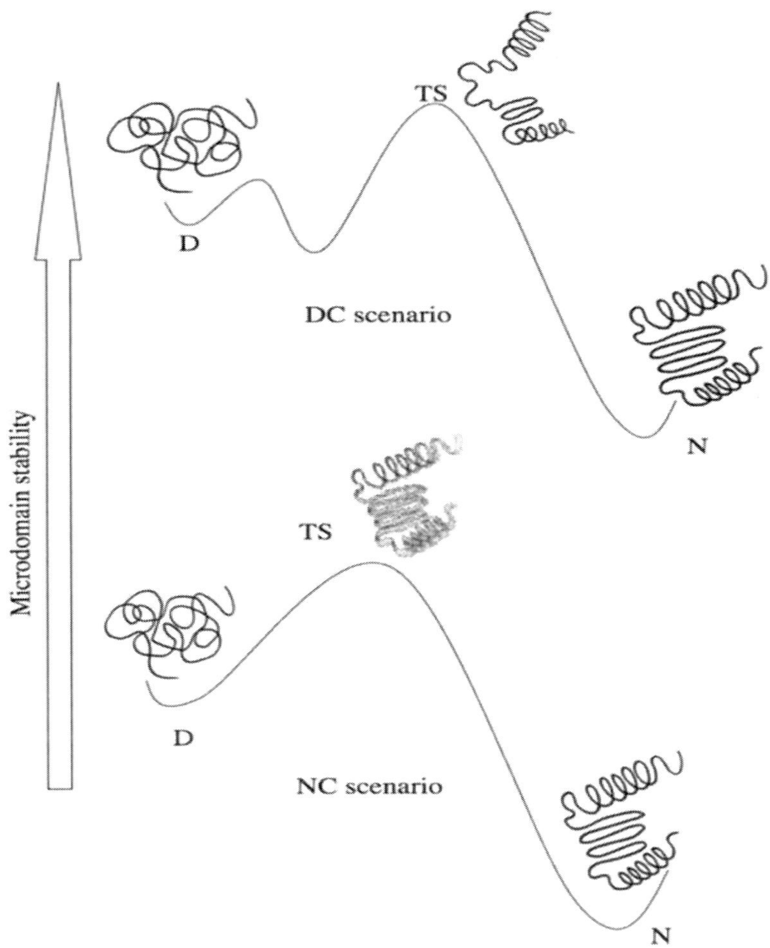

Figure 4. The classical diffusion–collision (*DC*) and nucleation–condensation (*NC*) mechanisms for protein folding. DC model (*top*) is based on the existence of micro-domains, involving segments of secondary structure, whose productive collision represents the rate-limiting step of folding. In*NC* model (*bottom*), the main folding TS is a distorted version of the native state and folding occurs via simultaneous formation of secondary and tertiary structure, around a weakly-structured folding nucleus. Reproduced from Ivarsson et al. [2008].

The mechanism of folding with helical elements fully preformed, concurrently with an increase in the inherent helical propensity in the homodomain family behavior showed the transformation from NC behavior to DC using experimental and computational approaches. A protein depending on the inherent stability of the secondary structure elements, may manifest itself as either NC or DC behavior [Gianni et al. 2003] involving Unifying mechanism of folding. The folding process of a PDZ domain involving the crossing of two consecutive TS barriers [Gianni et al. 2005] comprised elements of both the DC and NC mechanisms [Ivarsson et al. 2007; Gianni et al. 2007a]. Unifying folding mechanism involve three major events for the folding of small globular proteins: (1) formation of a weak nucleus that determines the native-like topology of the structure, (2) a global collapse of the entire polypeptide chain, and (3) consolidation of the remaining partially structured regions to achieve the native state conformations. The proteins can be rerouted through the energy landscape by mutational [Wright et al. 2003], topological [Lindberg and Oliveberg 2007] or solvent perturbations [Gianni et al. 2007b] according to the landscape theory, assuming that the trajectory taken by a protein molecule is determined by thermodynamic probabilities.

The existence of parallel folding pathways have been reported for a variety of small protein domains by molecular dynamic simulations [Lazaridis and Karplus 1997; Borreguero et al. 2004; Rao et al. 2005; Juraszek and Bolhuis 2006; Lam et al. 2007]. The major difference between apparent two-state and multi-state folding proteins is the relative stability of the partially folded intermediates. Small proteins often fold fast and without detectable folding intermediates [Krantz et al. 2002]. Studies of folding mechanism of homologous protein suggested that the structural mechanisms of folding may be conserved, even if the kinetic folding mechanism is different.

Methods for rapid initiation of protein folding can be roughly classified into three categories—photochemical triggering, temperature or pressure jump, and ultrarapid mixing methods. The photochemical trigger employed the photodissociation of carbon monoxide from denatured cytochrome*c* [Jones et al. 1993; Chan et al. 1996]. A different kind of photochemical trigger uses a photolabile disulfide [Lu et al. 1997; Volk et al. 1997], which does not require a metal site, so in principle it can be used as a trigger for a much wider range of proteins. A second class of optical triggers uses an intense laser pulse to produce a rapid temperature jump. This is a much more generally applicable method because it can be used to perturb the folding/unfolding equilibrium for any process that produces a significant enthalpy change. This was first done in a protein-folding experiment by heating a solution of a dye with a mode-locked picosecond laser operating at 532 nm [Philips et al. 1995].

Almost all proteins can be unfolded and remain soluble at sufficiently high denaturant concentrations of chemical denaturants such as urea and guanidinium chloride, so dilution of denaturants continues to be an extremely important way of initiating protein folding. The time-resolution in mixing experiments by using continuous flow methods have recently been applied to protein folding, one based on turbulent mixing [Chan et al. 1997; Takahashi et al. 1997; Shastry et al. 1998a; 1998b; 1998c, Park et al. 1999] and another based on hydrodynamic focusing [Knight et al. 1998; Pollack et al. 1999].

Studies of folding mechanism of homologous protein suggested that the structural mechanisms of folding may be conserved, even if the kinetic folding mechanism is different. The bacterial immunity proteins Im9 and Im7 apparently fold by two-state or three-state mechanisms, respectively [Ferguson et al. 1999]. However, the late transition state ensembles of the two proteins have similar properties [Friel et al. 2003].

i) Kinetics and Thermodynamics of Protein Folding

By systematically perturbing native interactions via mutagenesis while measuring the folding kinetics of the mutant protein, it is possible to identify interaction patterns presenting the folding transition state (Matouschek et al. 1990). The role of a given residue is measured by its θ value upon mutagenesis, which normalizes the change in stability of the activation barrier to that of the native state. The θ value is a structural index for a given residue in the transition states or folding intermediates; θ value of 1 suggests that the probed position is fully structured in the transition state where as θ value of 0 indicates that it is fully unstructured. Finally, protein-folding kinetics can be studied at equilibrium using dynamic nuclear magnetic resonance (NMR) methods [Huang and Oas 1995; Burton et al. 1996; 1997]. The method is useful for determining folding rates in the 10 μs-10 ms range under conditions where there is a significant population of both folded and unfolded states. Folding can be initiated by reduction of oxidized cytochrome *c* or dissociation of carbon monoxide in reduced cytochrome *c* [Hagen et al.1996; Hagen 2010].

The simplest elementary process in protein folding is the formation of a contact between two residues of an unfolded polypeptide chain. Time-resolved spectroscopy with nanosecond lasers was used to monitor heme absorption following photodissociation of the carbon monoxide complex of denatured reduced cytochrome*c* [Jones et al.1993]. Contact formation in peptides can be measured using long-lived triplet states. In the triplet-triplet energy transfer experiment, an organic donor (thioxanthone, T) attached at one end of a peptide is optically excited to its long-lived triplet state. It remains in this state until it forms a contact in a diffusion-limited process with an acceptor near the other end (naphthalene, N). Transfer of the excitation energy, raising the acceptor to its triplet state, is sufficiently fast that the diffusion-limited rate of contact formation is the same as the overall observed rate of energy transfer. In the triplet state quenching experiment tryptophan and cysteine are at two ends of the peptide, the contact formation was measured from the quenching of the triplet state of tryptophan at the C-terminus of a peptide by cysteine at the N-terminus [Eaton et al. 2000]. However, at least two factors contribute to the inconsistency of the results with this prediction from the two experiments. The contact radius*a* for the tryptophan-cysteine interaction is larger than for the methionine-heme encounter complex of cytochrome *c*, and the heme is only accessible to the methionine on one side, so the effective value of *a* is larger in the quenching experiments. Also, the peptides are rich in glycine and therefore have smaller $\langle r^2 \rangle$ compared to cytochrome *c*, which has only an average of 1 glycine per 6–7 residues between the heme and methionines [Szabo et al. 1980]. However, the tryptophan triplet lifetime measurements can provide a useful method for investigating the kinetics of forming a specific intra-molecular contact in an unfolded or folding protein. A maximum in the loop probability as a function of chain length has been predicted at about 10 residues for a generic polypeptide [Camacho and Thirumalai1995; Thirumalai 1999; Guo et al.2001].

Extensive equilibrium studies using fast kinetic techniques of α-helix formation in isolated peptides rich in alanine have been carried out because of their high helix-forming propensity [Marqusee et al. 1989; Chakrabartty and Baldwin 1995; Muñoz and Serrano 1995]. In a 21-residue peptide having the sequence X-$(A)_5$ $(AAARA)_3$-A-NH_2 (X = succinyl), a nano second laser was used to perturb the helix-coil equilibrium, and infrared absorption measurements in the amide I region were used to monitor the decrease in helix content. A simple nucleation/propagation model was developed to explain the fast relaxation results from helix propagation and partial melting of stretches of helix, while the slow relaxation corresponds to crossing a helix nucleation barrier [Thompson et al. 2000]. More recently the model has been modified to predict the kinetics of peptides having the length and composition found in helices of proteins incorporating the more detailed equilibrium description of the helix-coil transition contained in the program AGADIR [Muñoz and Serrano 1994; 1995]. In the first kinetic investigation of β-hairpins, the 16-residue C-terminal fragment of the protein GB1 showed that except for less cooperative thermal unfolding, the thermodynamic and kinetic behavior of this β-hairpin is very much like that of a small protein [Muñoz 1997; Muñoz 2007].

The reactions involving protein interactions, such as protein association, are different than those reactions that provided the original basis for the application of classical thermodynamics to chemistry (Weber 1999). The condensation reactions of proteins, that comprise protein association and protein folding, are endothermic chemical processes, taking place with absorption of heat from the environment. The classical chemical thermodynamics has been virtually confined to reactions of the exothermic variety and the relations applicable to them have been taken as generally valid for the endothermic case [Weber 1999]. Weber concluded that the energetics of protein association could not be simply interpreted by that of the exothermic reactions, particularly in what concerned the effects on temperature on the thermodynamic equilibrium [Weber 1993; 1999]. Among other consequences of the dissimilarity between these reactions is the fact that the condensation of proteins – such as folding, oligomerization and aggregation – would be always highly susceptible to pressure and to low temperatures [Privalov 1990; Silva 1993; Smeller 2002].

ii) Protein Self Assembly

The self-assembly mechanism of individual proteins is closely related to their function, it may be the key for rationalizing the underlying sequence-dependence of aggregation proteins as indicated in Alzheimer's and Parkinson's disease. Several studies were carried to carefully characterize the kinetics, thermodynamics, and effects of mutations in other small, single domain proteins [Jackson and Fersht 1991] to investigate the fundamental processes in protein folding, including formation of α-helices, β-sheets, and contacts between residues distant in sequence as well as overall collapse of the polypeptide chain and folding of the very fastest proteins. Simple statistical mechanical models, originally developed for explaining the fast kinetics of secondary structure formation in isolated peptides, has been remarkably successful in quantitatively explaining the kinetic behavior of small proteins [Callender et al. 1998; Gruebele 1999]. Novel theoretical and experimental approaches have shown that a key role in protein folding studies has been played by the description of folding transition states [Daggett and Fersht 2003; Fersht 2000]. The transition state (TS) theory observed kinetics of simple chemical inter-conversions [Eyring 1935] and was extended to protein folding studies contributing to the characterization of classical folding mechanisms. In analogy with the TS of chemical reactions, the transition state ensemble of folding is the ensemble of protein conformations with an equal probability to fold or unfold. Interactions formed in the TS of folding have been mapped out for several small proteins by analysis of θ value [Fersht et al. 1992], providing information on both native and non-native contacts formed in the TS [Fersht and Sato 2004; Weikl and Dill 2007].

The structural signatures of the denatured state ensemble (DSE), which show native contacts that are delocalized across the protein fold upon mutation should correlate with slower aggregation rates. The bacterial immunity proteins Im9 and Im7 apparently fold by two-state or three-state mechanisms, respectively [Ferguson et al. 1999]. However, the late transition state ensembles of the two proteins have similar properties [Friel et al. 2003]. In fact, under acidic conditions it was possible to stabilize a high-energy folding intermediate of Im9 so that it became kinetically detectable [Gorski et al. 2001]. Furthermore, the folding intermediate of Im7 involves formation of non-native contacts [Capaldi et al. 2002]. By rational engineering of Im9 it was possible to stabilize non-native interactions in the folding intermediate and thereby speed up the folding process [Friel et al. 2004]. Similar switch in the folding mechanism has been observed in the case of RNase H [Spudich et al. 2004]. In the case of c-type cytochromes, analyses of the folding mechanism of cytochromes from prokaryotes to eukaryotes indicated that the folding pathway of these proteins involves the formation of one and the same partially structured intermediate [Travaglini-Allocatelli et al. 2004; 2008]. In agreement with the proposed consensus mechanism, it was shown that the high-energy folding intermediate of *Pseudomonas aeruginosa*cyt *c*551 [Gianni et al. 2001] could be stabilized by rational mutagenesis so that it becomes kinetically detectable [Borgia et al. 2006].

5. Protein Aggregation and Amyloid Formation

Pathology, genetics, animal models, and biochemical, biophysical, and cell biological studies have demonstrated that protein aggregation contributes to neurodegeneration, does not necessarily result in neuronal death. Alzheimer's (AD), Huntington's (HD) and Parkinson's disease (PD), amyotrophic lateral sclerosis (ALS), and transmissible spongiform encephalopathies (TSEs or prion diseases), are characterized by the accumulation of intracellular or extracellular protein aggregates in tissue [Xu et al. 2002; Walsh and Selkoe 2004; Lee et al. 2008]. The aggregates may consist of fibrillar structures containing β-sheet-rich misfolded protein, termed amyloids. Protein aggregation is inevitable in living cells and may be brought about by partial unfolding during thermal or oxidative stress and by alterations in primary structure caused by mutation, RNA modification, or translational mis-incorporation. Their accumulation is tightly linked to neuronal degeneration or organ failure in many protein deposition diseases. However, healthy unstressed cells do not accumulate aggregates due to their clearance by the protein disaggregation machinery, which includes chaperones.

Aggregation of soluble polypeptides or proteins into insoluble amyloid fibrils with cross-ß structural motif has been observed in the progression of a great variety of diseases. Several diseases linked to excessive deposits of amyloid fibrils or plaques derived from different precursor proteins include Alzheimer's disease, Parkinson's disease, type II diabetes, and spongiform encephalopathies. A structured mass in human tissues considered to be a cellulose-containing substance due to its ability to be stained by iodine was termed as 'amyloid' [Virchow 1854].Amyloid fibrils share a common core filament structure, irrespective of the nature of their precursor proteins. X-ray [Sunde et al. 1997] and electron diffraction [Makin and Serpell, 2002] studies of amyloid fibrils have confirmed the generality of the cross-ß helical structure present in amyloid with ß-Strands separated by 4.7Å18 and ß-sheets separated by 9.8Å. The ß-sheet structure has the strands perpendicular to the long axis of the fibril and hydrogen bonded along the axis of the fibril [Sunde et al. 1997].The decrease in volume of proteins upon partial or complete disruption of native structure can be explained by hydration of exposed non-polar amino acid residues, electrostriction of exposed charges and the loss of free volume arising from packing defects in the completely folded structure

Amyloid fibril formation involves a structural rearrangement of the native state into aß -sheet rich fibrillar conformation [Sipe, 2005]. ß -sheets seem to provide a scaffold that is favourable for protein assembly: the edge strands of ß-sheet structures are unstable, and the sheet can grow by interacting with any other ß-strands it encounters [Finkelstein et al. 2007]. Natural ß-sheet proteins utilize a number of mechanisms to avoid the edge-to-edge aggregation of their ß–sheets [Richardson and Richardson 2002; Wang and Hecht 2002]. The assembly of misfolded proteins into amyloid fibrils and subsequently into IBs, plaques, NFTs or LBs is a complex process and could be similar among the various proteins that produce these structures. Research into the amyloid aggregation process starting from a partially folded peptide or the native protein to misfolded or unfolded monomeric α-synuclein, Aβ, tau and htt has revealed [Jerson etal. 2006], the production of several, distinct structures such as spherical or annular oligomers and amorphous aggregates and/or fibrils (Figure 5). The pathological depositionsof abnormal proteinsis associated with alterations in redox state homeostasis and mitochondrial dysfunction [Anderson 2004]. The quantity of such aggregates can be almost un-dectectable in some cases, whilst in systemic diseases kilograms of protein can be found in such deposits [Goedert 2004; Hirschfield 2004].

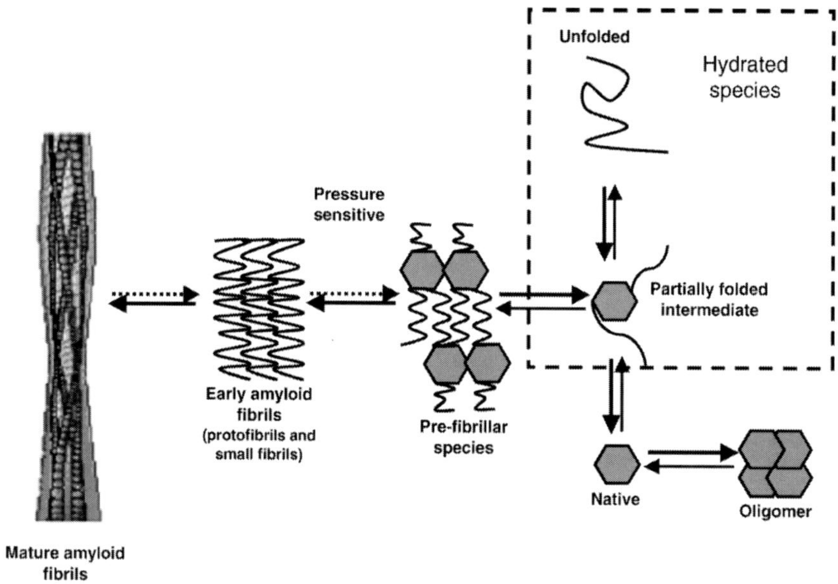

Figure 5. Representation of protein aggregates. A protein folding pathway, including formation of ordered aggregates originated from partially folded intermediate species. Reproduced from Jerson etal. 2006.

6. Protein Mis-Folding in the Cell

The term "misfolding" to describe processes that result in a protein acquiring a sufficient number of persistent non-native interactions to affect its overall architecture and/or its properties in a biologically significant manner. A monomeric intermediate populated during the normal folding process of a protein will not usually be described as misfolded, even though it may have some non-native contacts between its residues. In these non-native states, the peptide becomes loosely packed and hydrophobic cores become exposed to solvents enhancing the tendency to nucleate intitial oligomeric assemblies ("seeds") where the content of secondary beta structure is generally increased. In some of the diseases (e.g. cystic fibrosis) if proteins do not fold correctly they will not be able to exercise their proper functions. In other cases, misfolded proteins escape all the protective mechanisms and form intractable aggregates within cells or in the extracellular space.βAaccumulation is considered to play a central role in the pathogenesis of AD, with pre-amyloid deposits increasing in density over time and eventually developing into neurotoxic amyloid plaques and neurofibrillary tangles [Hardy1996]. Two different α-synuclein missense mutations have been found in dominant cases of PD both of which result in accelerated aggregate formation as compared with wild-type α-synuclein *in vitro* [Narhi etal.1999]. The aggregation process that leads to a peptide or protein to form an amyloid fibril has been described as"misfolding", as the interactions that determine the structure and properties of such fibrils are distinct from those that determine the structure and properties of the biologically active forms of the molecules concerned.

The presence of protein aggregates in the brain of PD patients could be due to dysfunction of molecular chaperone systems leading to inefficient clearance of the aggregates by the proteasome.The molecular chaperone systems normally responsible for prevention of protein misfolding. Dysfunction of the systems involved in detection and elimination of misfolded proteins, such as the HSPs and the ubiquitin-proteosome system (UPS) plays a role in the pathogenesis of neurodegenerative diseases.

The UPS itself has also been suggested to be disrupted by toxic proteins in what essentially amounts to a catastrophic feedback mechanism leading to accumulation of ever-increasing amounts of abnormal protein [Bence et al. 2001].Misfolding caused by errors in protein folding due to mutation or reduced chaperone function leads to aggregation of misfolded proteins with extensive β-sheet conformation or exposed hydrophobic residues (Figure 6).

Neurotoxicity caused by prefibrillar oligomeric intermediates by mediating cellular dysfunction and apoptosis show the way to the formation of inclusions as an end point of protein aggregation (thought to protect cells by sequestering toxic intermediates). An understanding of the mechanisms involved in disposal of aberrant proteins and of the effects of accumulation of such proteins on neuronal survival may allow rational drug design strategies for these diseases.

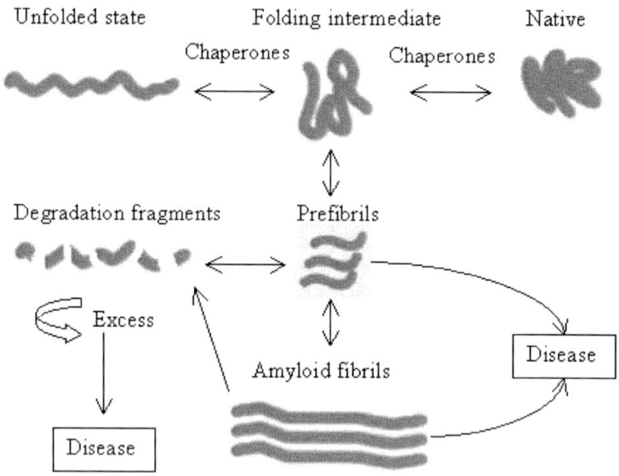

Figure 6. Misfolding caused by errors in protein folding due to mutation or reduced chaperone. Aggregation of misfolded proteins to prefibrillar oligomeric intermediates by mediating cellular dysfunction and protein aggregation leading to amyloid formation.Reproduced from Bence et al. [2001].

7. Mechanisms of Chaperone Protection in Models of Neurodegenerative Diseases

Chaperones are required for translocation of many proteins across cellular membranes, are involved in macromolecular assembly and disassembly, and facilitate the transfer of misfolded proteins to proteosome for degradation. Molecular chaperones provide a first line of defense against misfolded, aggregation-proneproteins, and are among the most potent suppressors ofneurodegeneration known for animal models of human disease. Molecular chaperones are neuroprotective because of their ability to modulate the earliest aberrantprotein interactions that trigger pathogenic cascades.A molecular chaperone is defined as any protein, which interacts, stabilizes or helps a non-native protein to acquire its native conformation but is not present in its final functional structure. Chaperones are involved in multitude of cellular functions such as de novo folding, refolding of stress-denatured proteins, oligomeric assembly, intracellular protein transport and assistance in proteolytic degradation. Binding to chaperone blocks aggregation and reduces the concentration of folding intermediate, whereas transient release of bound hydrophobic regions is necessary for folding to proceed [Hartl and Hartl

2009]. The chaperones act not by contributing steric information to folding process but rather by optimizing the efficiency of folding. Chaperones might alter the conformation of highly toxic protofibrils or oligomers — the intermediates of fibril formation — and reduce their neurotoxicity through changes in protein structure. By modulating the structure of α-synuclein, chaperones inhibit their interaction with other neurotoxic proteins that would activate cell death pathways. In the synucleinopathies, chaperone molecules become sequestered in Lewy bodies and Lewy neurites, leading to chaperone depletion, which might be directly responsible for cell death [Maries et al. 2003].

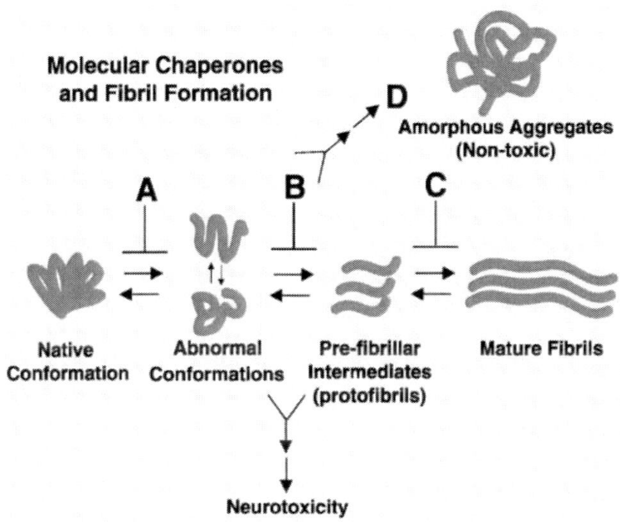

Figure 7. A Model for Molecular Chaperone Suppression of Neurotoxicity.Molecular chaperones may suppress neurotoxicity of amyloid-forming proteins by preventing their conversion between native conformation and toxic conformations (A), by preventing the formation of pre-fibrillar intermediates (B), by preventing the conversion between pre- fibrillar intermediates and mature fibrils (C), and/or by facilitating the conversion of toxic intermediates into nontoxic amorphous aggregates (D). Reproduced from Hartl and Hartl [2009].

Several cellular proteins undergo fibrillogenesis under special conditions and the accumulation of fibrils in specific organs and tissues can ultimately lead to death. The ordered fibrillar structures known as amyloid found inside and out side of diseased brains (PD, AD, HD etc.) implies an underlying incapacity in the cellular machinery of molecular chaperones that normally functions to prevent the accumulation of unfolded protein (**Fig. 7**).The chaperone pathways and networks acting in protein folding in the cytosol practice general organizational rules [Frydman 2001; Hartl and Hartl, 2002]. Two major principles of chaperone action have been proposed, which are represented by (i) machinery that functions in stabilizing nascent polypeptides on ribosomes and initiating folding and (ii) components that act downstream in completing the folding process [Langer 1992; Albane`se, 2006]. Both systems cooperate in coherent pathways. The number of interacting substrates and the degree of functional redundancy among chaperone components decreases from upstream to downstream [Hartl and Hartl 2009].

CONCLUSIONS

In summary, a systematic understanding of mechanism of folding of protein to native state or the formation of amyloid-assembly process will provide new probes for the physiological interactions that may give way to revert misfolded protein in native state or amyloidosis. The detailed knowledge of the mechanisms of amyloid growth and the factors that influence the (dis)aggregation rates at all stages of amyloid assembly will provide rational strategies based on interrupting or reversing amyloid aggregation at various points in amyloid assembly. Blocking and/or reversing amyloid formation will be an effective treatment for diseases involving organ failure due to amyloidosis.

Development of vaccines targeting small amyloidogenic aggregates (Jahn and Radford 2005; Englander et al. 2007) would benefit from understanding how the concentrations of amyloidogenic species will be influenced by the induced immunological response to and clearing of particular amyloid species. Chaperones may play a critical role in neurodegeneration and aging and this class of proteins holds much promise as a therapeutic target for the treatment of neurodegenerative disorders. The role of chaperones and prions in neuroprotection will shed an insight into the better approaches to the prevention of amyloid formation and new diagnostics for early detection of amyloid-related diseases. The identification of small molecules that can enhance chaperone expression or activities in brain cells may be an awesome process, however promises new molecular modulating switches.

REFERENCES

Abkevich VI, Gutin AM and Shakhnovich EI. Specific nucleus as the transition state for protein folding: evidence from the lattice model. *Biochemistry*33:10026–10036 (1994).

Albane`se, V, Yam AYW, Baughman J, Parnot C and Frydman, J. Systems analyses reveal two chaperone networks with distinct functions in eukaryotic cells. *Cell* 124:75–88 (2006).

Andersen JK. Oxidative stress in neurodegeneration: Cause or consequence? *Nat. Rev Neurosci.* 10:S18-25 (2004).

Bartlett AL and Radford SE. An expanding arsenal of experimental methods yields anexplosion of insights into protein folding mechanisms. *Nat. Struct.Mol. Biol.* 16:582-588 (2009).

Behl C, Davis JB, Lesley R and Schubert D. Hydrogen peroxide mediates amyloid-β toxicity. *Cell*77:817-827 (1994).

Bence NF, Sampat RM, and Kopito RR.Impairment of the ubiquitin-proteasome system by protein aggregation. *Science*292:1552-5 (2001).

Blanchard BJ, Chen A, Rozeboom LM, Stafford KA, Weigele P and Ingram VM.Efficient reversal of Alzheimer's disease fibril formation and elimination of neurotoxicity by a small molecule. *PNAS*101:14326-14332 (2004).

Borgia A, Bonivento D, Travaglini-Allocatelli C, Matteo AD, and Brunori M.Protein Structure and Folding:Unveiling a Hidden Folding Intermediate in c-Type Cytochromes by Protein Engineering. *J. Biol. Chem* ,281: 9331–9336 (2006).

Borreguero JM, Ding F, Buldyrev SV, Stanley HE, Dokholyan NV. Multiple folding pathways of the SH3 domain. *Biophys J.*, 87:521-533 (2004).

Brockwell DJ and Radford SE. Intermediates: ubiquitous species on folding energy landscapes? *Curr. Opin. Struct. Biol.* 17:30–37 (2007).

Browne SE, Ferrante RJ and Beal MF.Oxidative stress in Huntington's disease. *Brain Pathol. 9:*147-163 (1999).

Burton RE, Huang GS, Daugherty M A, Fullbright PW, Oas TG. Microsecond protein folding through a compact transition state. *J. Mol. Biol.* 263: 311–22 (1996).

Burton RE, Huang GS, Daugherty MA, Calderone T L and Oas T G. The energy landscape of a fast-folding protein mapped by Ala → Gly substitutions. *Nat Struct Biol* 4: 305–10 (1997).

Callender RH, Dyer RB, Gilmanshin R and Woodruff WH. Fast events in protein folding: the time evolution of primary processes. *Annu. Rev. Phys. Chem.* 49,173–202 (1998).

Camacho CJand Thirumalai D. Theoretical predictions of folding pathways by using the proximity rule, with applications to bovine pancreatic trypsin inhibitor.*PNAS* 92: 1277-81(1995).

Capaldi AP, Kleanthous C, and Radford SE. Im7 folding mechanism: misfolding on a path to the native state. *Nat. Struct .Biol.* 9(3): 209-16 (2002).

Chakrabartty A and Baldwin RL.Stability of α-helices.*Adv. Protein Chem.* 46:141–76 (1995).

Chan C-K, Hofrichter J and Eaton W A. Optical triggers in protein folding. *Science*274: 628–29 (1996).

Chan C-K, Hu Y, Takahashi S, Rousseau DL, Eaton WA, Hofrichter J. Sub-millisecond protein folding kinetics studied by ultrarapid mixing. *Proc. Natl. Acad. Sci. USA* 94:1779–84 (1997).

Chen S, Berthelier V, Yang W and Wetzel R. Polyglutamine aggregation behavior *in vitro* supports a recruitment mechanism of cytotoxicity. *J Mol Biol*311:173–182 (2001).

Clark JI and Muchowski PJ.Small heat-shockproteins and their potential role in human disease. *Curr. Opin. Struct .Biol.* 10(1): 52-9 (Feb 2000).

Cummings CJ, Mancini MA, Antalffy B, DeFranco DB, Orr HT and Zoghbi HY. Chaperone suppression of aggregation and altered subcellular proteasome localization imply protein misfolding in SCA1. *Nature Genet.*19:148–154 (1998).

Daggett V and Fersht AR.Is there a unifying mechanism for proteinfolding? *Trends Biochem. Sci.* 28(1):18-25 (2003).

Dobson CM. Protein folding and misfolding. *Nature* 426: 884–890 (2003).

Eanes ED and Glenner GG.X-ray diffraction studies on amyloid filaments. *J. Histochem Cytochem* 16:673–677 (1968).

Eaton WA ,Muñoz V, Hagen SJ,Jas GS,Lapidus LJ,Henry ER andHofrichter. *J. Annu. Rev. Biophys. Biomol. Struct.* 29:327-359 (2000).

Englander SW, Mayne L and Krishna MM.Proteinfolding and misfolding: mechanism and principles. *Q Rev. Biophys.* 40(4): 287-326 (2007).

Eyring H. The quantum theory of activation and absolute reaction rates of photochemical processes. *Cold Spring Harb. Symp.Quant .Biol.* 3:10-18 (1935).

Ferguson N, Capaldi AR, James R, Kleanthous C, and Radford SE. Rapid folding with and without populated intermediates in the homologous four-helix proteins Im7 and Im9. *J. Mol. Bio.* 286 (5): 1597-608 (1999).

Fersht AR, Matouschek A, Serrano L.The folding of an enzyme.I.Theory of protein engineering analysis of stability and pathway of protein folding. *J Mol Biol* 224:771-82 (1992).

Fersht AR. Optimization of rates of protein folding: the nucleation–condensation mechanism and its implications. *PNAS* 21:10869–10873 (1995).

Fersht AR.Transition-state structure as a unifying basis in protein-folding mechanisms: Contact order, chain topology, stability, and the extended nucleus mechanism. *PNAS* 97:1525-1529 (2000).

Fersht AR and Sato S.ΦValue analysis and the nature of protein-folding transition states *PNAS* 101: 7976 – 7981 (2004).

Finkelstein AV, Ivankov DN, SO Garbuzynskiy and OV Galzitskaya.Understanding the folding rates and folding nuclei of globular proteins.*Curr. Protein. Pept. Sci.* 8(6): 521-36 (2007).

Friel CT, Capaldi AP, and Radford SE Structural analysis of the rate-limiting transition states in the folding of Im7 and Im9: similarities and differences in the folding of homologous proteins. *J. Mol. Biol.* 326(1): 293-305 (2003).

Friel CT, Beddard GS and SE Radford.Switching two-state to three-state kinetics in the helical protein Im9 via the optimisation of stabilising non-native interactions by design. *J.Mol. Biol.* 342(1):261-73 (2004).

Frydman J. Folding of newly translated proteins in vivo: The role of molecular chaperones. *Annu. Rev. Biochem.*70:603–647 (2001).

Gianni S, Travaglini-Allocatelli C, Cutruzzola F, Bigotti MG and BrunoriM.Snapshots of proteinfolding. A study on the multiple transition state pathway of cytochromec(551) from Pseudomonas aeruginosa. *J. Mol. Biol.* 309(5).1177-87 (2001).

Gianni S, Guydosh NR, Khan F, Caldas TD, Mayor U, White GW, DeMarco ML, Daggett V, and Fersht AR. Unifying features in protein-folding mechanisms. *PNAS* 100:13286-13291(2003).

Gianni S, Engström A, Larsson M, Calosci N, Malatesta F, Eklund L, Ngang CC, Travaglini-Allocatelli C and JemthP.The Kinetics of PDZ Domain-Ligand Interactions and Implications for the Binding Mechanism.J Biol Chem280:34805-34812 (2005).

Gianni S, Geierhaas CD, Calosci N, Jemth P, Vuister GW, Travaglini-Allocatelli C, Vendruscolo M and Brunori M. A PDZ domain recapitulates a unifying mechanism for protein folding. *PNAS* 104:128–133 (2007a).

Gianni S, Ivarsson Y, Jemth P, Brunori M and Travaglini-Allocatelli C. Identifcation and characterization of protein folding intermediates. *Biophys Chem*128:105–113 (2007b).

Glenner GG and Wong CW. Alzheimer's disease and Down's syndrome: sharing of a unique cerebrovascular amyloid fibril protein. *Biochem. Biophys. Res. Commun.* 122:1131-1135 (1984).

Goedert MThe Neurofibrillary Pathology of Alzheimer's Disease. *Neuroscientist* 3:131-141 (1997).

Goedert M, Spillantini MG, Serpell LC, Berriman J, Smith MJ, Jakes R and Crowther AR.From genetics to pathology: tau and a–synuclein assemblies in neurodegenerative diseases. *Phil. Trans R. Soc. B.* 356: 213-227 (2001).

Goedert M. Tau protein and neurodegeneration. *Seminars in Cell & Developmental Biology* 15: 45-49(2004).

Gorski SA, Capaldi AP, Kleanthous C and Radford SE.Acidic conditions stabilise intermediates populated during the folding of Im7 and Im9. *J. Mol. Biol.* 312(4): 849-63 (2001).

Gruebele M. The fast protein folding problem. *Annu Rev. Phys. Chem.* 50: 485–516 (1999).

Guo M-L Rajamäki, Saarma M, and Jari PT. Valkonen.Towards a protein interaction map of potyviruses: protein interaction matrixes of two potyviruses based on the yeast two-hybrid system. *J. Gen. Virol.* 82:935-939 (2001).

Hardy J. New insights into the genetics of Alzheimer's disease.*Ann. Med.* 28:255-258(1996).

Hagen SJ, Hofrichter J, Szabo A and EatonWA.Diffusion-limited contact formation in unfolded cytochromec: Estimating the maximum rate of protein folding. *PNAS* 93: 11615-11617 (1996).

Hagen SJ.Solvent Viscosity and Friction in ProteinFolding Dynamics. *Curr. Protein. Pept. Sci*, (2010).

Hartl, F.U. & Hayer-Hartl, M. Molecular chaperones in the cytosol: from nascent chain to folded protein. *Science*295*:*1852–1858 (2002).

Hartl FU and Hayer-Hartl M., Converging concepts of protein folding in vitro and in vivo. *Nature Struct and Molecular Biol*16(60):574-581(2009).

Hirschfield GM. Amyloidosis: a clinico-pathophysiological synopsis. *Seminars in Cell & Developmental Biology* 15:39-44 (2004).

Huang GS and Oas TG. Submillisecond folding of monomeric λ repressor.*PNAS*92: 6878–82 (1995).

Huang H-C, Sherman MY, Kandror O and Goldberg AL. PROTEIN SYNTHESIS, POST-TRANSLATION MODIFICATION, AND DEGRADATION: The Molecular Chaperone DnaJ Is Required for the Degradation of a Soluble Abnormal Protein in Escherichia coli. *J. Biol. Chem.* 276:3920-3928 (2001).

Hsu LJ, Sagara Y, Arroyo A, Rockenstein E, Sisk A, Mallory M, Wong J, Takenouchi T, Hashimoto M and Masliah E. α-Synuclein promotes mitochondrial deficit and oxidative stress. *Am. J. Pathol.* 157:401-410 (2000).

Itzhaki LS, Otzen DE and Fersht AR The structure of the transition state for folding of chymotrypsin inhibitor 2 analysed by protein engineering methods: evidence for a nucleation–condensation mechanism for protein folding. *J. Mol. Biol.* 254:260–288 (1995).

Ivarsson Y, Travaglini-Allocatelli C, Jemth J, Malatesta F, Brunori M and Gianni S.An On-pathway Intermediate in the Folding of a PDZ Domain. J. Biol. Chem. 282:8568-8572 (2007).

Jackson SE and Fersht AR. Folding of chymotrypsin inhibitor 2.1.Evidence for a two-state transition. *Biochemistry* 30:10428-10435 (1991).

Jahn TR and Radford SE.The Yin and Yang of protein folding. *FEBS J.* 272:5962-5970 (2005).

Jerson LS, CordeiroY and Foguel D. Protein folding and aggregation: Two sides of the same coin in the condensation of proteins revealed by pressure studies. *Biochimica et Biophysica Acta* 1764 :443–451 (2006).

Jones CM, Henry ER, Hu Y, Chan CK, Luck SD, Bhuyan A, Roder H, Hofrichter J and Eaton WA. Fast events in protein folding initiated by nano second laser photolysis. *PNAS* 90:11860-64(1993).

Juraszek J and Bolhuis PG. Sampling the multiple folding mechanisms of Trp-cage in explicit solvent. *PNAS* 103:15859–15864 (2006).

Karplus M and Weaver DL.Protein-folding dynamics. *Nature* 260:404–406 (1976).

Karplus M and Weaver DL. Protcin folding dynamics: the diffusion– collision model and experimental data. *Protein Sci.* 3:650– 668 (1994).

Kazantsev A, Preisinger E, Dranovsky A, Goldgaber D and Housman D. Insoluble detergent-resistant aggregates form between pathological and nonpathological lengths of polyglutamine in mammalian cells. *PNAS* 96:11404–11409 (1999).

Knight JB, Vishwanath A, Brody JP and Austin RH Hydrodynamic focusing on a silicon chip: mixing nanoliters in microseconds. *Phys. Rev. Lett.* 80: 3863–66 (1998).

Krantz BA, Mayne L, Rumbley J, Englander SW and Sosnick TR. Fast and slow intermediate accumulation and the initial barrier mechanism in protein folding. *J. Mol. Biol.* 324:359–371(2002).

Lam AR, Borreguero JM, Ding F, Dokholyan NV, Buldyrev SV, Stanley HE and Shakhnovich E Parallel folding pathways in the SH3 domain protein. *J. Mol. Biol.* 373:1348–1360 (2007).

Langer T, Lu C, Echols H, Flanagan J, Hayer MK and Hartl DU.Successive action of DnaK, DnaJ and GroEL along the pathway of chaperone-mediated protein folding. *Nature* 356:683–689 (1992).

Lashuel HA, Hartley D, Petre BM, Walz T and Lansbury PT. Neurodegenerative disease: amyloid pores from pathogenic mutations. *Nature* 418:291 (2002).

Lazaridis T and Karplus M. "New view" of protein folding reconciled with the old through multiple unfolding simulations. *Science*278:1928–1931 (1997).

Lee HJ, Suk JE, Bae EJ and Lee SJ.Clearance and deposition of extracellular alpha-synucleinaggregatesin microglia. Biochem. Biophys.Res. Commun. 372(3): 423-8 (2008).

Lin MX, Mirzabekov T and Kagan BL. Channel formation by a neurotoxic prion protein fragment. *J. Biol. Chem.* 272: 44–47 (1997).

Lindberg MO and Oliveberg M. Malleability of protein folding pathways: a simplereason for complex behaviour. *Curr. Opin. Struct. Biol.* 17:21-29 (2007).

Lorenzetti D, Watase K, Xu B, Matzuk MM, Orr HT and Zoghbi HY.Repeat instability and motor incoordination in mice with a targeted expanded CAG repeat in the Sca1 locus. *Hum. Mol. Genet.* 9:779-785 (2000).

Lu HSM, Volk M and Kholodenko Y, Gooding E, Hochstrasser RM and DeGrado WF.Aminothiotyrosine disulfide, an optical trigger for initiation of protein folding.*J Am Chem Soc* 119:7173–80 (1997).

Makin OS and Serpell LC.Examining the structure of the mature amyloid fibril. *Biochem. Soc. Trans 30*:521(2002).

Makin OS and Serpell LC.X-ray diffraction studies of amyloid structure. *Methods Mol. Biol.* 299:67–80 (2005).

Maries E, Dass B, Collier TJ, Kordower JH and Steece-Collier K.The role of alpha-synuclein in Parkinson's disease: insights from animal models. *Nat. Rev. Neurosci.* 4(9): 727-38 (2003).

Marqusee S, Robbins VH and Baldwin RL.Unusually stable helix formation in short alanine based peptides. *PNAS.* 86:5286–90 (1989).

Matouschek A, Kellis Jr JT, Serrano L, Bycroft M and Fersht AR.Transient folding intermediates characterized by protein engineering. *Nature* 346: 440-5(1990).

McCampbell A, Taylor JP, Taye AA, Robitschek J, Li M, Walcott J, Merry D, Chai Y, Paulson H, Sobue G and Fischbeck KH.CREB-binding protein sequestration by expanded polyglutamine. *Hum. Mol. Genet.*9:2197–2202 (2000).

McNaught KS, Perl DP, Brownell ALand Olanow CW. Systemic exposure to proteasome inhibitors causes a progressive model of Parkinson's disease. *Ann. Neurol.* 56:149–162 (2004).

Muñoz V and Serrano L. Elucidating the folding problem of helical peptides using empirical parameters. *Nat. Struct Biol.* 1: 399–409 (1994).

Muñoz V and Serrano L. Elucidating the folding problem of helical peptides using empirical parameters. II. Helix macrodipole effects and rational modification of the helical content of natural peptides. *J. Mol .Biol.* 245:275–296 (1995).

Muñoz V, Thompson PA, Hofrichter J, Eaton WA. Folding dynamics and mechanism of β-hairpin formation. *Nature* 390: 196–99 (1997).

Munoz V.Conformational dynamics and ensembles in proteinfolding. *Annu. Rev. Biophys. Biomol. Struct.* 36:395-412 (2007).

Narhi L, Wood SJ, Steavenson S, Jiang Y, Wu GM, Anafi D, Kaufman SA, Martin F, Sitney K, Denis P, Louis J-C, Wypych J, Biere AL and Citron M. Both familial Parkinson's disease mutations accelerate alpha-synuclein aggregation. *J. Biol. Chem.* 274:9843-9846 (1999).

Neira JL, Davis B, Ladurner AG, Buckle AM, Gay Gde P and Fersht AR.Towards the complete structural characterization of a protein folding pathway: the structures of the denatured, transition and native states for the association/folding of two complementary fragments of cleaved chymotrypsin inhibitor 2. Direct evidence for a nucleation–condensation mechanism. *Fold Des.* 1:189–208 (1996).

Nucifora Jr. FC, Sasaki M, Peters MF, Huang H, Cooper JK, Yamada M, Takahashi H, Tsuji S, Troncoso J, Dawson VL, Dawson TM and Christopher A. Ross Interference by huntingtin and atrophin-1 with CBP-mediated transcription leading to cellular toxicity. *Science* 291:2423–2428 (2001).

Onuchic JN and Wolynes PG. Theory of protein folding.*Curr Opin Struct Biol*14, 70–75 (2004).

Park S-H, Shastry MCR and Roder H. Folding dynamics of the B1 domain of protein G explored by ultrarapid mixing. *Nature Struct. Biol.* 6: 943–47(1999).

Phillips CM, Mizutani Y and Hochstrasser RM. Ultrafast thermally induced unfolding of RNase A . *PNAS.* 92: 7292–96 (1995).

Pollack L, Tate MW, Darnton NC, Knight JB, Gruner S, Eaton WA and Austin RH. Compactness of the denatured state of a fast-folding protein measured by sub-millisecond small-angle x-ray scattering. *PNAS* 96:10115–17 (1999).

Preisinger E, Jordan BM, Kazantsev A and Housman D. Evidence for a recruitment and sequestration mechanism in Huntington's disease. *Phil Trans R Soc.* B. 354:1029–1034 (1999).

Privalov PL. Cold denaturation of proteins. *Crit. Rev. Biochem. Mol. Biol.* 25:281–305 (1990).

Quist A, Doudevski I, Lin H, Azimova R, Ng D, Frangione B, KaganB, Ghiso J and Lal R. Amyloid ion channels: A common structural link for protein-misfolding disease. *PNAS*102: 10427–10432 (2005).

Rao F, Settanni G, Guarnera E and CaXisch A. Estimation of protein folding probability from equilibrium simulations. *J. Chem. Phys.* 122:184901(2005).

Ravikumar B, Vacher C, Berger Z, Davies JE, Luo S, Oroz LG, Scaravilli F, Easton DF, Duden R, O'Kane CJ and Rubinsztein DC. Inhibition of mTOR induces autophagy and reduces toxicity of polyglutamine expansions in fly and mouse models of Huntington disease. *Nat. Genet* 36(6): 585–595 (2004).

Richardson JS and Richardson DC, Natural β -sheet proteins use negative design to avoid edge-to-edge aggregation. *PNAS*99:2754–2759 (2002).

Rochet JC and Lansbury Jr PT. Amyloid fibrillogenesis: themes and variations. *Curr. Opin. Struct .Biol.* 10(1): 60-8 (2000).

Ross CA andMichelle A. PoirierOpiniono n: What is the role of protein aggregation in neurodege-neration? *Nature Reviews Molecular Cell Biology 6(11):*891-8(2005). doi:10.1038/nrm1742.

Selkoe DJ. Alzheimer's Disease: Genes, Proteins, and Therapy. Physiol. Rev. 81: 741-766 (2001).

Szabo A, Schulten K and Schulten Z.The first passage time approach to diffusion-controlled reactions. *J. Chem. Phys.* 72: 4350–57 (1980).

Shastry MCR, Luck SD, Roder HA.Continuous-flow capillary mixing method to monitor reactions on the microsecond time scale. *Bioph. J.* 74:2714–21(1998a).

Shastry MCR and Roder H. Evidence for barrier-limited protein folding kinetics on the microsecond time scale. *Nat. Struct. Biol.* 5: 385–92 (1998b).

Shastry MCR, Sauder JM and Roder H. Kinetic and structural analysis of submil-lisecond folding events in cytochrome-*c*. *Acc. Chem. Res* 31: 717–25 (1998c).

Silva JL and Weber G. Pressure stability of proteins. *Annu Rev Phys. Chem.*44:89-113 (1993).

Sipe JC. Cladribine for multiple sclerosis: review and current status. *Expert. Rev. Neurother.* 5(6): 721-7 (2005).

Sisodia SS, Koo EH, Beyreuther K, Unterbeck A and Price DL. Evidence that beta-amyloid protein in Alzheimer's disease is not derived by normal processing. *Science* 248: 492-495 (1990).

Smeller L. Pressure–temperature phase diagrams of biomolecules. *Biochim. Biophys. Acta* 1595:11-29 (2002).

Spudich GM, Miller EJ and Marqusee S. Destabilization of the Escherichia coli RNase H kinetic intermediate: switching between a two-state and three-state folding mechanism. *J. Mol. Biol.* 335(2): 609-18 (2004).

Sunde M, Serpell LC, Bartlam M, Fraser PE, Pepys MB and Blake CC. Common core structure of amyloid fibrils by synchrotron X-ray diffraction. *J. Mol. Biol.* 273 (3): 729-39 (1997).

Sunde M and Blake CC.From the globular to the fibrous state: protein structure and structural conversion in amyloid formation. *Q Rev. Biophys.* 31(1):1-39 (1998).

Tabrizi SJ, Workman J, Hart PE, Mangiarini L, Mahal A, Bates G, Cooper JM, and Schapira AH. Mitochondrial dysfunction and free radical damage in the Huntington R6/2 transgenic mouse. *Ann. Neurol.* 47(1): 80–86 (2000).

Takahashi S, Yeh S R, Das T K, Chan C K, Gottfried D S, Rousseau D L. Folding of cytochromec initiated by submil-lisecond mixing. *Nat. Struct. Biol.* 1997; 4: 44–50.

Thirumalai D. Time scales for the formation of the most probable tertiary contacts in proteins with applications to cytochromec. *J. Phys. Chem. B.* 103: 608–10 (1999).

Thompson PA, Muñoz V, Jas GS, Henry ER, Eaton WA.The helix-coil kinetics of a heteropeptide. *J. Phys. Chem. B.* 104: 378–89 (2000).

Travaglini-Allocatelli C, Gianni S and Brunori M.A common folding mechanism in the cytochrome c family. *Trends Biochem. Sci.,* 29(10):535-41(2004).

Travaglini-Allocatelli C, Brunori M, Gianni, S Mechanisms of protein folding. Eur Biophys J (2008) 37:721–728.

Virchow R and Zur cellulose-frage.Virchows Arch. *Pathol.Anat.* 6, 416-4260 (1854).

Volk M, Lu HSM, Kholodenko Y, Gooding E, DeGrado WF and Hochstrasser RM. Peptide conformational dynamics and vibrational Stark effects following photinitiated disulfide cleavage. *J. Phys. Chem. B.* 101: 8607–16 (1997).

Walsh DM and Selkoe DJ.Oligomers on the brain: the emerging role of soluble proteinaggregatesin neurodegeneration. *Protein Pept Lett. 11*(3): 213-28 (2004).

Wang W and Hecht MH. Rationally designed mutations convert de novo amyloid-like fibrils into monomeric β -sheet proteins. *Proc. Natl. Acad. Sci. USA*, 2002, 99, 2760–2765.

Weber G. Thermodynamics of the association and the pressure dissociation of oligomeric proteins. *J. Phys. Chem.* 97: 7108–7115 (1993).

Weber G, Thermodynamic concepts in protein condensation. *Comments Mol. Cell Biophys.* 9: 201–218 (1999).

Weikl TR and Dill KA.Transition-states in proteinfolding kinetics: the structural interpretation of Phi values. *J. Mol. Biol.* 365(5): 1578-86 (2007).

White GW, Gianni S, Grossmann JG, Jemth P, Fersht AR and Daggett V. Simulation and experiment conspire to reveal cryptic intermediates and a slide from the nucleation–condensation to framework mechanism of folding. *J. Mol. Biol.* 350:757–775 (2005).

Wright CF, Lindorff-Larsen K, Randles LG and Clarke J. Parallelprotein-unfolding pathways revealed and mapped. *Nat. Struct .Biol.* 10:658–662 (2003).

Xu G, Gonzales V and BorcheltDR.Rapid detection of proteinaggregatesin the brains of Alzheimer patients and transgenic mouse models of amyloidosis. *Alzheimer Dis. Assoc. Disord.* 16 (3): 191-5 (2002).

Yan SD, Zhu H, Zhu A, Golabek A, Du H, Roher A, Yu J, Soto C, Schmidt AM, Stern D and Kindy M. Receptor-dependent cell stress and amyloid accumulation in systemic amyloidosis. *Nature Med.* 6, 643–651 (2000).

INDEX

A

B

C

D

E

F

G

H

I

J

K

N

T

Y

Z